Mechanisms and Novel Therapeutic Approaches for Gynecologic Cancer

Mechanisms and Novel Therapeutic Approaches for Gynecologic Cancer

Editor

Naomi Nakayama

MDPI • Basel • Beijing • Wuhan • Barcelona • Belgrade • Manchester • Tokyo • Cluj • Tianjin

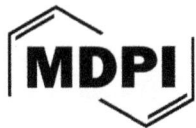

Editor
Naomi Nakayama
Hyogo Medical University
Japan

Editorial Office
MDPI
St. Alban-Anlage 66
4052 Basel, Switzerland

This is a reprint of articles from the Special Issue published online in the open access journal *Biomedicines* (ISSN 2227-9059) (available at: https://www.mdpi.com/journal/biomedicines/special_issues/gynecol_cancer).

For citation purposes, cite each article independently as indicated on the article page online and as indicated below:

LastName, A.A.; LastName, B.B.; LastName, C.C. Article Title. *Journal Name* **Year**, *Volume Number*, Page Range.

ISBN 978-3-0365-4383-3 (Hbk)
ISBN 978-3-0365-4384-0 (PDF)

Cover image courtesy of Naomi Nakayama

© 2022 by the authors. Articles in this book are Open Access and distributed under the Creative Commons Attribution (CC BY) license, which allows users to download, copy and build upon published articles, as long as the author and publisher are properly credited, which ensures maximum dissemination and a wider impact of our publications.

The book as a whole is distributed by MDPI under the terms and conditions of the Creative Commons license CC BY-NC-ND.

Contents

About the Editor vii

Naomi Nakayama
Mechanisms and Novel Therapeutic Approaches for Gynecologic Cancer
Reprinted from: *Biomedicines* **2022**, *10*, 1014, doi:10.3390/biomedicines10051014 1

**Naomi Nakayama, Gyosuke Sakashita, Takashi Nagata, Naohiro Kobayashi,
Hisashi Yoshida, Sam-Yong Park, Yuko Nariai, Hiroaki Kato, Eiji Obayashi,
Kentaro Nakayama, Satoru Kyo and Takeshi Urano**
Nucleus Accumbens-Associated Protein 1 Binds DNA Directly through the BEN Domain in a Sequence-Specific Manner
Reprinted from: *Biomedicines* **2020**, *8*, 608, doi:10.3390/biomedicines8120608 5

**Yue Liao, Susann Badmann, Till Kaltofen, Doris Mayr, Elisa Schmoeckel, Eileen Deuster,
Mareike Mannewitz, Sarah Landgrebe, Thomas Kolben, Anna Hester, Susanne Beyer,
Alexander Burges, Sven Mahner, Udo Jeschke, Fabian Trillsch and Bastian Czogalla**
Platelet-Activating Factor Acetylhydrolase Expression in BRCA1 Mutant Ovarian Cancer as a Protective Factor and Potential Negative Regulator of the Wnt Signaling Pathway
Reprinted from: *Biomedicines* **2021**, *9*, 706, doi:10.3390/biomedicines9070706 25

**Kuo-Min Su, Hong-Wei Gao, Chia-Ming Chang, Kai-Hsi Lu, Mu-Hsien Yu, Yi-Hsin Lin,
Li-Chun Liu, Chia-Ching Chang, Yao-Feng Li and Cheng-Chang Chang**
Synergistic AHR Binding Pathway with EMT Effects on Serous Ovarian Tumors Recognized by Multidisciplinary Integrated Analysis
Reprinted from: *Biomedicines* **2021**, *9*, 866, doi:10.3390/biomedicines9080866 45

**Aneta Popiel, Aleksandra Piotrowska, Patrycja Sputa-Grzegrzolka, Beata Smolarz,
Hanna Romanowicz, Piotr Dziegiel, Marzenna Podhorska-Okolow
and Christopher Kobierzycki**
Preliminary Study on the Expression of Testin, p16 and Ki-67 in the Cervical Intraepithelial Neoplasia
Reprinted from: *Biomedicines* **2021**, *9*, 1010, doi:10.3390/biomedicines9081010 75

**Rüdiger Klapdor, Shuo Wang, Michael A. Morgan, Katharina Zimmermann,
Jens Hachenberg, Hildegard Büning, Thilo Dörk, Peter Hillemanns and Axel Schambach**
NK Cell-Mediated Eradication of Ovarian Cancer Cells with a Novel Chimeric Antigen Receptor Directed against CD44
Reprinted from: *Biomedicines* **2021**, *9*, 1339, doi:10.3390/biomedicines9101339 87

**Ying-Cheng Chiang, Po-Han Lin, Tzu-Pin Lu, Kuan-Ting Kuo, Yi-Jou Tai, Heng-Cheng Hsu,
Chia-Ying Wu, Chia-Yi Lee, Hung Shen, Chi-An Chen and Wen-Fang Cheng**
A DNA Damage Response Gene Panel for Different Histologic Types of Epithelial Ovarian Carcinomas and Their Outcomes
Reprinted from: *Biomedicines* **2021**, *9*, 1384, doi:10.3390/biomedicines9101384 101

**Jacqueline Ho Sze Lee, Joshua Jing Xi Li, Chit Chow, Ronald Cheong Kin Chan,
Johnny Sheung Him Kwan, Tat San Lau, Ka Fai To, So Fan Yim,
Suet Ying Yeung and Joseph Kwong**
Long-Term Survival and Clinicopathological Implications of DNA Mismatch Repair Status in Endometrioid Endometrial Cancers in Hong Kong Chinese Women
Reprinted from: *Biomedicines* **2021**, *9*, 1385, doi:10.3390/biomedicines9101385 121

Tamer Soror, Ramin Chafii, Valentina Lancellotta, Luca Tagliaferri and György Kovács
Biological Planning of Radiation Dose Based on In Vivo Dosimetry for Postoperative Vaginal-Cuff HDR Interventional Radiotherapy (Brachytherapy)
Reprinted from: *Biomedicines* **2021**, *9*, 1629, doi:10.3390/biomedicines9111629 . . . . **135**

Momodou Cox, Apriliana E. R. Kartikasari, Paul R. Gorry, Katie L. Flanagan and Magdalena Plebanski
Potential Impact of Human Cytomegalovirus Infection on Immunity to Ovarian Tumours and Cancer Progression
Reprinted from: *Biomedicines* **2021**, *9*, 351, doi:10.3390/biomedicines9040351 . . . . **145**

Meng-Shin Shiao, Jia-Ming Chang, Arb-Aroon Lertkhachonsuk, Naparat Rermluk and Natini Jinawath
Circulating Exosomal miRNAs as Biomarkers in Epithelial Ovarian Cancer
Reprinted from: *Biomedicines* **2021**, *9*, 1433, doi:10.3390/biomedicines9101433 . . . . **161**

Maritza P. Garrido, Allison N. Fredes, Lorena Lobos-González, Manuel Valenzuela-Valderrama, Daniela B. Vera and Carmen Romero
Current Treatments and New Possible Complementary Therapies for Epithelial Ovarian Cancer
Reprinted from: *Biomedicines* **2022**, *10*, 77, doi:10.3390/biomedicines10010077 . . . . **181**

Sandrine Rousset-Rouviere, Philippe Rochigneux, Anne-Sophie Chrétien, Stéphane Fattori, Laurent Gorvel, Magali Provansal, Eric Lambaudie, Daniel Olive and Renaud Sabatier
Endometrial Carcinoma: Immune Microenvironment and Emerging Treatments in Immuno-Oncology
Reprinted from: *Biomedicines* **2021**, *9*, 632, doi:10.3390/biomedicines9060632 . . . . **213**

Elena-Codruța Dobrică, Cristina Vâjâitu, Carmen Elena Condrat, Dragoș Crețoiu, Ileana Popa, Bogdan Severus Gaspar, Nicolae Suciu, Sanda Maria Crețoiu and Valentin Nicolae Varlas
Vulvar and Vaginal Melanomas—The Darker Shades of Gynecological Cancers
Reprinted from: *Biomedicines* **2021**, *9*, 758, doi:10.3390/biomedicines9070758 . . . . **229**

About the Editor

Naomi Nakayama

Dr. Naomi Nakayama, MD, PhD, is an Associate Professor of the Department of General Medicine and Community Health Science at Hyogo Medical University School of Medicine. She graduated with an MD from Hyogo Medical University in 1996. She started her research in molecular biology and biochemistry and received her PhD in 2013 at Shimane University, School of Medicine. During her carrier as a research scientist, she finished a two-year research fellowship at Johns Hopkins University in 2007. From 2018 to 2022, she became a Professor at the University of Shimane, School of Nutrition Science. In 2022, she started working in her current position. She is actively involved in both experimental and clinical research in the field of gynecologic oncology, and she is continuously publishing her scientific research in international academic journals in this field.

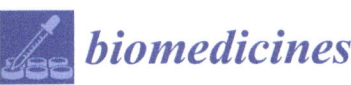

Editorial

Mechanisms and Novel Therapeutic Approaches for Gynecologic Cancer

Naomi Nakayama

Department of General Medicine and Community Health Science, School of Medicine, Hyogo Medical University, Hyogo 669-2321, Japan; na-nakayama@hyo-med.ac.jp; Tel.: +81-79-552-1181

The number of patients with gynecological cancers, such as ovarian and endometrial cancer, has been increasing worldwide. A possible cause of the high lethality of gynecological cancer is the lack of early detection tools and effective therapeutic interventions. In this regard, basic research on its pathophysiology and novel molecular-based therapeutic strategies is urgently required.

Recent research has focused on elucidating the tumor biology and molecular pathways that mediate cancer progression and drug resistance for the development of novel molecular-targeted therapies. These include monoclonal antibodies, small-molecule receptor tyrosine kinase inhibitors, and agents that block downstream signaling pathways in gynecological cancer. However, newly approved drugs for ovarian cancer are limited and the effectiveness of these incorporated therapies is limited. Therefore, further research is required to gain a better understanding of this phenomenon.

It was in this context that the Special Issue of *Biomedicines* entitled "Mechanisms and Novel Therapeutic Approaches for Gynecologic Cancer" was edited, focusing on how basic research, such as genomics, epigenomics, and proteomics, as well as clinical research can contribute to improving the mortality of patients with gynecological cancer.

This book, based on the aforementioned Special Issue of *Biomedicines*, contains a total of 13 papers (eight original research and five reviews) focusing on basic research of gynecologic cancer.

Among the original articles, the first study is an in vitro on ovarian cancer that focused on the novel ovarian cancer-related transcriptional factor, nucleus accumbens-associated protein 1 (NAC1). The researchers performed functional and structural analyses of its DNA-binding domain, the BEN domain, and clarified the target sequence using a PCR-assisted random oligonucleotide selection approach. The interaction between NAC1 and target DNA was validated using several novel techniques, including isothermal titration calorimetry (ITC), chromatin-immunoprecipitation assays, and NMR chemical shift perturbation (CSP). As NAC1 is significantly overexpressed in several types of carcinomas, including ovarian and cervical; is associated with tumor growth, survival and drug resistance; and is considered to be a target molecule for intervention, this study will contribute to novel molecular targeted therapies [1].

The second article describes a study of BRCA1 mutant ovarian cancer. They investigated the functional impact of platelet-activating factor acetylhydrolase (PAF-AH) and clarified its interaction with the Wnt signaling pathway. They then provided evidence that PAF-AH is a positive prognostic factor with functional impact mediated by the negative regulation of the Wnt/-catenin pathway in BRCA1 mutant ovarian cancer. This study shows the importance of PAF-AH as a biomarker for predicting disease risk in BRCA1 mutation carriers [2].

The third study incorporated gene ontology (GO)-based integrative approaches to explore the expression profiles of serous borderline ovarian tumors (BOTs) and serous ovarian carcinomas to identify common and meaningful dysregulated functions and dysfunctional pathways between these two groups. Then, they detected differentially expressed genes

(DEGs), such as SRC, ARNT, TBP, and SNAI2, which play a crucial role in the pathogenesis of both tumors, implying a gradual evolution from serous BOTs to ovarian carcinomas. These findings may contribute to the future development of targeted therapies [3].

The fourth study describes clinical research on cervical cancer, in which HPV DNA tests are highly sensitive, but the specificity of HPV tests is low. This study identified the potential role of this test in diagnosing cervical precancerous lesions (CIN) using archival paraffin-embedded specimens of CIN1 (31), CIN2 (75), and CIN3. The authors concluded that, based on HPV-induced oncogenesis, the expression profile of testin, Ki-67, and p16 would improve test sensitivity and specificity in diagnosing cervical intraepithelial changes [4].

The fifth study was an in vitro study to establish an effective treatment strategy that targeted ovarian cancer stem cells (CSCs), which are related to chemoresistance and cancer recurrence. They developed a codon-optimized third-generation chimeric antigen receptor (CAR) to specifically target CD44, a CSC marker. They showed that simultaneous treatment with CD44NK and cisplatin demonstrated excellent antitumor activity against CD44+ ovarian cancer cells in vitro. This study provides the basis for further in vivo studies and future clinical development [5].

In the sixth study, the authors investigated somatic mutations in DNA damage response (DDR) genes in ovarian cancer tissue using a multi gene panel with next-generation sequencing. They discovered that DDR gene somatic mutations is more relevant in serous carcinoma and are associated with recurrence and cancer-related death. They then clarified the clinical characteristics and outcomes of ovarian cancer based on the DDR gene mutation profile. This study provides a rationale for future studies on novel therapeutic targets for DNA damage response pathways [6].

The seventh study describes clinical research on endometrioid endometrial cancer, showing the role of DNA mismatch repair (MMR) status in survival and its correlation with clinical prognostic factors in a relatively large sample size. The authors recruited 238 patients with endometrioid endometrial cancer and demonstrated that MMR deficiency (dMMR) is present in a significant number of patients and is associated with poorer clinicopathological factors and worse prognosis, particularly in long term follow-up (5–10 years). They concluded that dMMR should be considered in the risk stratification of endometrial cancer to guide optimal therapeutic intervention and individualization for a longer follow-up plan [7].

The last retrospective clinical research article focused on radiation therapy for endometrial cancer. The authors used in vivo dosimetry (IVD) to measure the dose to organs at risk (OAR) ratio for patients receiving postoperative high-dose-rate (HDR) interventional radiotherapy in two different fractionation schedules, analyzed its efficacy on treatment-related toxicities retrospectively, and showed its safety and acceptability [8].

Three review papers in the field of ovarian cancer were included in this book. First, there is a review on the human cytomegalovirus (HCMV) infection and ovarian cancer. The authors highlighted the impact of immunomodulatory effects of HCMV infection on host immune responses to ovarian carcinogenesis [9]. The second review focuses on ovarian cancer and exosomes, which play important roles in cell–cell communication and the regulation of various biological processes in cancer progression. The authors reviewed the potential of exosomal miRNAs in the circulation as a good biomarker for non-invasive early detection of ovarian cancer, along with current clinical trials [10]. In the third review of ovarian cancer, the authors comprehensively reviewed the molecular characteristics of ovarian cancer and the recent evidence on approved molecular targeted drugs, such as immune checkpoint inhibitors, PARP inhibitors, and anti-angiogenic therapies, which have made great advances in EOC treatment. They summarized new possible complementary approaches in preclinical stages, focusing on drug repurposing, non-coding RNAs, and nanomedicine as new methods for drug delivery [11].

The next review is on endometrial carcinoma (EC) and focuses on immune microenvironment modifications and immune response activation. The authors summarized the current knowledge of the immune environment of EC, both for mismatch repair deficient and mismatch repair proficient tumors. They also reviewed clinical data on immune checkpoint inhibitors (ICI) and PD-1/PD-L1 inhibitors and discussed the future possibility of various ICI-based combination therapies to limit resistance to immunotherapy [12].

The last review is a comprehensive literature review of vulvovaginal melanomas, which are quite rare among gynecologic cancers. Due to the lack of a sufficient number of cases to conduct randomized clinical trials, specific treatment guidelines have not yet been established, and the prognosis of vulvovaginal melanomas is very poor without a standardized treatment strategy. In this regard, this review is significant in highlighting the increasing research on the future establishment of novel therapeutic schemes [13].

I believe that this book includes important advanced studies on gynecologic cancer and comprehensive reviews covering relatively frequent to rare tumors in gynecologic oncology.

Funding: This research received no external funding.

Institutional Review Board Statement: Not applicable.

Informed Consent Statement: Not applicable.

Conflicts of Interest: The author declares no conflict of interest.

References

1. Nakayama, N.; Sakashita, G.; Nagata, T.; Kobayashi, N.; Yoshida, H.; Park, S.; Nariai, Y.; Kato, H.; Obayashi, E.; Nakayama, K.; et al. Nucleus Accumbens-Associated Protein 1 Binds DNA Directly through the BEN Domain in a Sequence-Specific Manner. *Biomedicines* **2020**, *8*, 608. [CrossRef] [PubMed]
2. Liao, Y.; Badmann, S.; Kaltofen, T.; Mayr, D.; Schmoeckel, E.; Deuster, E.; Mannewitz, M.; Landgrebe, S.; Kolben, T.; Hester, A.; et al. Platelet-Activating Factor Acetylhydrolase Expression in BRCA1 Mutant Ovarian Cancer as a Protective Factor and Potential Negative Regulator of the Wnt Signaling Pathway. *Biomedicines* **2021**, *9*, 706. [CrossRef] [PubMed]
3. Su, K.; Gao, H.; Chang, C.; Lu, K.; Yu, M.; Lin, Y.; Liu, L.; Chang, C.; Li, Y.; Chang, C. Synergistic AHR Binding Pathway with EMT Effects on Serous Ovarian Tumors Recognized by Multidisciplinary Integrated Analysis. *Biomedicines* **2021**, *9*, 866. [CrossRef] [PubMed]
4. Popiel, A.; Piotrowska, A.; Sputa-Grzegrzolka, P.; Smolarz, B.; Romanowicz, H.; Dziegiel, P.; Podhorska-Okolow, M.; Kobierzycki, C. Preliminary Study on the Expression of Testin, p16 and Ki-67 in the Cervical Intraepithelial Neoplasia. *Biomedicines* **2021**, *9*, 1010. [CrossRef] [PubMed]
5. Klapdor, R.; Wang, S.; Morgan, M.; Zimmermann, K.; Hachenberg, J.; Büning, H.; Dörk, T.; Hillemanns, P.; Schambach, A. NK Cell-Mediated Eradication of Ovarian Cancer Cells with a Novel Chimeric Antigen Receptor Directed against CD44. *Biomedicines* **2021**, *9*, 1339. [CrossRef] [PubMed]
6. Chiang, Y.C.; Lin, P.; Lu, T.; Kuo, K.; Taiwan, Y.; Hsu, H.; Wu, C.; Lee, C.; Shen, H.; Chen, C.; et al. A DNA Damage Response Gene Panel for Different Histologic Types of Epithelial Ovarian Carcinomas and Their Outcomes. *Biomedicines* **2021**, *9*, 1384. [CrossRef] [PubMed]
7. Lee, J.H.S.; Li, J.J.X.; Chow, C.; Chan, R.C.K.; Kwan, J.S.H.; Lau, T.S.; To, K.F.; Yim, S.F.; Yeung, S.Y.; Kwong, J. Long-Term Survival and Clinicopathological Implications of DNA Mismatch Repair Status in Endometrioid Endometrial Cancers in Hong Kong Chinese Women. *Biomedicines* **2021**, *9*, 1385. [CrossRef] [PubMed]
8. Soror, T.; Chafii, R.; Lancellotta, V.; Tagliaferri, L.; Kovács, G. Biological Planning of Radiation Dose Based on In Vivo Dosimetry for Postoperative Vaginal-Cuff HDR Interventional Radiotherapy (Brachytherapy). *Biomedicines* **2021**, *9*, 1629. [CrossRef] [PubMed]
9. Cox, M.; Apriliana, E.R.; Kartikasari, P.; Gorry, R.; Flanagan, K.; Plebanski, M. Potential Impact of Human Cytomegalovirus Infection on Immunity to Ovarian Tumours and Cancer Progression. *Biomedicines* **2021**, *9*, 351. [CrossRef] [PubMed]
10. Shiao, M.; Chang, J.; Lertkhachonsuk, A.; Rermluk, N.; Jinawath, N. Circulating Exosomal miRNAs as Biomarkers in Epithelial Ovarian Cancer. *Biomedicines* **2021**, *9*, 1433. [CrossRef] [PubMed]
11. Garrido, M.P.; Fredes, A.N.; Lobos-González, L.; Valenzuela-Valderrama, M.; Vera, D.B.; Romero, C. Current Treatments and New Possible Complementary Therapies for Epithelial Ovarian Cancer. *Biomedicines* **2022**, *10*, 77. [CrossRef] [PubMed]
12. Rousset-Rouvière, S.; Rochigneux, P.; Chrétien, A.; Fattori, S.; Gorvel, L.; Provansal, M.; Lambaudie, E.; Olive, D.; Sabatier, R. Endometrial Carcinoma: Immune Microenvironment and Emerging Treatments in Immuno-Oncology. *Biomedicines* **2021**, *9*, 632. [CrossRef] [PubMed]
13. Dobrică, E.; Vâjâitu, C.; Condrat, C.E.; Crețoiu, D.; Popa, I.; Gaspar, B.S.; Suciu, N.; Crețoiu, S.M.; Varlas, V.N. Vulvar and Vaginal Melanomas—The Darker Shades of Gynecological Cancers. *Biomedicines* **2021**, *9*, 758. [CrossRef] [PubMed]

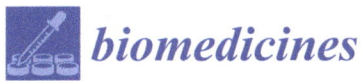

Article

Nucleus Accumbens-Associated Protein 1 Binds DNA Directly through the BEN Domain in a Sequence-Specific Manner

Naomi Nakayama [1,2], Gyosuke Sakashita [1], Takashi Nagata [3,4], Naohiro Kobayashi [5], Hisashi Yoshida [6], Sam-Yong Park [6], Yuko Nariai [1], Hiroaki Kato [1], Eiji Obayashi [1], Kentaro Nakayama [7], Satoru Kyo [7] and Takeshi Urano [1,*]

1. Department of Biochemistry, Shimane University School of Medicine, Izumo, Shimane 693-8501, Japan; n-nakayama@u-shimane.ac.jp (N.N.); gsakashi@med.shimane-u.ac.jp (G.S.); nariai@med.shimane-u.ac.jp (Y.N.); hkato@med.shimane-u.ac.jp (H.K.); eijioba@med.shimane-u.ac.jp (E.O.)
2. Department of Health and Nutrition, The University of Shimane, Izumo, Shimane 693-8550, Japan
3. Institute of Advanced Energy, Kyoto University, Kyoto 606-8501, Japan; nagata.takashi.6w@kyoto-u.ac.jp
4. Graduate School of Energy Science, Kyoto University, Kyoto 606-8501, Japan
5. Institute for Protein Research, Osaka University, Suita, Osaka 565-0871, Japan; naohiro@protein.osaka-u.ac.jp
6. Protein Design Laboratory, Graduate School of Medical Life Science, Yokohama City University, Yokohama, Kanagawa 230-0045, Japan; h-yosida@yokohama-cu.ac.jp (H.Y.); park@yokohama-cu.ac.jp (S.-Y.P.)
7. Department of Obstetrics and Gynecology, Shimane University School of Medicine, Izumo, Shimane 693-8501, Japan; kn88@med.shimane-u.ac.jp (K.N.); satoruky@med.shimane-u.ac.jp (S.K.)
* Correspondence: turano@med.shimane-u.ac.jp; Tel.: +81-853-20-2126

Received: 2 December 2020; Accepted: 10 December 2020; Published: 14 December 2020

Abstract: Nucleus accumbens-associated protein 1 (NAC1) is a nuclear protein that harbors an amino-terminal BTB domain and a carboxyl-terminal BEN domain. NAC1 appears to play significant and diverse functions in cancer and stem cell biology. Here we demonstrated that the BEN domain of NAC1 is a sequence-specific DNA-binding domain. We selected the palindromic 6 bp motif ACATGT as a target sequence by using a PCR-assisted random oligonucleotide selection approach. The interaction between NAC1 and target DNA was characterized by gel shift assays, pull-down assays, isothermal titration calorimetry (ITC), chromatin-immunoprecipitation assays, and NMR chemical shifts perturbation (CSP). The solution NMR structure revealed that the BEN domain of human NAC-1 is composed of five conserved α helices and two short β sheets, with an additional hitherto unknown N-terminal α helix. In particular, ITC clarified that there are two sequential events in the titration of the BEN domain of NAC1 into the target DNA. The ITC results were further supported by CSP data and structure analyses. Furthermore, live cell photobleaching analyses revealed that the BEN domain of NAC1 alone was unable to interact with chromatin/other proteins in cells.

Keywords: nucleus accumbens-associated protein 1 (NAC1); BEN (BANP, E5R and NAC1) domain; sequence-specific DNA-binding protein; solution NMR structure; isothermal titration calorimetry (ITC)

1. Introduction

Nucleus accumbens-associated protein 1 (NAC1), encoded by the NACC1 gene, is a nuclear protein that encompasses an amino-terminal BTB (broad complex, tramtrack, bric-à-brac) and a carboxyl-terminal BEN (BANP, E5R and NAC1) domain. NAC1 was originally identified and cloned as a cocaine-inducible transcript from the nucleus accumbens, a unique forebrain structure involved in reward motivation and addictive behavior [1]. NACC1 was also identified as a cancer-associated BTB gene by serial analysis of gene expression in ovarian cancer cells [2]. NAC1 is significantly overexpressed in several types of carcinomas, including ovarian, colorectal, breast, renal cell, cervical, and pancreatic carcinomas, is associated with tumor growth and survival, and increases the resistance of tumor cells to chemotherapy [2–14]. Furthermore, NAC1 was shown to be important for the pluripotency of embryonic stem cells [15,16] through direct transcriptional regulation of c-Myc [17]. In addition, it was recently demonstrated that NAC1 promotes mesendodermal and represses neuroectodermal fate selection in embryonic stem cells, in cooperation with the pluripotency transcription factors, Oct4, Sox2, and Tcf3 [18,19] and that NAC1 is critical for efficient iPSC generation [20]. NACC1 knockout mouse embryos and newborns exhibit a lower survival rate compared to wild-type embryos and newborns, and surviving mice showing defective bony patterning in the vertebral axis [21]. NAC1 has also been reported to be an important component of RIG-I-like receptor mediated innate immune responses against viral infection [22].

The BTB domain is a ~120-amino-acid highly conserved motif that mediates homodimerization and/or heterodimerization and interacts with other proteins [23,24]. NAC1 homodimerizes through its BTB domain [25,26] and heterodimerizes with Myc-interacting zinc-finger protein 1 through the respective BTB domains [27–29]. Most BTB proteins contain other C-terminal functional domains, such as DNA-binding C2H2/Krüppel-type zinc fingers.

The BEN domain (BEND) in metazoans and some viruses typically comprises 90–100 amino acid residues. Secondary structure analysis using multiple alignment predicted four α-helices with conserved hydrophobic residues [30]. The human genome encodes nine BEN domain-containing proteins. These proteins can be divided into two distinct groups: one group contains a BTB domain (NAC1 and NAC2 (also known as BTBD14A and RBB)), whereas the other group lacks other recognizable protein domains (i.e., they are BEN-solo proteins [31]) such as BANP (also known as BEND1 and SMAR1) and BEND2, -3, -4, -5, -6, and -7. BEND2 and BEND3 harbor tandem copies of two and four BEN domains, respectively. Based on characterized proteins possessing a BEN domain, it has been predicted that the BEN domain is involved in chromatin organization and transcriptional regulation by mediating protein–DNA and protein–protein interactions [30,32,33]. NAC1 functions as a transcriptional repressor through its association with REST corepressor 1 (also known as CoREST) [32] and with histone deacetylases HDAC3 and HDAC4 [17,34]. NAC2 functions as a transcriptional repressor through its association with nucleosome remodeling and deacetylase complex containing HDAC1 and HDAC2 [35]. The activity of BANP as a transcriptional repressor and candidate tumor suppressor involves the BEN domain in molecular interactions with SIN3-histone deacetylase complex containing HDAC1 [36]. BEND3, a quadruple BEN domain-containing protein, is a key factor that associates with chromatin remodeling complexes and modulates gene expression and heterochromatin organization [33,37,38]. BEND5, a neural BEN-solo protein, functions as a sequence-specific transcription repressor that regulates neurogenesis [39]. BEND6, a neural BEN-solo protein, acts as a corepressor of notch transcription factor [40].

2. Experimental Section

2.1. Cloning

For glutathione S-transferase (GST) fusion, NAC1 (2–527)/pMXs-FHG and NAC1 (2–250)/pMXs-FHG (41) were digested with BamHI and EcoRI. The fragments of human NAC1 cDNA encoding residues 2–527 (full-length, removal of the first methionine) and 2–250 were subcloned into pGEX-4T-2 (GE Healthcare, Piscataway, NJ, USA). The C-terminal fragment of human NAC1 cDNA encoding residues 251-527 was cloned into pGEX-4T-2 by polymerase chain reaction (PCR) using NAC1 (2–527)/pMXs-FHG as template. The NAC1(L432N) mutant was created by standard double PCR mutagenesis and subcloned into pGEX-4T-2. Human NPM1 full-length cDNA (CCDS4376.1) obtained by reverse transcribed PCR using the total RNA from HeLa cells was cloned into pGEX-4T-2.

To generate hexahistidine (His) tagged protein, NAC1 (2–527)/pGEX-4T-2 was digested with BamHI and EcoRI, then subcloned into pET28HisTEV [41]. The C-terminal fragment of human NAC1 cDNA encoding residues 322-485 was cloned into pET28HisTEV by PCR using NAC1 (2–527)/pMXs-FHG as template. All PCR-amplified cDNA products were fully sequenced using a 3130 genetic analyzer (Applied Biosystems/ThermoFisher Scientific, Waltham, MA, USA) to confirm their sequence and to verify the absence of secondary point mutations.

2.2. Screening of DNA-Binding Sequences

The random oligonucleotide pool N26 (5′-CAGGTCAGTTCAGCGGATCCTGTCG(N)26GAGGCG AATTCAGTGCAACTGCAGC-3′) contains a synthetic single-stranded random 26-base sequence flanked by two PCR primer sequences (N26-1S, 5′-CAGGTCAGTTCAGCGGATCCTGTCG-3′; N26-2AS, 5′-GCTGCAGTTGCACTGAATTCGCCTC-3′). The flanking sequences contain BamHI and EcoRI restriction sites to facilitate subsequent cloning. The random oligonucleotide pool (1.2 µg) was precleared with recombinant GST-NAC1(L432N), then incubated for 30 min at room temperature with GST-NAC1 in 500 µL of binding buffer (20 mM HEPES/KOH pH 7.9, 50 mM KCl, 2 mM $MgCl_2$, 0.5 mM EDTA, 10% glycerol, 1 mg/mL bovine serum albumin, 2 mM dithiothreitol, and 10 mg/mL poly(dI/dC)). After washing three times with the binding buffer, samples were resuspended in 100 µL distilled water and boiled for 10 min to elute bound DNA. Following centrifugation, 10 µL of the supernatant was used as template for PCR with the forward primer N26-1S and reverse primer N26-2AS using the following PCR conditions: 20 cycles of 1 min at 94 °C, 1 min at 62 °C, and 1 min at 72 °C. The PCR products were then purified using a PCR purification kit (Qiagen, Hilden, Germany), and resuspended in distilled water. Half the volume of each purified PCR product was subsequently used for the next cycle of selection. Four sequential repeats of selection were followed by PCR and the final selected DNA fragments were digested by BamHI and EcoRI, subcloned into pBluescript SK II (Stratagene, La Jolla, CA, USA), and the sequences were determined using T7 primer. The sequence data are shown aligned using the same orientation (as primed from the BamHI side) (Figure 1A).

2.3. Bioinformatics

Amino acid sequence alignment of the BEN domain from human BEN-domain containing proteins were conducted using Clustal Omega (http://www.ebi.ac.uk/Tools/msa/clustalo/).

PCR-assisted random oligonucleotide selection identified 18 independent clones that bound to GST-NAC1 and these sequences were entered into the MEME program (http://meme-suite.org/tools/meme) (Figure 1C). The relevant parameters were set such that each sequence was used once to generate a motif between 6–26 nucleotides long.

2.4. Oligonucleotide Pull-Down Assay

Sense oligonucleotides for the GADD45GIP1 promoter, with biotin added to their 5′-end, were synthesized by FASMAC (Kanagawa, Japan). The sequences for the oligonucleotides were as follows: Biotin-GP1, biotin-5′-TGTGTGTGTATGCATGTATGTATTTATT-3′ (wild type, sense) and 5′-AATAAATACATACATGCATACACACACA-3′ (wild type, antisense); Biotin-GP1 5′-mut, biotin-5′-TGTGTGTGTCATCATGTATGTATTTATT-3′ (sense) and 5′-AATAAA TACATACATGATGACACACACA-3′ (antisense); Biotin-GP1 mut, biotin-5′-TGTGTGTGTAT GGCATTATGTATTTATT-3′ (sense) and 5′-AATAAATACATAATGCCATACACACACA-3′ (antisense); Biotin-GP1 3′-mut, biotin-5′-TGTGTGTGTATGCATGACGGTATTTATT-3′ (sense) and 5′-AATA AATACCGTCATGCATACACACACA-3′ (antisense). Each pair of oligonucleotides was annealed following standard protocols. Bacterially expressed and purified GST-NAC1 (5 µg) were precleared using streptavidin-magnetic beads (20 µL/sample, Dynabeads M-280, ThermoFisher Scientific) for 1 h at 4 °C. The precleared supernatant was incubated with 100 pmol of biotinylated double-stranded DNA (dsDNA) oligonucleotides and 10 µg of poly(dI/dC) for 30 min at 4 °C. DNA-bound proteins were collected using 30 µL of streptavidin-magnetic beads for 1 h at 4 °C. After washing three times, the bound proteins were eluted from the beads in SDS-PAGE sample buffer and resolved by SDS-PAGE, followed by Coomassie blue staining of the gel.

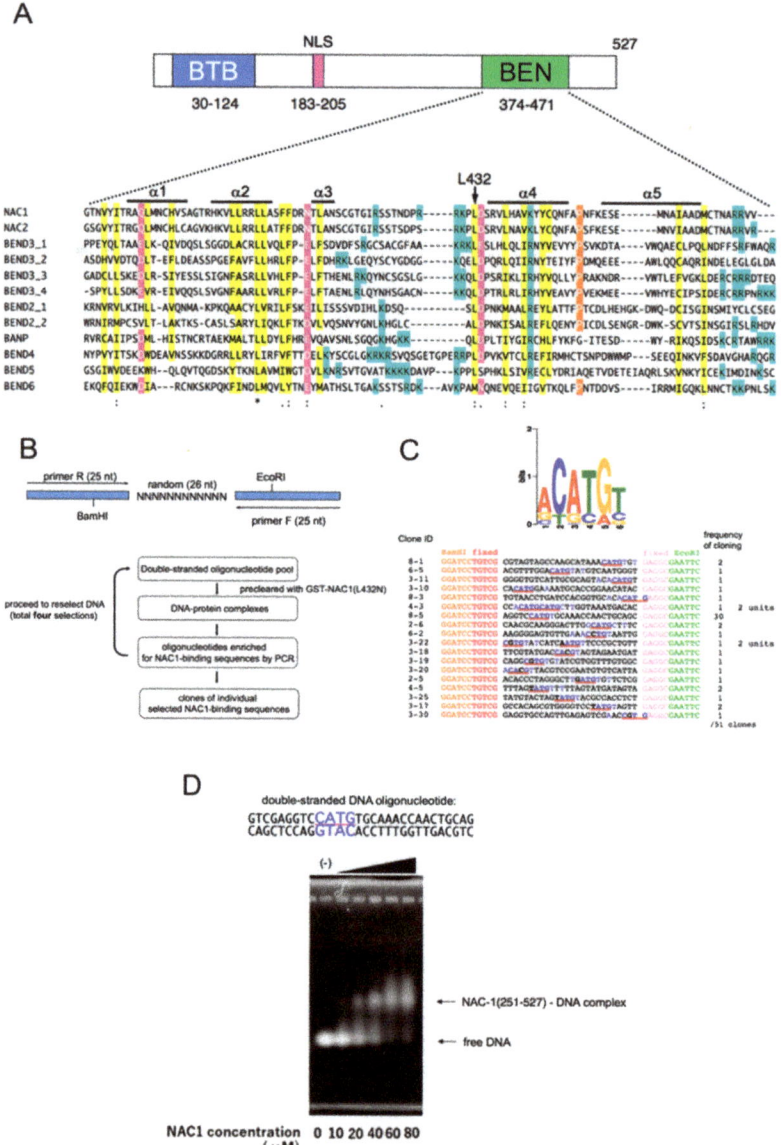

Figure 1. Identification of the consensus DNA-binding sequence of NAC1. (**A**) Schematic representation of human NAC1 protein showing the BTB domain, nuclear localization signal (NLS) and the BEN domain. Clustal Omega alignment of human BEN domain-containing proteins showing highly conserved residues. Color coding reflects the conservation of amino acid types: yellow, blue and magenta for hydrophobic, positively and negatively charged amino acids, respectively. Symbols are as follows: (*), identical residues; (:), highly conserved residues; (.) lower but significant conservation between all members. α-Helical regions are labeled above and are based on Figure 3A. The source and corresponding UniProt accession numbers are indicated. NAC1, Q96RE7; NAC2, Q96BF6; BANP, Q8N9N5; BEND2, Q4V9S2; BEND3, Q5T5 × 7; BEND4, Q6ZU67; BEND5, Q7L4P6; BEND6, Q5SZJ8;

BEND7, Q8N7W2. (**B**) Construction of the dsDNA oligonucleotide pool containing a random 26 bp core flanked by 25 nucleotide (nt) primer sequences (upper panel). Lower panel, outline of the selection procedure conducted to determine the DNA-binding motif of NAC1. (**C**) MEME graphical representation of the oligonucleotides selected by NAC1 after four rounds of selection (upper panel). The MEME program parameters were set to use each nucleotide once and to generate a motif with a maximum length of 26 nucleotides. The horizontal axis represents the position of each base. The height of each stack on the vertical axis indicates nucleotide conservation at that position (in bits) and the height of each nucleotide symbol within a stack corresponds to how frequently that nucleotide occurs. Lower panel, sequences of the 18 oligonucleotides used to generate the motif in the upper panel. Only the random portion of the oligonucleotide sequence flanked by the BamHI and EcoRI sites is shown. Sequences corresponding to CATG are underlined in red, and conserved sequences are highlighted with blue characters. The numbers at the left indicate the clone ID. Numbers showing the frequency of cloning are indicated on the right. (**D**) Band shift assay using a biotin-labeled dsDNA oligonucleotide probe corresponding to the #8-5 sequence (Upper panel). Lower panel, the probe (20 µM) was mixed with increasing amounts of bacterially expressed and purified NAC1 without GST (-, 0 µM; 10 µM, 20 µM, 40 µM, 60 µM and 80 µM) and analysed by band shift assay.

2.5. Antibody and Chromatin Immunoprecipitation (ChIP) Assay

To generate rabbit polyclonal antibodies, the region encompassing amino acids 251-527 of human NAC1 was expressed as His-tagged proteins in Escherichia coli. The anti-NAC1 antibodies were affinity-purified on protein coupled to CNBr-activated Sepharose 4B (GE Healthcare, Buckinghamshire, UK).

Human ovarian OV207 cells were cross-linked with a final concentration of 1% (*v/v*) formaldehyde for 10 min at 37 °C, then the cells were incubated for 5 min at 37 °C in 0.125 M glycine to stop the cross-linking reaction. After washing twice with ice-cold PBS, the cells were lysed with 200 µL of SDS-lysis buffer (1% SDS, 10mM EDTA, 50mM Tris-HCl, pH 8.1) and protease inhibitors for 10 min on ice, then 1800 µL of ChIP buffer (0.01% SDS, 1.1% Triton X-100, 1.2mM EDTA, 16.7mM Tris-HCl, pH 8.1, 167mM NaCl) was added. A Branson sonifier 250 was used to shear the genomic DNA by sonification. After removal of cellular debris by centrifugation and digestion of the RNA with RNase A, equal amounts of DNA were incubated with 3 µg of anti-NAC1 antibody or control IgG antibodies previously bound to anti-rabbit IgG-coupled magnetic beads (Dynabeads M-280, ThermoFisher Scientific). After extensive washing, the precipitated DNA fragments were eluted. Precipitated DNA was analyzed by PCR using the following primers: PSAT1, 5′-GGCAGGTGGTCAACTTTGG-3′ (forward) and 5′-GAACACTAATGCCAACTCC-3′ (reverse); AZU1, 5′-TTTCCATCAGCAGCATGAGC-3′ (forward) and 5′-TATCGTCACGCTGCTGGTG-3′ (reverse); β-actin, 5′-CCAACCGCGAGAAGATGACCC-3′ (forward) and 5′-CGTCACCGGAGTCCATCACGA-3′ (reverse). Each PCR product was quantified using a Takara Thermal Cycler Dice RealTime System (Kusatsu, Shiga, Japan). ChIP experiments were performed at least in triplicate on independent biological samples. The value for each sample, as shown in Figure 2C, was normalized using the value for β-actin.

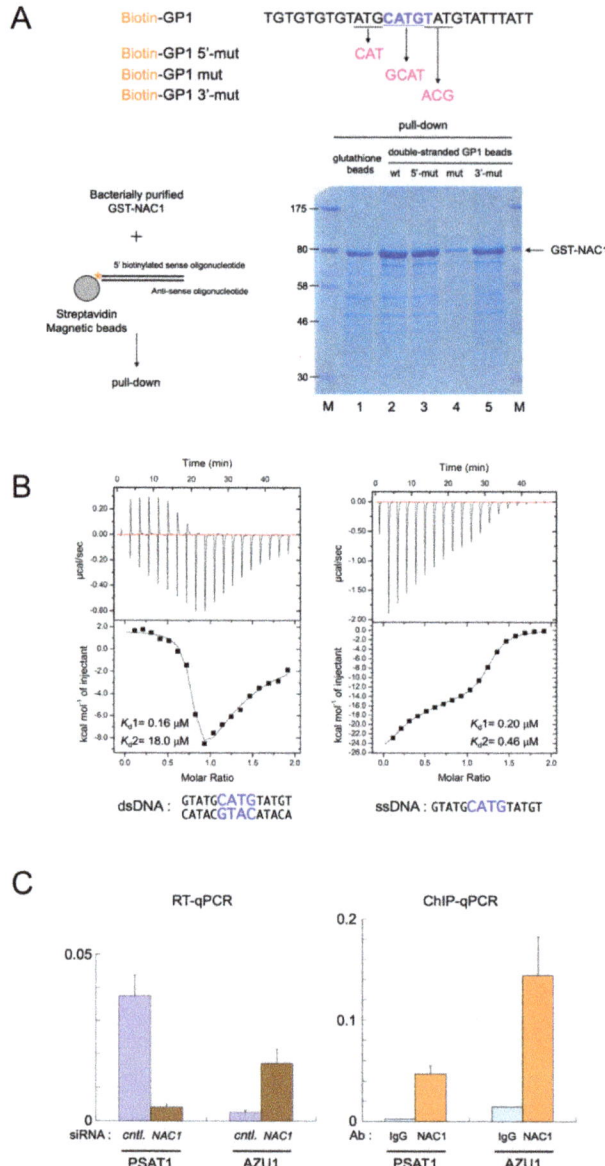

Figure 2. Characterization of the consensus DNA-binding sequence of NAC1. (**A**) Pull-down assay using dsDNA oligonucleotides for wild type and mutant probes against GADD45GIP1 promoter (Upper panel, only sense oligonucleotides are shown). Lower left panel, outline of the pull-down procedure. Lower right panel, 5 μg of bacterially expressed and purified GST-NAC1 was mixed with biotin-labeled dsDNA oligonucleotides for wild type and mutant probes, and pull-down assays were performed. The gel was stained with Coomassie blue to detect NAC1 in the dsDNA-protein complexes pulled down by the oligonucleotides. (**B**) Isothermal titration calorimetry. Upper panels are raw titration data plotted as heat (μcal/s) versus time (min). Each experiment consisted of 28 injections of 10 μL of 50 μM

dsDNA (left panel) or of ssDNA (right panel) into a solution of 500 μM NAC-1 (322–485) at 25 °C. The lower panels are integrated heat responses plotted as normalized heat per mole of injectant. Smooth curves represent best fits of the data to the equation as described under "Materials and methods" using software provided by the instrument manufacturer. Data shown is representative of three independent experiments. (**C**) Left panel, RT-qPCR of PSAT1 and AZU1 mRNAs in control (cntl.) and NAC1 knockdown OV207 cells. Right panel, qPCR of ChIP analysis for control IgG (IgG) and NAC1 in OV207 cells.

2.6. Isothermal Titration Calorimetry (ITC) Experiments

All calorimetric titrations were carried out on iTC200 calorimeters (MicroCal, Malvern Biosciences, Columbia, MD, USA). Protein samples were dialyzed against the buffer containing 20 mM HEPES (pH 7.0) and 0.1M NaCl with 1mM Tris (2-carboxyethyl)phosphine. The sequences for the oligonucleotides were as follows: GP1 [14], 5′-GTATGCATGTATGT-3′ (wild type, sense) and 5′-ACATACATGCATAC-3′ (wild type, antisense), GP1 mut, 5′-GTATGGCATTATGT-3′ and 5′-ACATAATGCCATAC-3′, de novo motif 1, 5′-AACCGCCGCCAA-3′ and 5′-TTGGCGGCGGTT-3′, de novo motif 2, 5′- AACCCCGCCCCAA-3′ and 5′- TTGGGGCGGGGTT-3′. The sample cell was filled with a 50 μM solution of dsDNA or ssDNA of GP1, dsDNA of GP1 mut, de novo motif 1 and motif 2, and the injection syringe was filled with 500 μM titrating NAC-1322-485. For iTC200, each titration typically consisted of a preliminary 0.4-μL injection followed by 19 subsequent 2-μL injections every 150 s. All of the experiments were performed at 20 °C. Data for the preliminary injection, which were affected by diffusion of the solution from and into the injection syringe during the initial equilibration period, were discarded. Binding isotherms were generated by plotting heats of reaction normalized by the moles of injected protein versus the ratio of the total injected one to total DNA per injection. The data were fitted using Origin software (Northampton, MA, USA).

2.7. NMR Spectroscopy

Escherichia coli strain BL21 (DE3) RIPL CodonPlus was transformed with NAC1 (322–485)/pET28HisTEV. Cells were induced with 0.5 mM IPTG, then grown overnight at 15 °C in M9 minimal medium containing 1 g/L 15N-NH4Cl (ISOTEC, Canton, GA, USA) and 5 g/L 13C-glucose (ISOTEC) as nitrogen and carbon sources, respectively. Harvested cells were resuspended in Ni-NTA binding buffer (20 mM Tris-HCl, pH 8.0, 1M NaCl, 25 mM imidazole, 10 mM β-mercaptoethanol) and lysed using an EmulsiFlex homogeniser (Avestin, Ottawa, ON, Canada). After centrifugation, the supernatant was loaded onto Ni-NTA agarose (Qiagen, Hilden, Germany) columns equilibrated with the same buffer. Protein was eluted using a 25–500 mM linear gradient of imidazole. Peak fractions were incubated overnight with His-tagged TEV protease at room temperature while dialyzing against Ni-NTA low-salt buffer (20mM Tris-HCl, pH 8.0, 150 mM NaCl, 25 mM imidazole, 10 mM β-mercaptoethanol). After complete cleavage, the sample was loaded onto a Ni-NTA agarose column to remove the His-tag, His-tagged TEV protease, and minor protein contaminants.

13C, 15N-labeled NAC1322-485 was concentrated to 500 μM and dissolved in 20 mM sodium phosphate buffer (pH 6.0) prepared using 95% 1H2O/5% 2H2O and containing 50 mM NaCl and 1 mM 1,4-DL-dithiothreitol (DTT). All NMR data were collected at 298 K on a Bruker AVANCE 600 MHz NMR spectrometer (Billerica, MA, USA) equipped with a cryogenic probe. NMR spectra were processed with NMRPipe/NMRDraw program [42]. Spectral analysis was performed with KUJIRA 0.984 [43], a program suite for interactive NMR analysis that works in conjunction with NMRView [44], and SPARKY 3, according to the methods described previously [45]. The backbone 1H, 15N, and 13C resonances of NAC1322-485 were assigned by standard double- and triple-resonance NMR experiments [46,47]: 2D 1H–15N heteronuclear single quantum correlation (HSQC), and 3D HNCO, 3D HN(CA)CO, 3D CBCA(CO)NH, and 3D HNCACB spectra.

Assignments of side chain resonances for nonaromatic residues were obtained by 2D 1H-13C HSQC and 3D HBHA(CO)NH, HC(CCO)NH, C(CCO)NH, H(C)CH correlation spectroscopy (COSY),

H(C)CH-total correlated spectroscopy (TOCSY), and (H)CCH-TOCSY, whereas assignments for aromatic residues were performed using H(C)CH COSY, aided by 13C-edited nuclear Overhauser effect spectroscopy (NOESY)-HSQC spectra obtained using a mixing time of 80 ms. Distance restraints were derived from 3D 15N-edited and 13C-edited NOESY-HSQC spectra, and each was measured using a mixing time of 80 ms. Protein backbone φ, ψ and side chain χ_1, χ_2 torsion angle restraints were determined by chemical shift database analysis using the program TALOS+ [48] and by inspecting the pattern of intraresidual NOE intensities [49], respectively. The chemical shift data were deposited in BioMagResDB (BMRB ID: 36342).

An NMR titration experiment on NAC1322-485 with dsDNA was performed by recording 2D 1H–15N HSQC spectra at 298 K. The sequences for the 14-mer oligonucleotides derived from GP1 were 5′-GTATGCATGTATGT-3′ (sense) 5′-ACATACATGCATAC-3′ (antisense) and the oligonucleotide pair was annealed following standard protocols. Increasing amounts of unlabeled dsDNA were added to 75 µM 15N-labeled NAC1322-485 to obtain molar ratios of 1:0, 1:0.2, 1:0.4, 1:0.6, 1:0.8, 1:1, 1:1.2, and 1:1.5. The weighted chemical shift perturbations for backbone 15N and 1HN resonances at a ratio of [protein]:[dsDNA] = 1:1.5 were calculated as: $\Delta\delta = [(\Delta\delta HN)^2 + (\Delta\delta N/6.5)^2]^{1/2}$ [50].

2.8. Structure Calculation

Structure calculations for NAC1322-485 were performed using CYANA 2.1 [51–53]. The standard CYANA simulated annealing schedule was used with 40,000 torsion angle dynamics steps per conformer with 200 initial randomized conformers. The 40 conformers exhibiting the lowest final CYANA target function values were further energy minimized with AMBER 12 [54] using the AMBER 2003 force field and a generalized Born model, as described previously [45]. The force constants for distance, torsion angle, and ω angle restraints were set to 32 kcal mol-1 Å-2, 60 kcal mol-1 rad-1, and 50 kcal mol-1 rad-2, respectively. The 20 conformers that were most consistent with the experimental restraints were then used for further analyses. The final structures were validated and visualized by using the Ramachandran plot web server [55] and CHIMERA software [56,57]. Detailed experimental data and structural statistics are summarized in Table S1. The final ensembles of 20 conformers were deposited in the Protein Data Bank (PDB ID: 7BV9).

2.9. Cell Culture and siRNA Transfection

The human ovarian cell line OV207 was a kind gift from Dr. Ie-Ming Shih (Johns Hopkins Medical Institutions, Baltimore, MD, USA). Cells were grown in Dulbecco's modified Eagle's medium (DMEM; Nissui Pharmaceutical, Tokyo, Japan) supplemented with 10% fetal bovine serum (Sigma, St. Louis, MO, USA). Stealth small interfering RNA (siRNA) against NAC1 (5′-CCGGCUGAACUUAUCAACCAGAUUG-3′) and control siRNA (5′-CACAUGAAGCAGCACGACUUCUUCA-3′) were purchased from ThermoFisher Scientific [12]. Cells were transfected with siRNA using Oligofectamine (ThermoFisher Scientific), according to the manufacturer's instructions.

2.10. FRAP and FLIP Analyses

Fluorescent images were acquired using an FV1000 laser scanning confocal unit coupled to an inverted microscope (model IX81; Olympus, Tokyo, Japan) equipped with a ×100 oil immersion objective (UPLSAPO 100XO, NA 1.40, Olympus) and analysed using Fluoview software (Olympus). Cells were maintained at 37 °C in a Tokai Hit incubation system for microscopes (Tokai Hit, Shizuoka, Japan). Cells were analyzed on 35 mm glass-bottom dishes (IWAKI, Tokyo, Japan) in CO2-independent medium (ThermoFisher Scientific) to avoid medium acidification in the CO2-free atmosphere. A 473 nm laser (laser power: 0.1%) was used to excite GFP. A square region of interest (ROI) of 150 × 150 pixels (1 pixel = 0.124 µm) was scanned with a 2-line Kalman filter to obtain a noise-free image ideal for intensity measurements.

For FRAP experiments, five and 95 images (scanning time: 456 ms/frame) were acquired before and after bleaching, respectively. Photobleaching was performed by creating a bleach spot of 8×8 pixels using the Tornado mode of the FV1000 confocal unit (bleaching time: 250 ms; laser power: 100%). Using this bleaching condition, the bleaching constant (K) and the half width of the beam (w) were estimated to be 3.56 ± 0.432 and 1.63 ± 0.145, respectively. The intensities of the bleached area (B), unbleached area (U), and the background (bg) in each post-bleach image were measured to obtain the intensity ratio (Rn): $Rn = (B - bg)/(U - bg)$. Rn values were divided by the average intensity ratio (R0) of the five pre-bleach images to obtain the normalized FRAP values (R): $R = Rn/R0$. We defined the time point when R reached 0.5 as t1/2. For each condition, the mean and SD of at least 35 individual FRAP values were calculated to draw the plots. Welch's two sample t test was used in the FRAP analysis to calculate the p-values; ***, $p < 0.001$.

FLIP experiments were conducted using the time controller function of the FV1000, according to the manufacturer's instructions. Five pre-bleach images were acquired before beginning 50 bleach-scan cycles. In a bleach-scan cycle, half of the ROI (150×75 pixels) was bleached once (laser power: 100%) before scanning a post-bleach image (150×150 pixels). Intensity ratios of the pre- and post-bleach images were calculated to obtain normalized FLIP values, as in the FRAP experiments. For each condition, the mean and SD values of at least 8 individual FLIP values were calculated to draw the plots.

2.11. Accession Numbers

Detailed experimental data and structural statistics have been deposited with the Protein Data bank under accession number 7BV9. The chemical shift data have been deposited in BioMagResDB (BMRB ID: 36342).

3. Results

3.1. NAC1 Binds DNA through Its BEN Domain

We have recently shown that NAC1 harbors an unusual bipartite-type nuclear localization signal to endow transcriptional regulator functions (Figure 1A) [58], and used live cell photobleaching analysis to show that a substantial fraction of NAC1 in the nucleus is associated with or interacts with nuclear proteins or chromatin [59]. However, whether NAC1 directly binds DNA, and if so, which domain of NAC1 is involved in binding, remains unknown. We performed gel mobility shift assays to investigate whether NAC1 protein directly binds DNA, using nucleophosmin (NPM1) as a positive control [60]. Linearized pBluescript SK II plasmid DNA was incubated with bacterially expressed and purified glutathione S-transferase (GST)-NAC1 protein. We found that the mobility of SKII DNA was slower than that of free plasmid DNA, whereas there was no difference in the mobility of SK II DNA following incubation with proteins such as GST alone or BSA, as shown in Figure S1A. During the experiments, we noticed that bacterially expressed and purified NAC1 proteins are contaminated with the bacterial genome (Figure S1A, lane 3). The size distribution of the bacterial genome was likely the result of physical shearing by sonication during cell lysis. For subsequent experiments we therefore used a simple and convenient assay without linearized plasmid DNA as a screening tool and denoted this assay 'bacterial genome carry-over assay'.

To determine which domain of NAC1 is responsible for its DNA-binding properties, we divided NAC1 protein into two parts: the N-terminal half containing the BTB domain and nuclear localization signal (NLS), and the C-terminal half harboring the BEN domain (Figure 1A). Bacterial genome carry-over assays clearly showed that the C-terminal, but not the N-terminal half of NAC1 is contaminated with the bacterial genome (Figure S1B). The BEN domain was identified by computational analysis and may mediate protein–DNA and/or protein–protein interactions during chromatin organization and transcription [30]. We hypothesized that the BEN domain directly binds DNA. We therefore attempted to generate full-length NAC1 protein mutants with amino acid substitutions of highly conserved residues in the BEN domain (Figure 1A). Full-length NAC1 carrying the L432N substitution was expressed in E. coli, purified, and then subjected to bacterial genome carry-over analysis. As shown in Figure S1C, NAC1 (L432N) showed severely impaired carry-over activity. DNase or RNase treatment of the carry-over materials revealed that NAC1 exhibited a clear preference for DNA over RNA (Figure S1D). These findings suggest that NAC1 directly binds DNA via the BEN domain.

3.2. Identification of the Consensus DNA-Binding Sequence of NAC1

We used a PCR-assisted random oligonucleotide selection approach to identify the consensus DNA-binding sequence for human NAC1 [61] (Figure 1B). Bacterially expressed GST-NAC1 protein on beads was washed with an excess volume of washing buffer containing 500 mM NaCl to prevent contamination by the bacterial genome. The purified protein was used to select preferred binding sequences from a random pool of dsDNA. Following precipitation of the NAC1-DNA complex using glutathione beads, we washed away unbound oligonucleotides, eluted the NAC1-DNA complex, and then PCR amplified the selected fragments through four rounds of selection. The background of oligonucleotides precipitated due to non-specific binding was reduced by preclearing the oligonucleotide pool with GST-NAC1 (L432N) beads in each round. We then cloned and sequenced all 51 oligonucleotide fragments (18 different clones) (Figure 1C, lower panel). All 18 oligonucleotides were used to generate a binding motif using MEME software [62]. Our results show that NAC1 selects the palindromic 6-bp motif ACATGT containing the core sequence CATG (Figure 1C, upper panel).

GST is known to form stable dimers. To eliminate the influence of GST-fusion, we checked the binding of NAC1 (251-527) without GST to the most frequently cloned sequence #8-5 using band shift experiments. As shown in Figure 1D, the dsDNA oligonucleotide derived from #8-5 was avidly bound by NAC1 without GST, clarifying that the binding of NAC1 to DNA is direct.

NAC1 has been reported to repress the transcriptional activity of human GADD45GIP1 [3,6]. In our hands, siRNA-mediated knockdown of endogenous NAC-1 resulted in increased levels of GADD45GIP1 protein [41]. The promoter region of human GADD45GIP1 was predicted by searching the Ensembl regulatory build database (ENSR00000343712) [63]. Visual examination of the promoter region upstream of ATG in human GADD45GIP1 revealed only one motif-like sequence within the region (Figure S2). We investigated whether NAC1 directly binds to the site detected on the GADD45GIP1 promoter using the NAC1 consensus in the context of its surrounding sequence by performing oligonucleotide pull-down assays. We incubated bacterially expressed and purified GST-NAC1 with biotin-labeled dsDNA oligonucleotides for wild type and mutant probes against GADD45GIP1 promoter, then performed pull-down assays and Coomassie blue staining to detect NAC1 in the DNA-protein complexes pulled down by the oligonucleotides. As shown in Figure 2A, we detected binding of NAC1 to wild type dsDNA oligonucleotide GP1. The core sequence mutation of CATG to GCAT in GP1 (GP1 mut) decreased the binding of the probe to NAC1, whereas mutations outside the core sequence, such as ATG to CAT (GP1 5′-mut) or TAT to ACG (GP1 3′-mut) in GP1, retained binding activity. These results indicate that the palindromic core sequence CATG is necessary to affect binding, whereas mutations outside the core sequence are not sufficient to decrease binding activity.

Next, we performed isothermal titration calorimetry (ITC) experiments to measure the binding affinity of NAC1322-485 to dsDNA oligonucleotide GP1. The titration curve clearly indicated the presence of two sequential and non-equivalent binding events (Figure 2B and Table S2). The thermodynamic data of the first binding event showed that the positive binding enthalpy ($\Delta H1$ = 1.8 kcal/mol) is compensated by entropy contribution ($\Delta S1$ = 37.1 cal/mol/deg), which corresponds to the binding affinity (Kd1, 0.16 µM). This suggests that the interaction between protein and DNA is formed by hydrophobic contacts through base unspecific manner. The ITC data of the second event showed the negative binding enthalpy ($\Delta H1$ = −30.4 kcal/mol) and entropy contribution ($\Delta S1$ = −80.2 kcal/mol/deg), which corresponds to the binding affinity (Kd2, 18.0 µM), indicating the sequence specific base recognition involving in structural conformational change of protein. Titration of the ssDNA into the protein (Figure 2B, right panel) elucidated a double exothermic binding event as well as the case of that using GP1 dsDNA, but in contrast, both are similar binding manner, corresponding to that of Kd1 for GP1 dsDNA, with binding affinity (Kd1, 0.2 µM, Kd2, 0.46 µM). These results clarified the binding preference of NAC1 to dsDNA over ssDNA. Also, ITC experiment was performed using GP1 (mut) dsDNA. Although binding of GP1 (mut) dsDNA to NAC1 was weaker than that of GP1 shown by pull down assay (Figure 2A, lane 4), ITC data elucidated that GP1 (mut) dsDNA binds to NAC1 in similar binding manner showing two phase interactions. Binding affinity of first event is 135 µM, ~840-fold larger binding affinity than that of Kd1 for GP1, whether that of second one is 0.37 µM, ~48-fold smaller binding affinity than that of Kd2 for GP1. These results indicate that NAC1 binds DNA, especially recognizing a palindromic core sequence CATG involved in protein structural change. Furthermore, binding experiments were measured using two different motifs dsDNA reported by Malleshaiah et al. as NAC1 binding motifs elucidated by ChIP methods [18]. Both binding curves show interactions through base unspecific manner corresponding to that of Kd1 for GP1 (Kd for de novo motif 3.0 µM, Kd for de novo motif 2, 0.82 µM) (Figure S3). Therefore, the preferable sequence for NAC1 is GP1 more than de novo motif 1 and motif 2.

We conducted a chromatin immunoprecipitation (ChIP) assay to verify whether NAC1 binds to promoter regions in cells to regulate gene expression using the NAC1 consensus sequence. We were unable to generate suitable primers for the ChIP assay against GADD45GIP1 promoter because of composition, complexity and interspersed repeats content. The promoter regions of the PSAT1 and AZU1 genes were therefore chosen for further analyses for several reasons. First, one of the top ten could be selected from genes by microarray experiments upon NAC1 knockdown in the human ovarian OV207 cell line compared with control siRNA treated OV207 cells (data not shown). Second, promoter regions (PSAT1, ENSR00001306399; AZU1, ENSR00000341277, Figure S2) predicted by the Ensembl regulatory build database harbored the consensus DNA-binding sequence of NAC1. Third, we could construct appropriate primers for the ChIP assay against these promoters. Fourth, as detected by real-time quantitative PCR (RT-qPCR), the expression of PSAT1 mRNA was significantly reduced upon NAC1 knockdown in OV207 cells. However, the expression of AZU1 mRNA was up-regulated (Figure 2C, left panel). ChIP assay using NAC1 antibody detected the binding of NAC1 to the promoter regions of PSAT1 and AZU1 (Figure 2C, right panel). These results confirm the in vitro and in cell validity of the NAC1-binding consensus sequence determined by our selection procedure.

3.3. Solution NMR Structure of the BEN Domain of NAC1

The solution structure of NAC1322-485, a construct encompassing the BEN domain, was determined by multidimensional heteronuclear NMR [47]. Nearly complete resonance assignments were obtained for this construct using standard double and triple resonance experiments. NMR structures were generated using a combination of CYANA distance geometry calculations [51–53] and restrained molecular dynamics refinements in AMBER [54]. The 20 conformers with the lowest restraint violation energy were selected for the final representative ensemble and are shown in Figure 3A and Figure S4. The BEN domain of human NAC1 was determined to be composed of five conserved α helices and two short β sheets, with one additional N-terminal α helix (hereafter abbreviated α0).

NMR chemical shifts are very sensitive to changes in protein structure, and their variation upon titration of a protein with its binding partner allows accurate mapping of the binding site [47]. A dsDNA 14-mer GP1S was gradually titrated into a 75 µM solution of 15N-labeled NAC1322-485 to a final ratio of 1.5:1 of GP1S to NAC1. Binding was monitored by collecting the 1H–15N HSQC spectra of NAC1 at each titration point. An overlay of eight spectra, one for each titration point in the series, is shown in Figure 3B, where the free NAC1 spectrum is shown in grey, and the NAC1 spectrum in the presence of a 1.5× molar excess of dsDNA is shown in red. The five insets depict five selected spectral regions and clearly show the disappearance of peaks or large chemical shift changes (color gradient from grey to red) upon the addition of GP1S dsDNA oligonucleotide.

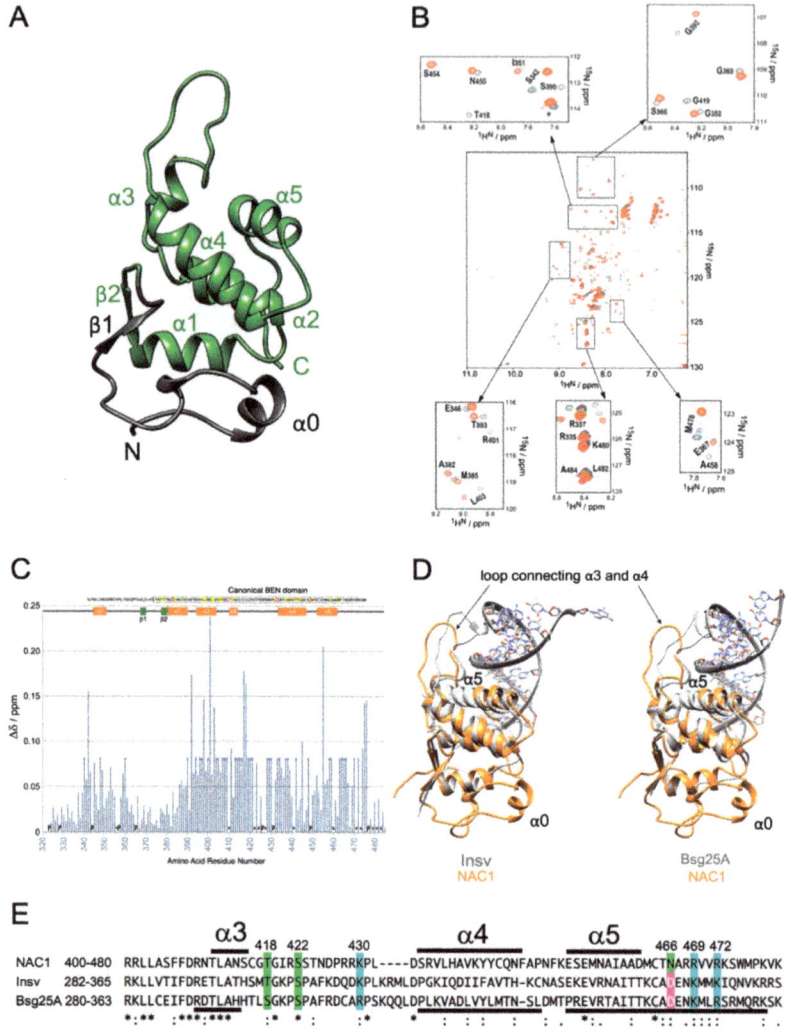

Figure 3. NMR experiments of NAC1. (**A**) Ribbon representation of the lowest-energy solution structure of the BEN domain from human NAC1 (residues 322–485), determined by NMR spectroscopy. The secondary structure elements are shown with arrows (β-strand) and helices (α-helix). The predicted BEN domain is colored green. (**B**) NMR titration experiments of NAC1 with the NAC1 consensus dsDNA oligonucleotide. Overlay of the 1H–15N HSQC spectra of NAC1(322-485) alone (grey) and in the presence of 0.2 (purple), 0.4 (cyan), 0.6 (magenta), 0.8 (green), 1.0 (yellow), 1.2 (pink), and 1.5 (red) equivalents of dsDNA oligonucleotide. The five insets show peaks that disappeared or gradually changed position (from grey to red) in selected spectral regions upon the addition of dsDNA oligonucleotide. (**C**) Total changes in 1HN and 15N chemical shifts (Δδ) for NAC1(322-485) upon the addition of dsDNA oligonucleotide to a ratio of [protein]:[dsDNA] = 1:1.5 are plotted versus residue number. Δδ is given by $\Delta\delta = [(\Delta\delta HN)^2 + (\Delta\delta N/6.5)^2]^{1/2}$, where ΔδHN and ΔδN are the chemical shift differences for 1HN and 15N, respectively. Residues that were not assigned (asterisks) or whose 1H-15N resonances disappeared upon the addition of dsDNA oligonucleotide (arrows) are indicated. "P" indicates proline residues. Highly conserved residues of human BEN domain-containing proteins identified by Clustal Omega alignment are highlighted and shown at the top of the plot. See Figure 1A.

The canonical BEN domain is boxed. Color coding reflects the conservation of amino acid types: yellow and magenta for hydrophobic and negatively charged amino acids, respectively. (**D**) Structural alignment of the BEN domain of human NAC1 and Drosophila BEN-solo proteins. NAC1 (322-485) is shown as a gold ribbon, and the Insv-BEN domain with dsDNA (PDB ID: 4IX7) (left panel) and Bsg25A (Elba1) with dsDNA (PDB ID: 4 × 0 G) (right panel) are shown in grey. (**E**) Clustal Omega alignment of the BEN domains of human NAC1, Drosophila Insv and Drosophila Bsg25A proteins. Color coding reflects the conservation of amino acid types: green, blue and magenta for hydrophilic, positively and negatively charged amino acids, respectively. Symbols are as follows: (*), identical residues; (:), highly conserved residues; (.) lower but significant conservation between all members. The α-helical regions labeled above are based on Figure 3A and those labeled below are based on PDB 4IX7 and 4 × 0 G. The source and corresponding UniProt accession numbers are indicated. NAC1, Q96RE7; Insv, Q8SYK5; Bsg25A (ELBA1), Q9VR17.

The weighted CSPs of the backbone amide nitrogens and protons between the free and bound forms of NAC1 were plotted versus the residue number (Figure 3C). Most residues whose peaks disappeared or showed a large change in frequency ($\Delta\delta > 0.13$ ppm) upon the addition of GP1S dsDNA oligonucleotide were in the BEN domain, and particularly in the region connecting α3 and α4 (residues 413–434). It is noteworthy that the residues in this region except Leu-432 and Asp-433, are not conserved between human BEN domain-containing proteins, whereas the regions of human BEN domain-containing proteins harbor one to seven positively charged residues (Arg-421, Arg-428, Arg-429, and Lys-431 in human NAC1) (Figure 1A). As seen in Figure 3B,C, only a subset of peaks changed position upon the addition of dsDNA, indicating a specific interaction between the BEN domain of NAC1 and the GP1S dsDNA oligonucleotide.

3.4. The BEN Domain of NAC1 Alone Cannot Interact with Chromatin/Other Proteins in Living Cells

To study the dynamics and function of the BEN domain of NAC1 in living cells, we generated HeLa cell lines stably expressing GFP-NAC1 (251-527) or GFP-NAC1 (251-527, L432N) (Figure S5). NAC1 (L432N), in which a conserved leucine residue within the BEN domain of NAC1 is replaced with asparagine, severely impaired DNA-binding activity (Figure S1C). Asynchronized HeLa cells stably expressing GFP-NAC1 (251-527) or GFP-NAC1 (251-527, L432N) were subjected to fluorescence recovery after photobleaching (FRAP) analysis (Figure 4A). In parallel, HeLa cells stably expressing a freely diffusing GFP, GFP-NAC1, or a very stable chromatin binding histone H3 fused with GFP (GFP-histone H3), were analyzed for comparison [59]. NAC1 (251-527) showed significantly faster recovery kinetics ($t_{\frac{1}{2}} = 1.06 \pm 0.52$ s) compared to full-length NAC1 ($t_{\frac{1}{2}} = 3.19 \pm 1.21$ s) (Figure 4B,C). In contrast, there was no difference in the nuclear mobility and kinetic properties of NAC1 (251-527) and NAC1 (251-527, L432N).

We next employed a complementary approach, fluorescence loss in photobleaching (FLIP) (Figure 4D). Repetitive bleaching of the GFP-NAC1 signal in one half of the nucleus led to gradual fluorescence loss in the other half of the nucleus, and resulted in a complete loss of fluorescence from the entire nucleus within 3 min (Figure 4E, GFP-NAC1, compare GFP and GFP-histone H3). Consistent with the FRAP data, this result indicates that NAC1 in the nucleus is highly mobile and rapidly exchanges with unbleached GFP-NAC1 molecules in the nucleus, although its diffusion is slower than that of freely diffusing GFP. GFP-NAC1 (251-527) showed a considerably faster loss of fluorescence in the unbleached half of the nucleus compared to wild-type GFP-NAC1, and there was no difference between NAC1 (251-527) and NAC1 (251-527, L432N) (Figure 4E). Taken together, these findings suggest that the BEN domain of NAC1 alone is likely to not interact with chromatin/other proteins as avidly as full-length protein.

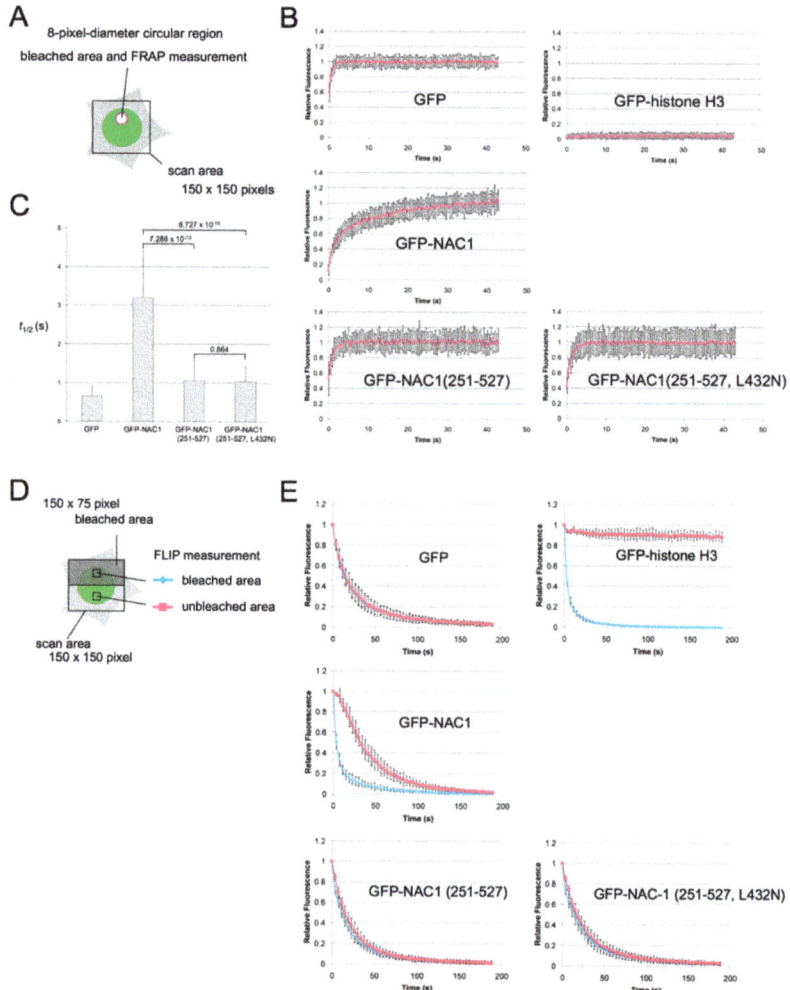

Figure 4. Intranuclear dynamics of the BEN domain of NAC1 in living cells. (**A**) Schematic drawing of FRAP analysis. Quantitative FRAP analysis (FRAP recovery curves) (**B**) and t1/2 analysis (**C**) of stably expressed GFP, GFP-histone H3, GFP-NAC1, GFP-NAC1(251-527) and GFP-NAC1(251-527, L432N) in HeLa cells. Each value is the mean ± SD. Calculated with Welch's two sample *t* test. (**D**) Schematic drawing of FLIP analysis. (**E**) Quantitative FLIP analysis of stably expressed GFP, GFP-histone H3, GFP-NAC1, GFP-NAC1(251-527) and GFP-NAC1(251-527, L432N) in HeLa cells. The fluorescence loss was monitored in the bleached (blue) and control unbleached (magenta) regions. Each value is the mean ± SD.

4. Discussion

On the basis of the contextual conservation of BEN domain-containing proteins, the BEN domain has been predicted to mediate chromatin organization and transcriptional regulation by mediating protein–DNA and protein–protein interactions [30]. The Drosophila genome encodes three BEN domain-containing proteins: Insensitive (Insv), Bsg25A (Elba1), and CG9883 (Elba2). All three Drosophila proteins lack other recognizable biochemical function protein domains. To date, two crystal structures of the BEN domains of Drosophila proteins complexed with target DNA have been determined: Insv (PDB 4IX7) [39] and Bsg25A (Elba1) (PDB 4 × 0 G) [52]. Analyses revealed the association between the BEN domains and specific DNA binding through extensive nucleotide contacts with their α helices and C-terminal loop, suggesting that the BEN domain functions in a DNA sequence-specific manner. On the other hand, recently, the Drosophila BEN-solo protein Elba2, but not Insv, was shown to rescue the deficiency of histone H1 protein in early larvae [53], supporting the sequence-recognition specificity and sequence-specific function of BEN domains.

The human genome encodes nine BEN domain-containing proteins; NAC1 and NAC2 also contain a BTB domain, whereas the seven other proteins lack other recognizable domains. Human NAC1 and NAC2 are similar (55/64% identity/similarity in overall amino acid sequence), and their BEN domains share 86/92% identity/similarity. Xuan et al. clearly showed that human NAC2 protein binds to non-palindromic TGTCA/GG/CT/AT/AC/TT/CGA/TC sequences through the BEN domain [35]. Immunofluorescence microscopy of human MCF-7 cells with anti-NAC2 polyclonal antibody yields homogeneous uniform staining throughout the nucleus, with the exception of the nucleoli [35]. On the other hand, immunofluorescence analysis of human HeLa cells using a specific monoclonal antibody revealed that endogenous NAC1 is almost exclusively localized with a fine granular pattern in the nucleus, excluding the nucleoli [41]. This fine granular appearance strongly suggests that NAC1 is not uniformly distributed along the chromatin fiber, and our live cell photobleaching analyses revealed that a substantial fraction of NAC1 in the nucleus is associated with or interacts with nuclear proteins or chromatin [42]. These observations prompted us to investigate whether NAC1 directly binds DNA, and if so, which domain of NAC1 is responsible for binding and which consensus DNA-binding sequence human NAC1 binds to. Our bacterial genome carry-over assays revealed that NAC1 directly binds DNA via the BEN domain (Figure S1), similar to NAC2 [35]. In vitro PCR-assisted random oligonucleotide selection experiments showed that monomeric NAC1 preferentially binds ACATGT palindromes containing the core sequence CATG (Figure 1), revealing a DNA-binding property distinct from that of NAC2. Interestingly, the Drosophila BEN-solo proteins Insv and Bsg25A (Elba1) efficiently bind the palindromic CCAATTGG motif in vitro [39,52].

Currently, genome-wide binding data from chromatin immunoprecipitation followed by sequencing (ChIP-seq) experiments provide optimum information for inferring the DNA-binding affinity of transcription factors [54,64]. The NAC1 DNA-binding motif determined from in vitro PCR-assisted random oligonucleotide selection experiments does not match the de novo consensus sequence of the motif identified by DREME and TOMTOM programs in the NAC1 ChIP-seq data of mouse ES cells [18]. This discrepancy is likely due to binding being affected by the specific cell type, condition, developmental stage or tissue, since transcription factors primarily bind DNA in conjunction with one or more other DNA-binding transcription factor and nuclear proteins in cells. Genome-wide binding data from NAC1 ChIP-seq experiments, when coupled with information on the in vitro DNA-binding motif, provide insights into the physical mechanisms of transcriptional modulation of NAC1.

Surprisingly, we observed isotherms for the binding of BEN domain of NAC1 (322-485) with dsDNA oligonucleotide GP1 that show two sequential and non-equivalent binding events (Figure 2b and Table S2). A molecular interpretation of the two binding events is that the second binding invokes the sequence specific base recognition involving in structural conformational change of protein. We found supportive results for this observation in the NMR structure of BEN domain of NAC1 without target DNA compared with two crystal structures of the BEN domains of Drosophila BEN-sole proteins with target DNA. The superimpositions clearly showed three structural differences (Figure 3D). First, NAC1 has an additional N-terminal α helix, α0 (345-351), outside the canonical BEN domain (374-471). Second, superimposition of the loops connecting α3 and α4 with or without target DNA fit poorly. The loops of Insv and Bsg25A are positioned in the minor grove of the target DNA. Thr300 and Lys312 in Drosophila Insv and Ser298 and Arg310 in Drosophila Bsg25A contact the sugar-phosphate backbone of the target DNA, and Ser304 in Insv and Ser302 in Bsg25A make base-specific contacts (PDB 4IX7 and 4 × 0 G). The loop of NAC1 contains at least three residues (Thr418, Lys430, and Ser422) that can interact with DNA (Figure 3E). Third, the α5 helices of Insv and Bsg25A positioned within the major groove are longer than the α5 helix of the BEN domain of NAC1 in the absence of target DNA. The C-terminal half of α5 helix of Insv harbors Asp351 and Lys352, and Asp349 and Lys352 in Bsg25A: the C-terminal halves of both proteins make base-specific contacts. Furthermore, Lys357 in Insv and Arg355 in Bsg25A form contacts with the sugar-phosphate backbone (PDB 4IX7 and 4 × 0 G). The short α5 helix of NAC1 is followed by Asn466, Arg469, and Arg472 (Figure 3E). The latter two structural differences on the basis of the superimpositions and NMR CSPs (Figure 3C) suggest that α2, α3, and the short α5 helices of NAC1 are involved in the first binding event with the target DNA, and that this first binding facilitates the fixation of the loop connecting α3 and α4 to the target DNA and the formation of a longer α5 helix during the second binding event.

Live cell photobleaching analyses clearly showed that there was no difference in the nuclear mobility and kinetic properties of the BEN domain of NAC1 (251-527) and NAC1 (251-527, L432N) carrying a mutation which abolishes DNA-binding activity (Figure 4). The BEN domain of NAC1 alone could bind the target DNA in vitro (Figures 1–3) but was unable to interact with chromatin/other proteins in cells. Our previous study showed that NAC1 in the nucleus is associated with or interacts with nuclear proteins or chromatin [59]. Additional, uncharacterized binding partners may be required for the function of NAC1 in cells. The results also suggest caution in the general and indiscriminate use of the BEN domains of BEN-domain containing proteins in reporter assays in cells.

In summary, NAC1 is a sequence-specific DNA-binding protein that binds the target DNA through the BEN domain. We used molecular and structural biology approaches to clarify the two-step binding model. Furthermore, the results of live cell photobleaching analyses suggest that the BEN domains of BEN-domain containing proteins must be used with caution in reporter assays in cells.

Supplementary Materials: The following are available online at http://www.mdpi.com/2227-9059/8/12/608/s1, Figure S1: Bacterial genome carry-over assay of the bacterially expressed and purified proteins, Figure S2: The promoter region of human GADD45GIP1, PSAT1 and AZU1 genes harbored the consensus DNA-binding sequence of NAC1, Figure S3: Isothermal titration calorimetry, Figure S4: The 20 conformers representing the solution conformation of the BEN domain of NAC1322-485, c: A representative HeLa cell stably expressing GFP, GFP-NAC1, GFP-NAC1(251-527) or GFP-NAC1(251-527, L432N). Table S1: Structural Statistics for NAC1 (322-485), Table S2: Thermodynamic parameters (average of three experiments) for the interactions between oligonucleotides and NAC1 (322-485).

Author Contributions: T.U. conceived the study and designed the experiments. N.N., G.S., Y.N., H.K., K.N. and S.K. performed gel mobility shift assays, bacterial genome carry-over assays, in vitro oligonucleotide selections, pull-down assays and chromatin-immunoprecipitation assays. H.Y. and S.-Y.P. performed band shift assays and ITC experiments. T.N., N.K. and E.O. performed soluble NMR experiments. T.U. and H.K. performed live cell photobleaching analyses. All authors discussed the results. T.U. wrote the manuscript with comments from all authors. All authors have read and agreed to the published version of the manuscript.

Funding: This study was funded by Grants-in-Aid for Scientific Research (25893136 to N. N., 17K07307, 17H05878 and 26440026 to T. N.) and the SUIGAN project of Shimane University [1b01 to T. U.]. The authors declare no competing financial interests.

Acknowledgments: The authors thank Forte Science Communications for editing this manuscript. We would like to acknowledge the technical expertise of the Interdisciplinary Center for Science Research Organization for Research and Academic Information, Shimane University.

Conflicts of Interest: The authors declare no conflict of interest. The funders had no role in the design of the study; in the collection, analyses, or interpretation of data; in the writing of the manuscript, or in the decision to publish the results.

References

1. Cha, X.Y.; Pierce, R.C.; Kalivas, P.W.; Mackler, S.A. NAC-1, a rat brain mRNA, is increased in the nucleus accumbens three weeks after chronic cocaine self-administration. *J. Neurosci.* **1997**, *17*, 6864–6871. [CrossRef]
2. Nakayama, K.; Nakayama, N.; Davidson, B.; Sheu, J.J.; Jinawath, N.; Santillan, A.; Salani, R.; Bristow, R.E.; Morin, P.J.; Kurman, R.J.; et al. A BTB/POZ protein, NAC-1, is related to tumor recurrence and is essential for tumor growth and survival. *Proc. Natl Acad. Sci. USA* **2006**, *103*, 18739–18744. [CrossRef]

3. Nakayama, K.; Nakayama, N.; Wang, T.-L.; Shih Ie, M. NAC-1 controls cell growth and survival by repressing transcription of Gadd45GIP1, a candidate tumor suppressor. *Cancer Res.* **2007**, *67*, 8058–8064. [CrossRef] [PubMed]
4. Yeasmin, S.; Nakayama, K.; Ishibashi, M.; Katagiri, A.; Iida, K.; Purwana, I.N.; Nakayama, N.; Miyazaki, K. Expression of the bric-a-brac tramtrack broad complex protein NAC-1 in cervical carcinomas seems to correlate with poorer prognosis. *Clin. Cancer Res.* **2008**, *14*, 1686–1691. [CrossRef] [PubMed]
5. Ishibashi, M.; Nakayama, K.; Yeasmin, S.; Katagiri, A.; Iida, K.; Nakayama, N.; Fukumoto, M.; Miyazaki, K. A BTB/POZ gene, NAC-1, a tumor recurrence-associated gene, as a potential target for Taxol resistance in ovarian cancer. *Clin. Cancer Res.* **2008**, *14*, 3149–3155. [CrossRef] [PubMed]
6. Jinawath, N.; Vasoontara, C.; Yap, K.L.; Thiaville, M.M.; Nakayama, K.; Wang, T.-L.; Shih Ie, M. NAC-1, a potential stem cell pluripotency factor, contributes to paclitaxel resistance in ovarian cancer through inactivating Gadd45 pathway. *Oncogene* **2009**, *28*, 1941–1948. [CrossRef]
7. Ishibashi, M.; Nakayama, K.; Yeasmin, S.; Katagiri, A.; Iida, K.; Nakayama, N.; Miyazaki, K. Expression of a BTB/POZ protein, NAC1, is essential for the proliferation of normal cyclic endometrial glandular cells and is up-regulated by estrogen. *Clin. Cancer Res.* **2009**, *15*, 804–811. [CrossRef]
8. Ishikawa, M.; Nakayama, K.; Yeasmin, S.; Katagiri, A.; Iida, K.; Nakayama, N.; Miyazaki, K. NAC1, a potential stem cell pluripotency factor expression in normal endometrium, endometrial hyperplasia and endometrial carcinoma. *Int. J. Oncol.* **2010**, *36*, 1097–1103.
9. Nakayama, K.; Rahman, M.T.; Rahman, M.; Yeasmin, S.; Ishikawa, M.; Katagiri, A.; Iida, K.; Nakayama, N.; Miyazaki, K. Biological role and prognostic significance of NAC1 in ovarian cancer. *Gynecol. Oncol.* **2010**, *119*, 469–478. [CrossRef]
10. Shih Ie, M.; Nakayama, K.; Wu, G.; Nakayama, N.; Zhang, J.; Wang, T.-L. Amplification of the ch19p13.2 NACC1 locus in ovarian high-grade serous carcinoma. *Mod. Pathol.* **2011**, *24*, 638–645. [CrossRef]
11. Yeasmin, S.; Nakayama, K.; Rahman, M.T.; Rahman, M.; Ishikawa, M.; Katagiri, A.; Iida, K.; Nakayama, N.; Otuski, Y.; Kobayashi, H.; et al. Biological and clinical significance of NAC1 expression in cervical carcinomas: A comparative study between squamous cell carcinomas and adenocarcinomas/adenosquamous carcinomas. *Hum. Pathol.* **2012**, *43*, 506–519. [CrossRef] [PubMed]
12. Nishi, T.; Maruyama, R.; Urano, T.; Nakayama, N.; Kawabata, Y.; Yano, S.; Yoshida, M.; Nakayama, K.; Miyazaki, K.; Takenaga, K.; et al. Low expression of nucleus accumbens-associated protein 1 predicts poor prognosis for patients with pancreatic ductal adenocarcinoma. *Pathol. Int.* **2012**, *62*, 802–810. [CrossRef] [PubMed]
13. Nakayama, N.; Sakashita, G.; Nariai, Y.; Kato, H.; Sinmyozu, K.; Nakayama, J.I.; Kyo, S.; Urano, T.; Nakayama, K. Cancer-related transcription regulator protein NAC1 forms a protein complex with CARM1 for ovarian cancer progression. *Oncotarget* **2018**, *9*, 28408–28420. [CrossRef] [PubMed]
14. Liu, Y.; Du, M.; Song, Y.; Liu, H.; Xiang, S. NAC1/HMGB1 Signaling Pathway Is Associated with Epithelial-mesenchymal Transition, Invasion, and Metastasis of Lung Cancer Cell Line. *Ann. Clin. Lab. Sci.* **2018**, *48*, 559–564. [PubMed]
15. Wang, J.; Rao, S.; Chu, J.; Shen, X.; Levasseur, D.N.; Theunissen, T.W.; Orkin, S.H. A protein interaction network for pluripotency of embryonic stem cells. *Nature* **2006**, *444*, 364–368. [CrossRef]
16. Kim, J.; Chu, J.; Shen, X.; Wang, J.; Orkin, S.H. An extended transcriptional network for pluripotency of embryonic stem cells. *Cell* **2008**, *132*, 1049–1061. [CrossRef]
17. Ruan, Y.; He, J.; Wu, W.; He, P.; Tian, Y.; Xiao, L.; Liu, G.; Wang, J.; Cheng, Y.; Zhang, S.; et al. Nac1 promotes self-renewal of embryonic stem cells through direct transcriptional regulation of c-Myc. *Oncotarget* **2017**, *8*, 47607–47618. [CrossRef]
18. Malleshaiah, M.; Padi, M.; Rué, P.; Quackenbush, J.; Martinez-Arias, A.; Gunawardena, J. Nac1 coordinates a sub-network of pluripotency factors to regulate embryonic stem cell differentiation. *Cell Rep.* **2016**, *14*, 1181–1194. [CrossRef]
19. Choi, H.; Park, H.J.; Kim, H.; Kim, J.; Lee, Y.K.; Kim, J. Nac1 facilitates pluripotency gene activation for establishing somatic cell reprogramming. *Biochem. Biophys. Res. Commun.* **2019**, *518*, 253–258. [CrossRef]
20. Faiola, F.; Yin, N.; Fidalgo, M.; Huang, X.; Saunders, A.; Ding, J.; Guallar, D.; Dang, B.; Wang, J. NAC1 Regulates Somatic Cell Reprogramming by Controlling Zeb1 and E-cadherin Expression. *Stem Cell Rep.* **2017**, *9*, 913–926. [CrossRef]

21. Yap, K.L.; Sysa-Shah, P.; Bolon, B.; Wu, R.C.; Gao, M.; Herlinger, A.L.; Wang, F.; Faiola, F.; Huso, D.; Gabrielson, K.; et al. Loss of NAC1 expression is associated with defective bony patterning in the murine vertebral axis. *PLoS ONE* **2013**, *8*, e69095. [CrossRef] [PubMed]
22. Xia, Z.; Xu, G.; Nie, L.; Liu, L.; Peng, N.; He, Q.; Zuo, Q.; Zhou, Y.; Cao, Z.; Liu, S.; et al. NAC1 Potentiates Cellular Antiviral Signaling by Bridging MAVS and TBK1. *J. Immunol.* **2019**, *203*, 1001–1011. [CrossRef] [PubMed]
23. Maeda, T. Regulation of hematopoietic development by ZBTB transcription factors. *Int. J. Hematol.* **2016**, *104*, 310–323. [CrossRef] [PubMed]
24. Chaharbakhshi, E.; Jemc, J.C. Broad-complex, tramtrack, and bric-à-brac (BTB) proteins: Critical regulators of development. *Genesis* **2016**, *54*, 505–518. [CrossRef]
25. Stead, M.A.; Carr, S.B.; Wright, S.C. Structure of the human Nac1 POZ domain. *Acta. Crystallogr. Sect. F Struct. Biol. Cryst. Commun.* **2009**, *65*, 445–449. [CrossRef]
26. Wang, X.; Ji, C.; Zhang, H.; Shan, Y.; Ren, Y.; Hu, Y.; Shi, L.; Guo, L.; Zhu, W.; Xia, Y.; et al. Identification of a small-molecule compound that inhibits homodimerization of oncogenic NAC1 protein and sensitizes cancer cells to anticancer agents. *J. Biol. Chem.* **2019**, *294*, 10006–10017. [CrossRef]
27. Stead, M.A.; Wright, S.C. Nac1 interacts with the POZ-domain transcription factor, Miz1. *Biosci. Rep.* **2014**, *34*, e00110. [CrossRef]
28. Stead, M.A.; Wright, S.C. Structures of heterodimeric POZ domains of Miz1/BCL6 and Miz1/NAC1. *Acta Crystallogr. F Struct. Biol. Commun.* **2014**, *70*, 1591–1596. [CrossRef]
29. Wu, T.; He, P.; Wu, W.; Chen, Y.; Lv, F. Targeting oncogenic transcriptional corepressor Nac1 POZ domain with conformationally constrained peptides by cyclization and stapling. *Bioorg. Chem.* **2018**, *80*, 1–10. [CrossRef]
30. Abhiman, S.; Iyer, L.M.; Aravind, L. BEN: A novel domain in chromatin factors and DNA viral proteins. *Bioinformatics* **2008**, *24*, 458–461. [CrossRef]
31. Duan, H.; Dai, Q.; Kavaler, J.; Bejarano, F.; Medranda, G.; Nègre, N.; Lai, E.C. Insensitive is a corepressor for Suppressor of Hairless and regulates Notch signalling during neural development. *EMBO J.* **2011**, *30*, 3120–3133. [CrossRef] [PubMed]
32. Korutla, L.; Degnan, R.; Wang, P.; Mackler, S.A. NAC1, a cocaine-regulated POZ/BTB protein interacts with CoREST. *J. Neurochem.* **2007**, *101*, 611–618. [CrossRef] [PubMed]
33. Sathyan, K.M.; Shen, Z.; Tripathi, V.; Prasanth, K.V.; Prasanth, S.G. A BEN-domain-containing protein associates with heterochromatin and represses transcription. *J. Cell Sci.* **2011**, *124*, 3149–3163. [CrossRef] [PubMed]
34. Korutla, L.; Wang, P.J.; Mackler, S.A. The POZ/BTB protein NAC1 interacts with two different histone deacetylases in neuronal-like cultures. *J. Neurochem.* **2005**, *94*, 786–793. [CrossRef] [PubMed]
35. Xuan, C.; Wang, Q.; Han, X.; Duan, Y.; Li, L.; Shi, L.; Wang, Y.; Shan, L.; Yao, Z.; Shang, Y. RBB, a novel transcription repressor, represses the transcription of HDM2 oncogene. *Oncogene* **2013**, *32*, 3711–3721. [CrossRef] [PubMed]
36. Rampalli, S.; Pavithra, L.; Bhatt, A.; Kundu, T.K.; Chattopadhyay, S. Tumor suppressor SMAR1 mediates cyclin D1 repression by recruitment of the SIN3/histone deacetylase 1 complex. *Mol. Cell. Biol.* **2005**, *25*, 8415–8429. [CrossRef]
37. Saksouk, N.; Barth, T.K.; Ziegler-Birling, C.; Olova, N.; Nowak, A.; Rey, E.; Mateos-Langerak, J.; Urbach, S.; Reik, W.; Torres-Padilla, M.-E.; et al. Redundant Mechanisms to Form Silent Chromatin at Pericentromeric Regions Rely on BEND3 and DNA Methylation. *Mol. Cell* **2014**, *56*, 580–594. [CrossRef]
38. Khan, A.; Giri, S.; Wang, Y.; Chakraborty, A.; Ghosh, A.K.; Anantharaman, A.; Aggarwal, V.; Sathyan, K.M.; Ha, T.; Prasanth, K.V.; et al. BEND3 represses rDNA transcription by stabilizing a NoRC component via USP21 deubiquitinase. *Proc. Natl Acad. Sci. USA* **2015**, *112*, 8338–8343. [CrossRef]
39. Dai, Q.; Ren, A.; Westholm, J.O.; Serganov, A.A.; Patel, D.J.; Lai, E.C. The BEN domain is a novel sequence-specific DNA-binding domain conserved in neural transcriptional repressors. *Genes* **2013**, *27*, 602–614. [CrossRef]
40. Dai, Q.; Andreu-Agullo, C.; Insolera, R.; Wong, L.C.; Shi, S.H.; Lai, E.C. BEND6 is a nuclear antagonist of Notch signaling during self-renewal of neural stem cells. *Development* **2013**, *140*, 1892–1902. [CrossRef]
41. Yoshida, H.; Park, S.Y.; Oda, T.; Akiyoshi, T.; Sato, M.; Shirouzu, M.; Tsuda, K.; Kuwasako, K.; Unzai, S.; Muto, Y.; et al. A novel 3′ splice site recognition by the two zinc fingers in the U2AF small subunit. *Genes Dev.* **2015**, *29*, 1649–1660. [CrossRef]

42. Delaglio, F.; Grzesiek, S.; Vuister, G.W.; Zhu, G.; Pfeifer, J.; Bax, A. NMRPipe: A multidimensional spectral processing system based on UNIX pipes. *J. Biomol. NMR* **1995**, *6*, 277–293. [CrossRef] [PubMed]
43. Kobayashi, N.; Iwahara, J.; Koshiba, S.; Tomizawa, T.; Tochio, N.; Güntert, P.; Kigawa, T.; Yokoyama, S. KUJIRA, a package of integrated modules for systematic and interactive analysis of NMR data directed to high-throughput NMR structure studies. *J. Biomol. NMR* **2007**, *39*, 31–52. [CrossRef] [PubMed]
44. Johnson, B.A. Using NMRView to visualize and analyze the NMR spectra of macromolecules. *Methods Mol. Biol.* **2004**, *278*, 313–352. [PubMed]
45. Nagata, T.; Suzuki, S.; Endo, R.; Shirouzu, M.; Terada, T.; Inoue, M.; Kigawa, T.; Kobayashi, N.; Guntert, P.; Tanaka, A.; et al. The RRM domain of poly(A)-specific ribonuclease has a noncanonical binding site for mRNA cap analog recognition. *Nucleic Acids Res.* **2008**, *36*, 4754–4767. [CrossRef] [PubMed]
46. Clore, G.M.; Gronenborn, A.M. Determining the structures of large proteins and protein complexes by NMR. *Trends Biotechnol.* **1998**, *16*, 22–34. [CrossRef]
47. Cavanagh, J.; Fairbrother, W.J.; Palmer, A.G.R.; Rance, M.; Skelton, N.J. *Protein NMR Spectroscopy, Second Edition: Principles and Practice*; Academic Press, Inc.: San Diego, CA, USA, 2006.
48. Shen, Y.; Delaglio, F.; Cornilescu, G.; Bax, A. TALOS+: A hybrid method for predicting protein backbone torsion angles from NMR chemical shifts. *J. Biomol. NMR* **2009**, *44*, 213–223. [CrossRef]
49. Powers, R.; Garrett, D.S.; March, C.J.; Frieden, E.A.; Gronenborn, A.M.; Clore, G.M. The high-resolution, three-dimensional solution structure of human interleukin-4 determined by multidimensional heteronuclear magnetic resonance spectroscopy. *Biochemistry* **1993**, *32*, 6744–6762. [CrossRef]
50. Mulder, F.A.; Schipper, D.; Bott, R.; Boelens, R. Altered flexibility in the substrate-binding site of related native and engineered high-alkaline Bacillus subtilisins. *J. Mol. Biol.* **1999**, *292*, 111–123. [CrossRef]
51. Case, D.A.; Cheatham, T.E., 3rd; Darden, T.; Gohlke, H.; Luo, R.; Merz, K.M., Jr.; Onufriev, A.; Simmerling, C.; Wang, B.; Woods, R.J. The Amber biomolecular simulation programs. *J. Comput. Chem.* **2005**, *26*, 1668–1688. [CrossRef]
52. Dai, Q.; Ren, A.; Westholm, J.O.; Duan, H.; Patel, D.J.; Lai, E.C. Common and distinct DNA-binding and regulatory activities of the BEN-solo transcription factor family. *Genes Dev.* **2015**, *29*, 48–62. [CrossRef] [PubMed]
53. Xu, N.; Lu, X.W.; Kavi, H.; Emelyanov, A.V.; Bernardo, T.J.; Vershilova, E.; Skoultchi, A.I.; Fyodorov, D.V. BEN domain protein Elba2 can functionally substitute for linker histone H1 in Drosophila in vivo. *Sci. Rep.* **2016**, *6*, 34354. [CrossRef] [PubMed]
54. Bailey, T.L.; Machanick, P. Inferring direct DNA binding from ChIP-seq. *Nucleic Acids Res.* **2012**, *40*, e128. [CrossRef] [PubMed]
55. Lovell, S.C.; Davis, I.W.; Arendall, W.B., 3rd; de Bakker, P.I.; Word, J.M.; Prisant, M.G.; Richardson, J.S.; Richardson, D.C. Structure validation by Cα geometry: φ,ψ and Cβ deviation. *Proteins* **2003**, *50*, 437–450. [CrossRef] [PubMed]
56. Meng, E.C.; Pettersen, E.F.; Couch, G.S.; Huang, C.C.; Ferrin, T.E. Tools for integrated sequence-structure analysis with UCSF Chimera. *BMC Bioinform.* **2006**, *7*, 339.
57. Pettersen, E.F.; Goddard, T.D.; Huang, C.C.; Couch, G.S.; Greenblatt, D.M.; Meng, E.C.; Ferrin, T.E. UCSF Chimera—A visualization system for exploratory research and analysis. *J. Comput. Chem.* **2004**, *25*, 1605–1612. [CrossRef]
58. Okazaki, K.; Nakayama, N.; Nariai, Y.; Kato, H.; Nakayama, K.; Miyazaki, K.; Maruyama, R.; Kosugi, S.; Urano, T.; Sakashita, G. Nuclear localization signal in a cancer-related transcriptional regulator protein NAC1. *Carcinogenesis* **2012**, *33*, 1854–1862. [CrossRef]
59. Nakayama, N.; Kato, H.; Sakashita, G.; Nariai, Y.; Nakayama, K.; Kyo, S.; Urano, T. Protein complex formation and intranuclear dynamics of NAC1 in cancer cells. *Arch. Biochem. Biophys.* **2016**, *606*, 10–15. [CrossRef]
60. Wang, D.; Baumann, A.; Szebeni, A.; Olson, M.O. The nucleic acid binding activity of nucleolar protein B23.1 resides in its carboxyl-terminal end. *J. Biol. Chem.* **1994**, *269*, 30994–30998.
61. Pollock, R.M. Determination of protein-DNA sequence specificity by PCR-assisted binding-site selection. *Curr. Protoc. Mol. Biol.* **2001**, *12*. [CrossRef]
62. Bailey, T.L.; Elkan, C. Fitting a mixture model by expectation maximization to discover motifs in biopolymers. *Proc. Int. Conf. Intell. Syst. Mol. Biol.* **1994**, *2*, 28–36.

63. Zerbino, D.R.; Wilder, S.P.; Johnson, N.; Juettemann, T.; Flicek, P.R. The ensembl regulatory build. *Genome Biol.* **2015**, *16*, 56. [CrossRef] [PubMed]
64. Boeva, V. Analysis of Genomic Sequence Motifs for Deciphering Transcription Factor Binding and Transcriptional Regulation in Eukaryotic Cells. *Front. Genet.* **2016**, *7*, 24. [CrossRef] [PubMed]

Publisher's Note: MDPI stays neutral with regard to jurisdictional claims in published maps and institutional affiliations.

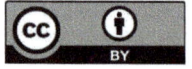

© 2020 by the authors. Licensee MDPI, Basel, Switzerland. This article is an open access article distributed under the terms and conditions of the Creative Commons Attribution (CC BY) license (http://creativecommons.org/licenses/by/4.0/).

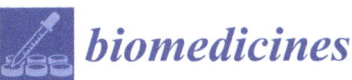

Article

Platelet-Activating Factor Acetylhydrolase Expression in BRCA1 Mutant Ovarian Cancer as a Protective Factor and Potential Negative Regulator of the Wnt Signaling Pathway

Yue Liao [1,2,†], Susann Badmann [1,†], Till Kaltofen [1], Doris Mayr [3], Elisa Schmoeckel [3], Eileen Deuster [1], Mareike Mannewitz [1], Sarah Landgrebe [3], Thomas Kolben [1], Anna Hester [1], Susanne Beyer [1], Alexander Burges [1], Sven Mahner [1], Udo Jeschke [1,4], Fabian Trillsch [1] and Bastian Czogalla [1,*]

[1] Department of Obstetrics and Gynecology, University Hospital, Ludwig Maximilians University (LMU) Munich, 81377 Munich, Germany; yue.liao@med.uni-muenchen.de (Y.L.); susann.badmann@med.uni-muenchen.de (S.B.); till.kaltofen@med.uni-muenchen.de (T.K.); eileen.deuster@med.uni-muenchen.de (E.D.); mareike.mannewitz@med.uni-muenchen.de (M.M.); thomas.kolben@med.uni-muenchen.de (T.K.); anna.hester@med.uni-muenchen.de (A.H.); susanne.beyer@med.uni-muenchen.de (S.B.); alexander.burges@med.uni-muenchen.de (A.B.); sven.mahner@med.uni-muenchen.de (S.M.); udo.jeschke@med.uni-muenchen.de (U.J.); fabian.trillsch@med.uni-muenchen.de (F.T.)

[2] Department of Breast Surgery, Zhujiang Hospital Affiliated to Southern Medical University, Guangzhou 510515, China

[3] Institute of Pathology, Faculty of Medicine, Ludwig Maximilians University (LMU) Munich, 81377 Munich, Germany; doris.mayr@med.uni-muenchen.de (D.M.); elisa.schmoeckel@med.uni-muenchen.de (E.S.); sarah.landgrebe@med.uni-muenchen.de (S.L.)

[4] Department of Obstetrics and Gynecology, University Hospital Augsburg, 86156 Augsburg, Germany

* Correspondence: bastian.czogalla@med.uni-muenchen.de; Tel.: +49-89-4400-74775

† These authors contributed equally to this work.

Abstract: Aberrantly activated Wnt/β-catenin signaling pathway, as well as platelet-activating factor (PAF), contribute to cancer progression and metastasis of many cancer entities. Nonetheless, the role of the degradation enzyme named platelet-activating factor acetylhydrolase (PLA2G7/PAF-AH) in ovarian cancer etiology is still unclear. This study investigated the functional impact of platelet-activating factor acetylhydrolase on BRCA1 mutant ovarian cancer biology and its crosstalk with the Wnt signaling pathway. PAF-AH, pGSK3β, and β-catenin expressions were analyzed in 156 ovarian cancer specimens by immunohistochemistry. PAF-AH expression was investigated in ovarian cancer tissue, serum of BRCA1-mutated patients, and in vitro in four ovarian cancer cell lines. Functional assays were performed after PLA2G7 silencing. The association of PAF-AH and β-catenin was examined by immunocytochemistry. In an established ovarian carcinoma collective, we identified PAF-AH as an independent positive prognostic factor for overall survival (median 59.9 vs. 27.4 months; $p = 0.016$). PAF-AH correlated strongly with the Wnt signaling proteins pGSK3β (Y216; nuclear: cc = 0.494, $p < 0.001$; cytoplasmic: cc = 0.488, $p < 0.001$) and β-catenin (nuclear: cc = 0.267, $p = 0.001$; cytoplasmic: cc = 0.291, $p < 0.001$). In particular, high levels of PAF-AH were found in tumor tissue and in the serum of BRCA1 mutation carriers. By in vitro expression analysis, a relevant gene and protein expression of PLA2G7/PAF-AH was detected exclusively in the BRCA1-negative ovarian cancer cell line UWB1.289 ($p < 0.05$). Functional assays showed enhanced viability, proliferation, and motility of UWB1.289 cells when PLA2G7/PAF-AH was downregulated, which underlines its protective character. Interestingly, by siRNA knockdown of PLA2G7/PAF-AH, the immunocytochemistry staining pattern of β-catenin changed from a predominantly membranous expression to a nuclear one, suggesting a negative regulatory role of PAF-AH on the Wnt/β-catenin pathway. Our data provide evidence that PAF-AH is a positive prognostic factor with functional impact, which seems particularly relevant in BRCA1 mutant ovarian cancer. For the first time, we show that its protective character may be mediated by a negative regulation of the Wnt/β-catenin pathway. Further studies need to specify this effect. Potential use of PAF-AH as a biomarker for predicting the disease risk of BRCA1 mutation carriers and for the prognosis of patients with BRCA1-negative ovarian cancer should be explored.

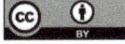

Keywords: platelet-activating factor acetylhydrolase (PAF-AH; PLA2G7); BRCA1 mutant ovarian cancer; Wnt signaling; pGSK3β; β-catenin; prognosis

1. Introduction

Ovarian cancer is one of the five leading causes of cancer-related death in females [1]. Because of minor symptoms at the beginning and limited screening methods for early diagnosis of epithelial ovarian cancer (EOC), the relative 5-year survival rate is less than 45% [2]. Among clinically used prognostic markers, such as the disease stage at diagnosis (FIGO), grading, ascites volume, and patients' age, the volume of residual disease after surgery is the most relevant [3–5]. However, widely accepted non-invasive prognostic biomarkers are rare.

In 15–20% of EOC patients, there is a mutation in the tumor suppressor genes breast cancer 1/2 (BRCA1/2), leading to a familial accumulation of ovarian and breast cancer [6,7]. BRCA genes encode essential caretaker proteins for DNA surveillance and damage repair [8]. When those genes are mutated, damaged DNA may not be repaired correctly via homologous recombination and transcriptional regulation, probably leading to cancer [7,9]. Consequently, BRCA1 mutation carriers have a 40–60% risk of developing ovarian cancer in their lifetime, while BRCA2 mutation carriers' cumulative risk is up to 25% [10]. Therefore, a genetic examination of BRCA mutation status is indicated in case of positive family history, and close medical care as well as prevention strategies are required.

Platelet-activating factor (PAF) plays a crucial role in inflammation, oncogenic transformation, and metastasis of various tumor entities [11–13]. PAF is a lipid second messenger secreted into the tumor microenvironment by circulating cells and cancer cells mediating its effect through a specific G-protein-coupled receptor (PTAFR) [11,14]. Several studies report that PAF and its receptor enhance cancer progression and invasiveness of EOC [15–18]. Consequently, inhibition of PTAFR leads to sensitization to cisplatin chemotherapy and a reduction in tumor growth [19]. On the basis of this evidence, we hypothesize that an increased degradation of PAF may have protective effects. Therefore, we investigated the role of platelet-activating factor acetylhydrolase (PAF-AH), the degradation enzyme of PAF, in ovarian cancer. PAF-AH is a lipoprotein-bound, calcium-independent phospholipase that is involved in various physiological and pathological processes that influence cell signaling and metabolism [20]. Apart from this, two other PAF-AH types are known in mammals, namely, intracellular type I and II. Even though the PAF-AH isoforms show a low sequence homology, they share a function in PAF catabolism [21]. While intracellular PAF-AH I shows antiapoptotic effects and has often been described as a critical driver in cancer pathogenesis [22–25], for plasma type PAF-AH, both pro- and anti-tumorigenic effects have been reported. On the one hand, high PLA2G7/PAF-AH expression was associated with aggressive disease and poor prognosis in prostate cancer and in triple-negative breast cancer [26,27]. On the other hand, mouse models of Kaposi's sarcoma and melanoma with PAF-AH overexpression showed reduced tumor growth and more prolonged survival. In situ, the inactivation of PAF by PAF-AH impaired metastasis through inhibition of neoangiogenesis and tumor cell motility [28].

The canonical Wnt/β-catenin signaling is one of the major pathways involved in tumorigenesis, cancer progression, and the development of therapy resistance to platinum-based chemotherapies or even poly ADP ribose polymerase inhibitors [29–31]. The cascade regulates many cellular processes, including development, stemness, cell fate decisions, and cell proliferation [32]. Aberrant activation promotes a wide range of human malignancies, including EOC [33–35]. Although mutations in Wnt-related genes are relatively rare in EOC, except for the endometrioid subtype, expression profiling data prove constitutive activation of Wnt signaling in ovarian cancer, most likely by alterations in the subcellular localization of β-catenin [36–38]. β-catenin plays a central role in Wnt signaling through its nuclear translocation and activation of β-catenin-responsive genes. It is tightly regulated by its degradation and nuclear translocation [8]. In this context, glycogen synthase kinase-3β (GSK3β) represents an important molecular hub. In its active form (phosphorylated at Y216), GSK3β phosphorylates β-catenin, leading to its ubiquitination and proteasomal degradation [8,39]. Conversely, in the presence of canonical Wnt ligands, GSK3β kinase activity is inhibited by phosphorylation at S9 and nuclear β-catenin levels increase initiating epithelial–mesenchymal transition (EMT) programs [40].

Taken together, the biological consequences of signaling events mediated by PLA2G7/PAF-AH seem to be tissue- and context-dependent and need to be specified in EOC [41]. Beyond the cellular function, we aimed to assess a possible influence of PAF-AH on the Wnt signaling pathway for a better understanding of ovarian cancer pathophysiology, taking into account differences between BRCA1 mutation carriers and BRCA wildtype (WT) patients.

2. Materials and Methods

2.1. Ethical Approval

The tissue samples used in this study were initially obtained for pathological diagnosis, completed prior to the current study. Patients' data were fully anonymized and encoded for observers during the analysis procedure. The study was approved by the Ethics Committee of Ludwig Maximilians University, Munich, Germany (approval numbers 227-09, 17-471, 17-527, and 19-972). All experiments were carried out with respect to the standards of the Declaration of Helsinki (1975).

2.2. Patients and Specimens

In this study, 156 tissue samples from patients who underwent EOC surgery at the Department of Obstetrics and Gynecology, Ludwig-Maximilian University of Munich, from 1990 to 2002 were analyzed. Patients with benign or borderline tumors were excluded, and no patient had been treated with neoadjuvant chemotherapy. The follow-up data were obtained from the Munich Cancer Registry (Munich Tumor Center, Munich, Germany). The tissue specimens were fixed in 4% buffered formalin and embedded in paraffin for immunohistochemical analysis. Staging and grading of EOC were assessed by gynecological pathologists. Detailed information about the clinical characteristics of patients enrolled in this study, including tumor grading, histology, and staging, was available. The staging was performed according to the WHO and FIGO classification (2014).

Unfortunately, the BRCA mutation status of this EOC collective is not available. Therefore, the BRCA mutation status was defined as unknown, with a BRCA mutation probability of 10–20% [6,7]. To investigate PAF-AH expression levels in BRCA1 mutation carriers, we stained additional tumor tissue of 107 patients with a genetically confirmed BRCA1 mutation (Table 1): 15 patients with a single BRCA1 mutation, and 92 patients with a combined BRCA1/2 mutation.

Table 1. BRCA mutation status of analyzed patients.

BRCA Mutation Status	n	Percentage (%)
Mutation unknown	141	56.9
BRCA1 mutation	107	43.1
BRCA1	15	6
BRCA1 + 2	92	37

All mutation carriers showed a proven pathogenic variant and no variant of uncertain significance according to the classification recommended by the IARC Unclassified Genetic Variants Working Group (IARC) and endorsed by the Evidence-based Network for the Interpretation of Germline Mutant Alleles (ENIGMA) Consortium. The specific mutations were identified and evaluated by next-generation sequencing in our genetic laboratory.

Furthermore, blood samples of EOC patients with pathogenic BRCA1 mutation or BRCA WT were used in this study. BRCA mutations were identified by next-generation sequencing in our genetic laboratory. The characteristics of the patients included in blood analysis are shown in Table 2.

Table 2. Patient characteristics of the blood analysis.

BRCA Mutation Status	n	Percentage (%)	Overall Survival (Months; Median)	Progression-Free Survival (Months; Median)
No mutation	17	73.9	25.0	17.0
BRCA1 mutation	6	26.1	34.5	28.0

2.3. Immunohistochemistry and Immunocytochemistry

As previously described, tissue microarrays of formalin-fixed, paraffin-embedded tissue specimens (three spots/patient) were prepared [42]. For immunohistochemistry (IHC) staining, the tissue slides were dewaxed in xylol, washed in 100% ethanol, incubated in methanol with 3% H_2O_2 for 20 min, and rehydrated in a descending ethanol gradient. The samples were demasked in a pressure cooker using sodium citrate buffer (pH = 6.0) containing 0.1 M citric acid and 0.1 M sodium citrate in distilled water. After cooking for 5 min, the slides were cooled down and washed in phosphate-buffered saline (PBS). All slides were incubated with a blocking solution for 30 min to prevent the non-specific binding of the primary antibody (Reagent 1; Zytochem-Plus HRP-Polymer-Kit (mouse/rabbit); Zytomed, Berlin, Germany). Primary antibodies against PAF-AH, pGSK3β, and β-catenin (Table S1) were applied for 16 h at 4 °C. The slides were washed with PBS and incubated with a complex of the secondary antibody and an HRP polymer (Reagent 3; Zytochem-Plus HRP Polymer-kit (mouse/rabbit); Zytomed, Berlin, Germany). In order to visualize the immunostaining, we applied the substrate and chromogen-3,3'-diaminobenzidine (DAB; Dako, Hamburg, Germany) for 10 min. The slides were counterstained with Mayer's hemalum and dehydrated in an ascending series of alcohol. Healthy colon tissue or metastatic colon carcinoma tissue served as positive and negative controls (Figure S1) for the IHC staining to test antibody function and choose the adequate dilution of the antibody.

For immunocytochemistry (ICC), 5×10^3 UWB1.289 cells/cm^2 were seeded on chamber slides (Merck, Darmstadt, Germany). PLA2G7 silencing of UWB1.289 cells was performed after 48 h incubation. Untreated cells served as reference (basal expression). After treatment, slides were washed with PBS 0.1 M, fixed in 100% ethanol and methanol (1:1) for 15 min at room temperature (RT), and air dried. To reduce non-specific background staining, we treated slides with a protein block solution (Dako, Glostrup, Denmark) for 20 min at RT. The slides were incubated with primary antibodies against PAF-AH and β-catenin (Table S1) for 16 h at 4 °C. After washing with PBS, the slides were incubated with a biotinylated secondary anti-mouse or anti-rabbit antibody (Vector Laboratories, Burlingame, CA, USA) for 30 min at RT. Again, the slides were washed in PBS and incubated with an avidin–biotin peroxidase complex (Vectastain-Elite; Vector Laboratories, Burlingame, CA, USA) for 30 min at RT. The antigen–antibody complex was visualized with the chromogen 3-amino-9-ethylcarbazole (AEC; Dako, Hamburg, Germany) and counterstained with Mayer's hemalum. Finally, the slides were washed with water and cover slipped using Kaiser's glycerin gelatin (Merck, Darmstadt, Germany).

2.4. Staining Evaluation and Statistical Analysis

For evaluation of PAF-AH, pGSK3β, and β-catenin staining, the semi-quantitative immunoreactive score (IRScore) was used [43], which is calculated by multiplying the optical staining intensity (0 = no, 1 = weak, 2 = moderate, and 3 = strong staining) by the percentage of positive stained cells (0 = no staining, $1 \leq 10\%$, 2 = 11–50%, 3 = 51–80% and $4 \geq 81\%$ stained cells). All slides were analyzed by two independent observers in a double-blind process using a photomicroscope (Leitz, Wetzlar, Germany). The median of IRScores resulting from the three spots of one patient was calculated and used for further analyses.

Data processing and statistical analysis of patient data, IHC results, and blood analysis were performed with SPSS 25.0 (v26; IBM, Armonk, NY, USA). The Mann–Whitney U test was applied to compare IRScores or serum concentrations of PAF-AH between two independent subgroups (no/unknown mutation vs. BRCA1) [44]. Spearman's analysis was used to calculate bivariate correlations between PAF-AH and the Wnt signaling proteins pGSK3β and β-catenin [45]. Survival times were compared using log-rank testing and visualized in Kaplan–Meier plots [46]. To identify appropriate cut-off values ROC analysis, we performed a widely accepted method for cut-off point selection. The Youdan index, defined as the maximum (sensitivity + specificity^{-1}) [47], is determined to ensure the optimal cut-off, which maximizes the sum of sensitivity and specificity [48,49]. A Cox regression model was established for multivariate analysis [50]. p-values ≤ 0.05 were considered significant. Ct values of the investigated genes were obtained by qPCR and the relative expression was calculated applying the 2-$\Delta\Delta$Ct formula [51]. For data visualization and statistical analysis of in vitro-generated data, Graph Pad Prism 7.03 (v7; San Diego, CA, USA) was used.

2.5. PAF-AH ELISA

To determine the PAF-AH concentration in serum samples, we conducted an enzyme-linked immunosorbent assay (ELISA; R&D Systems, Minneapolis, MN, USA) according to the instructions of the manufacturer. The standard curve was created using a four-parameter logistic curve fit. The assay range was 0.8–50 ng/mL with a sensitivity of 0.284 ng/mL.

2.6. Cell Lines

The human ovarian cancer cell lines ES-2 (clear cell; ATCC, Rockville, MD, USA), SKOV3 (serous, BRCA WT; ATCC, Rockville, MD, USA), TOV112D (endometrioid; ATCC, Rockville, MD, USA), and UWB1.289 (serous, BRCA1-negative; ATCC, Rockville, MD, USA) were maintained in culture with RPMI 1640 GlutaMAX medium (Gibco, Gibco, Paisley, UK) supplemented with 10% fetal bovine serum (FBS; Gibco, Paisley, UK) in a humified incubator at 37 °C under 5% CO_2. The benign ovarian cell line HOSEpiC (served as the reference; ATCC, Rockville, MD, USA) was maintained in culture in Ovarian Epithelial Cell Medium (OEpiCM) (ScienCell, Carlsbad, CA, USA,) in a humidified incubator at 37 °C under 5% CO_2. The benign breast cell line MCF10A (served as the reference; ATCC, Rockville, MD, USA) was maintained in a special growth and assay medium in a humidified incubator at 37 °C under 5% CO_2.

2.7. qPCR

Isolation of mRNA was performed according to the manufacturer's protocol using the RNeasy Mini Kit (Qiagen, Venlo, The Netherlands). A total of 1 µg RNA was converted into cDNA with the MMLV Reverse Transcriptase 1st-Strand cDNA Synthesis Kit (Epicentre, Madison, WI, USA). qPCR was performed using FastStart Essential DNA Probes Master and gene-specific primers (Roche, Basel, Switzerland). Relative expression was calculated by the 2−$\Delta\Delta$Ct method using β-actin and GAPDH as housekeeping genes (primer sequences are available in the Table S2) [51].

2.8. siRNA Knockdown

Lipofectamine RNAiMAX reagent (Invitrogen, Carlsbad, CA, USA) was used to transfect small interfering RNA (siRNA; 4 different sequences for PLA2G7: siRNA 1 (SI00072198): CACCCTTTGGATCCCAAATAA, siRNA 2 (SI00072191): TCAGGACACTTTATTCTGCTA, siRNA 3 (SI00072184): TCCGTTGGTTGTACAGACTTA, siRNA 4 (SI00072177): AAGGACTCTATTGATAGGGAA; Qiagen Sciences, Germantown, MD, USA) into UWB1.289 cells. A scrambled negative control siRNA (Qiagen, Hilden, Germany) was used as a reference. UWB1.289 cells were seeded into 6-well plates, and the transfection was performed when cell density reached 60–70%. The cells were treated with Opti-MEM Reduced

Serum Medium (Thermo Fisher Scientific, Waltham, MA, USA) containing siRNA-PLA2G7 and Lipofectamine RNAiMAX. After 36 h, cells were harvested and used for further experiments.

2.9. Western Blot

The Western blot analysis was performed as previously reported [52]. In short, adherent cells were lysed for 15 min at 4 °C with 200 µL RIPA buffer (Sigma-Aldrich Co., St. Louis, MO, USA), containing a protease inhibitor (1:100 dilution; Sigma-Aldrich Co., St. Louis, MO, USA). The protein concentration of the lysates was determined with Bradford protein assay. Protein extracts (65 µg) were separated according to their molecular weight using 12% sodium dodecyl sulfate–polyacrylamide gel and transferred onto a polyvinylidene fluoride membrane (EMD Millipore, Billerica, MA, USA). The membrane was blocked for 1 h with casein (Vector Laboratories, Burlingame, CA, USA) to prevent nonspecific binding of the antibodies. After casein saturation, the membrane was incubated with diluted primary antibodies gently shaken overnight at 4 °C. As primary antibodies, a rabbit polyclonal antibody against PAF-AH (1:200 dilution; Cayman, Ann Arbor, MI, USA), a mouse monoclonal antibody against GAPDH (1:1000 dilution; GeneTex Co., Eching, Germany), and a mouse monoclonal antibody against β-actin (1:1000 dilution; Sigma, St. Louis, MO, USA) were used. GAPDH/β-actin Western blots served as controls. Afterwards, membranes were washed with 1:10 casein three times and subjected to biotinylated anti-mouse/anti-rabbit IgG secondary antibodies and ABC-AmP reagent (VECTASTAIN ABC-AmP Kit for rabbit IgG; Vector Laboratories, Burlingame, CA, USA). The antibody complexes were visualized with 5-bromo-4-chloro-3-indolylphosphate/nitroblue tetrazolium chromogenic substrate (Vectastain ABC-AmP Kit; Vector Laboratories, Burlingame, CA, USA). Western blotting detection and analysis was performed with Bio-Rad Universal Hood II and the corresponding software Quantity One (Bio-Rad Laboratories Inc., Hercules, CA, USA). Each Western blot experiment was validated nine times ($n = 9$, three times in three lanes).

2.10. Cell Viability Assay and Proliferation Assay

3-(4,5-Dimethylthiazol-2-yl)-2,5-diphenyltetrazolium bromide (MTT) colorimetric assay was performed to measure the cell viability, while 5-bromo-2-deoxyuridine (BrdU) incorporation assay (Roche, Basel, Switzerland) was used to determine cell proliferation. For both assays, 5×10^3 UWB1.289 cells/100 µL were seeded on 96-well plates. The cells were incubated in RPMI 1640 GlutaMAX medium with 10% FBS for 48 h before transfection (PLA2G7 gene knockdown) was performed, as described above. After PLA2G7 36 h gene knockdown, MTT and BrdU assay were conducted according to manufacturer's protocol. The optical density (OD) was measured with an Elx800 universal Microplate Reader (BioTek, Winooski, VT, USA) at 595 nm (MTT) and 450 nm (BrdU). Each experiment was validated three times ($n = 3$).

2.11. Wound Healing Assay

UWB1.289/HCC1937 cells were seeded on a 24-well plate (2×10^5 cells/mL). After 24 h, a vertical line was scratched into the middle of the monolayer with a 100 µL pipet tip to create an artificial wound. Subsequently, the transfection was performed, and digital images of the scratch assays were taken exactly 0 h and 36 h after PLA2G7 gene knockdown. The cell migration was monitored using an inverse phase contrast microscope (Leica Dmi1; Leica, Wetzlar, Germany) with a camera (LEICA MC120 HD; Leica, Wetzlar, Germany). Microphotographs of wounded areas and areas covered with cells were analyzed by ImageJ. Available online: https://imagej.nih.gov/ij/ (accessed on 12 April 2020). The cell migration area is defined as the difference of the area covered with cells at 36 h and 0 h.

3. Results

3.1. PAF-AH Is an Independent Positive Prognostic Factor in EOC and Correlated with the Wnt Signaling Proteins pGSK3β and β-Catenin

To understand the role of PAF-AH in aberrant cell signaling, we investigated PAF-AH's expression patterns in 156 EOC specimens by IHC. Similarly, the expression of the Wnt signaling proteins pGSK3β and β-catenin were examined. For PAF-AH, 86.52% of all successfully stained tissue samples were positive with a median (range) IRScore of 3 (0–12). The expression profile of PAF-AH regarding clinical characteristics and pathological data is shown in Table 3. Differences in staining intensity between the histological subtypes were detected. EOC tissue with serous and endometrioid histology showed higher PAF-AH levels than clear cell and mucinous specimens. However, there were no relevant differences regarding subcellular localization of PAF-AH. A total of 98.57% showed cytoplasmatic pGSK3β (Y216; median IRScore = 4 (0–12)), and all specimens showed membranous β-catenin (median IRScore = 8 (2–12)) expression. Strong positive correlations between nuclear/cytoplasmatic PAF-AH, cytoplasmic pGSK3β, and membranous β-catenin were found (Table 4).

Table 3. Expression profile of PAF-AH regarding clinical and pathological characteristics.

Clinicopathological Parameters	PAF-AH Total			PAF-AH Nucleus			PAF-AH Cytoplasm		
	n	Median IRScore	p	n	Median IRScore	p	n	Median IRScore	p
Histology			<0.001 *			<0.001 *			<0.001 *
Serous	102	3		102	3		102	3	
Clear cell	11	1		11	1		11	1	
Endometrioid	19	3		19	2		19	3	
Mucinous	10	0.5		10	0.5		10	1	
Lymph node			NS			NS			NS
pN0/X	94	3		94	2		94	3	
pN1	48	3		48	2		48	3	
Distant Metastasis			NS			NS			NS
pM0/X	137	3		137	2		137	3	
pM1	5	4		5	2		5	3	
FIGO			NS			NS			NS
I/II	39	3		39	2		39	3	
III/IV	98	3		98	2		98	3	
Age			0.047 *			0.022 *			0.047 *
≤60 years	75	3		75	2		75	3	
>60 years	67	3		67	3		67	3	
Serous Grading			NS			NS			NS
Low	22	3		22	3		22	3	
High	74	3.5		74	3		74	3	
Clear cell, endometrioid, mucinous grading			NS			NS			NS
G1	10	2.5		10	1		10	2.5	
G2	10	2		10	1		10	2.5	
G3	15	2		15	1		15	2	

Differences in IRScores of PAF-AH (total, nucleus and cytoplasm) staining were detected regarding clinical and pathological characteristics using Mann–Whitney U test. Significant results are indicated by asterisks (*: $p \leq 0.05$). p = two-tailed significance, n = number of patients, NS = not significant.

Table 4. Correlations between PAF-AH and Wnt signaling proteins pGSK3β and β-catenin.

	PAF-AH Nucleus	PAF-AH Cytoplasm	pGSK3β Cytoplasm	β-Catenin Membrane
PAF-AH nucleus				
Cc	1	0.469	0.494	0.267
p	-	<0.001 *	<0.001 *	0.001 *
n	141	141	135	140
PAF-AH cytoplasm				
Cc	0.469	1	0.448	0.291
p	<0.001 *	-	<0.001 *	<0.001 *
n	141	141	135	140
pGSK3β cytoplasm				
Cc	0.494	0.448	1	0.224
p	<0.001 *	<0.001 *	-	0.008 *
n	135	135	140	139
β-Catenin membrane				
Cc	0.267	0.291	0.224	1
p	0.001 *	<0.001 *	0.008 *	-
n	140	140	139	147

IRScores of PAF-AH (nucleus and cytoplasm), pGSK3β (cytoplasma) and β-catenin (membrane) staining were correlated to each other using Spearman's correlation analysis. Significant correlations are indicated by asterisks (*: $p \leq 0.05$). Cc = correlation coefficient, p = two-tailed significance, n = number of patients.

In our patients' collective, the median age was 58.7 (±31.4) years with a total range of 31–88 years, while the median overall survival (OS) time was 34.4 (±57.8) months. Univariate survival analysis revealed that high levels of all studied proteins are associated with a significantly longer OS (at least twice as long; Figure 1a–c).

Combined survival analysis of the investigated proteins showed an even longer survival time (median OS 199.8 months vs. 35.2 months, $p = 0.044$; Figure S2). However, the subgroup with high expression levels of all factors (total PAF-AH, cytoplasmatic pGSK3β, and membranous β-catenin) was quite small ($n = 11$).

A multivariate Cox regression model was established to assess whether the prognostic factors were independent. Age (>60 vs. ≤60 years, $p = 0.039$), FIGO stage (III/IV vs. I/II, $p = 0.004$), grading (high/G2-3 vs. low/G1, $p = 0.002$), and tumoral PAF-AH expression (high vs. low, $p = 0.021$) turned out to be independent prognostic factors for OS in the present cohort. In contrast, cytoplasmatic pGSK3β ($p = 0.645$) and membranous β-catenin ($p = 0.745$) were not independent (Table 5). Due to insufficient data, the residual disease after primary surgery was not included in the multivariate analysis.

Table 5. Multivariate analysis confirmed the independency of tumoral PAF-AH expression as a positive prognostic factor for OS.

Covariate	p	Hazard Ratio (95% CI)
Age > 60 vs. ≤60	0.039 *	1.637 (1.026–2.612)
FIGO III/IV vs. I/II	0.004 *	2.585 (1.366–4.891)
Grading high/G2-3 vs. low/G1	0.002 *	2.797 (1.436–5.449)
Total PAF-AH expression high (>2) vs. low (≤2)	0.021 *	0.583 (0.369–0.921)
Cytoplasmatic pGSK3β (Y216) expression high (>6) vs. low (≤6)	0.645	0.877 (0.501–1.535)
Membranous β-catenin expression high (>8) vs. low (≤8)	0.745	0.736 (0.545–1.544)

Significant independent factors are indicated by asterisks (*: $p \leq 0.05$). CI: confidence interval.

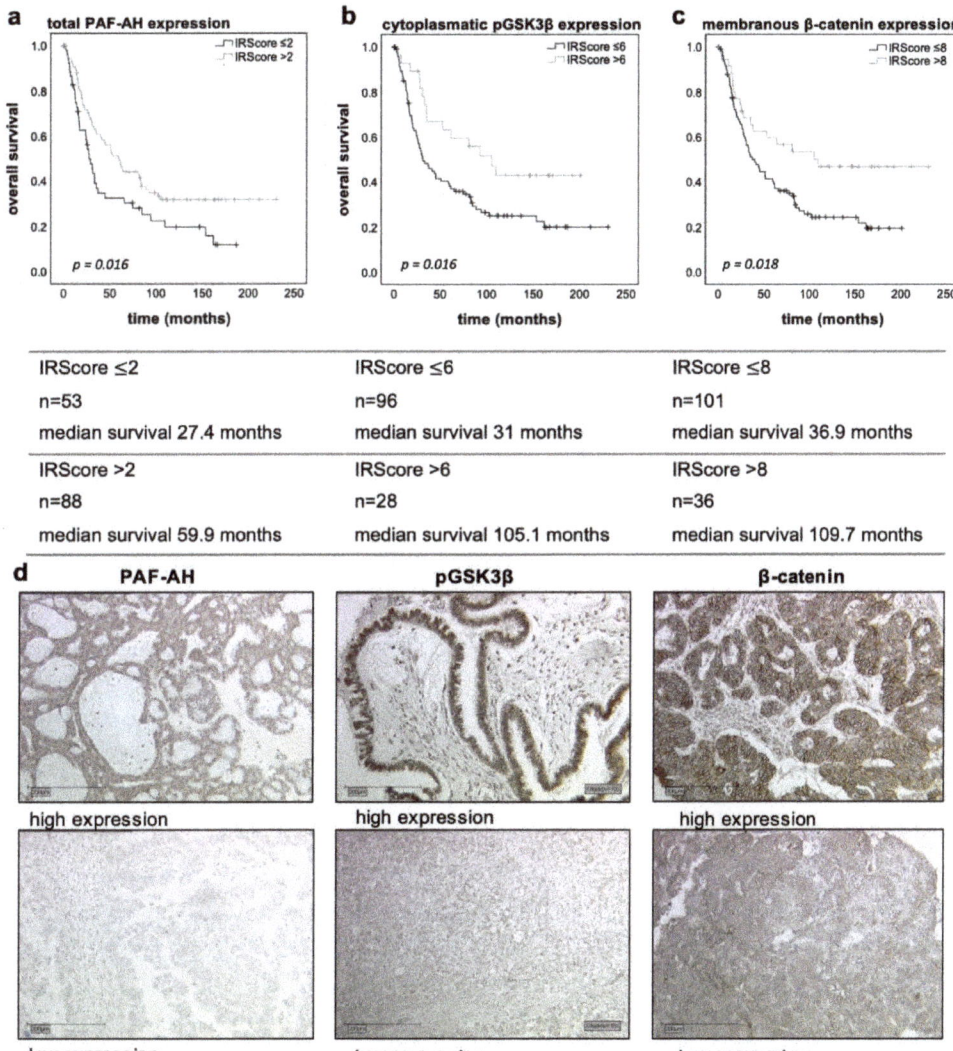

Figure 1. Univariate analyses and representative microphotographs of the immunostainings. The Kaplan–Meier estimates (log-rank testing) show that high tumoral PAF-AH (IRScore > 2; (**a**)) expression as well as high levels of cytoplasmatic pGSK3β (IRScore > 6; (**b**)) and membranous β-catenin (IRScore > 8; (**c**)) are associated with prolonged OS. Censoring events have been marked in the graphs (+). Representative microphotographs of the immunostainings (10× magnification, scale bar = 200 μm; (**d**)) show the difference between high expression (top) and low expression (bottom).

3.2. BRCA1 Mutant Patients Had Higher PAF-AH Levels in Tumor Tissue and in Serum

PAF-AH expression was also investigated by IHC in tumor tissue of BRCA1 mutation carriers (n = 107; Table 2). Interestingly, patients with BRCA1 mutation or BRCA1 + 2 mutations showed significantly higher tumoral expression levels of PAF-AH (median IRScore = 4) compared to patients with unknown BRCA mutation status (n = 141; median IRScore = 3), for which a mutation probability of 10–20% can be assumed (Figure 2) [6,7].

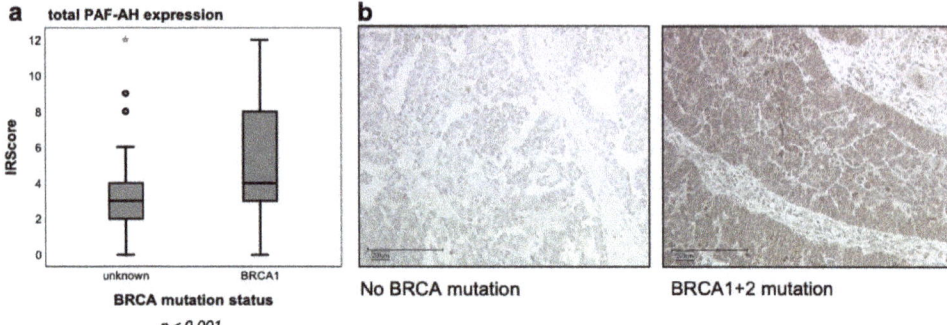

Figure 2. BRCA1 mutation carriers showed higher tumoral PAF-AH expression. PAF-AH expression was significantly higher in tumor tissue of BRCA1 mutation carriers (median IRScore = 4; $p < 0.001$ indicated by asterisk *; (**a**)), when compared (Mann–Whitney U test) to patients with unknown BRCA mutation status (median IRScore = 3). Representative microphotographs of PAF-AH immunostaining of patients with BRCA WT and BRCA1 + 2 mutation are shown on the right (**b**) in 10× magnification (scale bar = 200 µm).

On the basis of the results of IHC, the question arose as to whether differences in PAF-AH expression between BRCA WT and BRCA mutation carriers can be detected in blood samples. In a preliminary analysis, PAF-AH serum concentrations of six BRCA1-mutated and 17 BRCA WT EOC patients were determined (Table 2). Indeed, patients with a genetically confirmed BRCA1 mutation had significantly higher PAF-AH serum concentrations (median = 264.56 ng/mL) than BRCA WT patients (median = 176.35 ng/mL, Mann–Whitney U test, $p = 0.012$) (Figure 3).

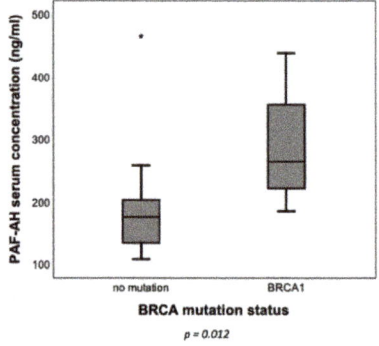

Figure 3. BRCA1 mutation carriers showed higher PAF-AH serum concentrations. PAF-AH serum concentrations were determined with ELISA. Higher levels of PAF-AH were detected in blood samples of BRCA1 mutation carriers ($n = 6$) when compared to patients with BRCA WT ($n = 17$) (Mann–Whitney U test, $p = 0.012$ indicated by asterisk *).

3.3. Only BRCA1-Negative UWB1.289 Cell Line Showed Relevant Expression of PLA2G7/PAF-AH

The basal mRNA and protein expression of PLA2G7/PAF-AH in four ovarian cancer cell lines were compared to the benign ovarian epithelial cell line HOSEpiC. Both PLA2G7 expression on mRNA level ($p < 0.05$; Figure 4A) and PAF-AH expression on protein level ($p < 0.05$; Figure 4B) were significantly increased in the BRCA1 mutant ovarian cancer cell line UWB1.289 compared to HOSEpiC and other ovarian cancer cell lines. The results derived from qPCR and Western blot were consistent with the results of IHC.

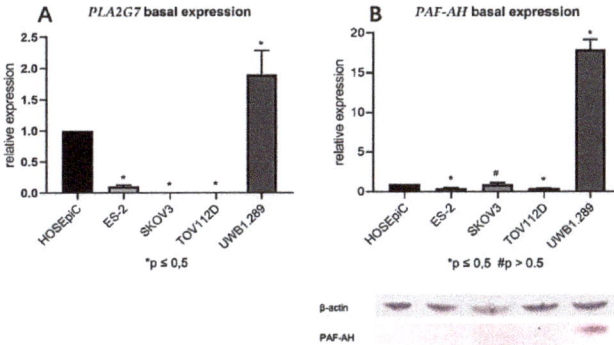

Figure 4. Only the BRCA1 mutant ovarian cancer cell line UWB1.289 showed a relevant expression of PLA2G7/PAF-AH. Basal mRNA (qPCR; (**A**)) and protein (Western blot analysis; (**B**)) expression of PLA2G7/PAF-AH in four ovarian cancer cell lines were compared to the expression in the benign ovarian cell line HOSEpiC. Significant results are indicated by asterisks (*: $p \leq 0.05$), no significant results by diamonds (#: $p > 0.05$).

3.4. PLA2G7 Knockdown Enhanced Viability, Proliferation, and Motility of UWB1.289 Cells

To assess the functional role of PLA2G7/PAF-AH and its possible impact on the Wnt/β-catenin signaling pathway in ovarian cancer, we performed in vitro experiments in the BRCA1-negative ovarian cancer cell line UWB1.289. Firstly, siRNA was transfected into UWB1.289 for PLA2G7 silencing. A successful downregulation of PLA2G7 and its protein PAF-AH was confirmed by qPCR and Western blot analysis (Figure S3). As a degradation enzyme of PAF, we hypothesized that PAF-AH is a protective factor in ovarian cancer biology. Concordantly, the IHC results showed a positive association of PAF-AH expression with OS. To characterize the cellular function of PAF-AH, we investigated viability, proliferation, and migration of UWB1.289 cells. Results of UWB1.289 cells under PLA2G7 knockdown with the siRNAs described above were compared with the results of an untreated control group (pseudo-knockdown with scrambled siRNA). As shown in Figure 5A, the viability of UWB1.289 cells was increased by PLA2G7 silencing. Furthermore, PLA2G7-downregulated UWB1.289 cells exhibited significantly higher proliferation rates in comparison to the control group, which indicates that PLA2G7 knockdown induces the proliferation of EOC cells (Figure 5B). Results from the wound healing assay showed that after transfection of PLA2G7 siRNA, the migration ability of UWB1.289 was significantly activated compared to the control group (Figure 5C). These results indicate that PLA2G7 silencing causes cancer progression by activation of viability, proliferation, and migration.

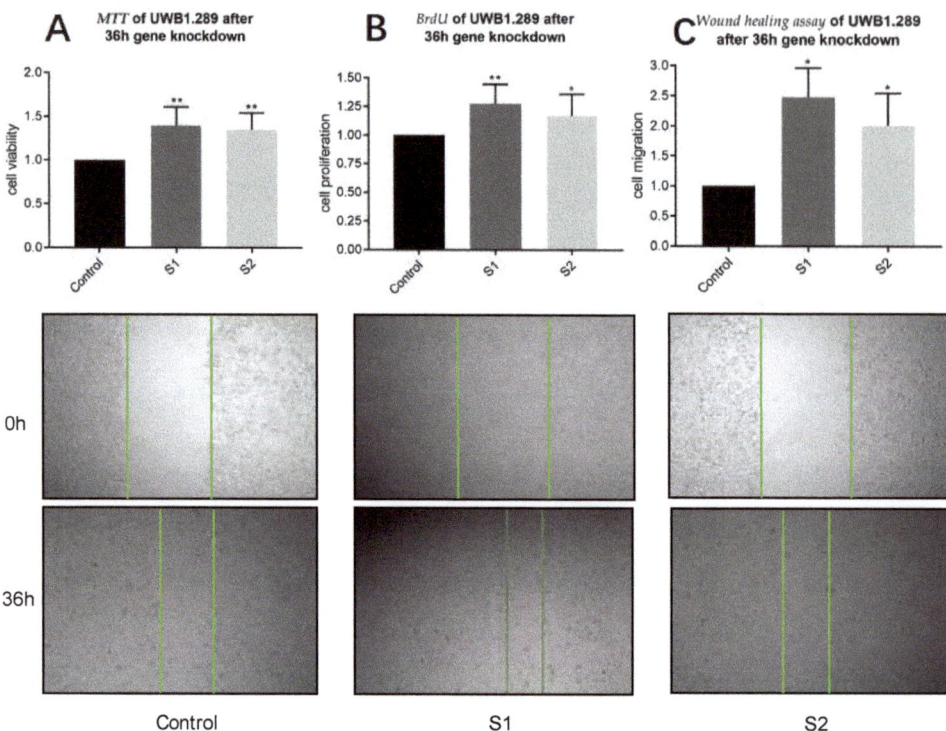

Figure 5. PLA2G7 silencing favored cancer progression by an activation of viability, proliferation, and migration. MTT results show that after 36 h siRNA (sequence S1 and S2) knockdown of PLA2G7, the viability of UWB1.289 increased significantly ((**A**); $p < 0.001$). DNA incorporation of BrdU was also significantly higher in the PLA2G7 downregulated group, indicating an increasing proliferation rate (**B**). The wound healing assay proved that the migration ability of PLA2G7-downregulated UWB1.289 cells was significantly activated compared to the control group ((**C**); $p < 0.05$). Significant results are indicated by asterisks (*: $p \leq 0.05$) and double asterisks (**: $p \leq 0.001$).

3.5. The Cellular Distribution Pattern of β-Catenin Changed by PLA2G7 Knockdown from the Membrane to Nucleus

After demonstrating the functional impact of PLA2G7 and its protein PAF-AH on cancer progression, we aimed to validate how PLA2G7 affects the Wnt/β-catenin signaling pathway. On the basis of the correlation of PAF-AH and β-catenin found in IHC, we carried out a series of ICCs to prove an interplay of PAF-AH and β-catenin. As expected, PAF-AH staining was downregulated after knockdown of PLA2G7 compared to the control with pseudo-knockdown (Figure 6A). Interestingly, the distribution of β-catenin also changed by PLA2G7 knockdown. While membrane expression was weakened compared to the control group, the nuclear expression was enhanced (Figure 6B).

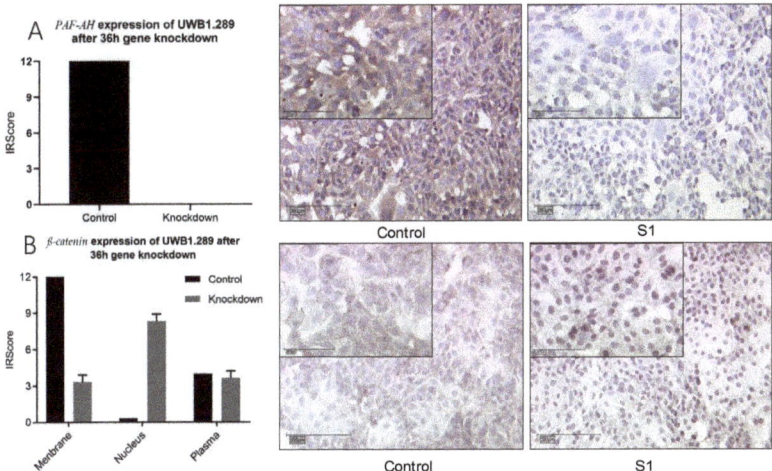

Figure 6. PLA2G7 silencing caused a shift of β-catenin from the membrane to nucleus. ICC staining of PAF-AH and β-catenin changed after 36 h silencing of PLA2G7 with siRNA (representative pictures 1. 10× magnification, scale bar = 200 μm and 25× magnification, scale bar = 100 μm). The expression of PAF-AH was downregulated as expected (**A**). The distribution of β-catenin changed by PLA2G7 knockdown from a predominantly membranous expression to a nuclear one (**B**).

4. Discussion

In this study, PLA2G7/PAF-AH's role in ovarian cancer and its influence on the Wnt signaling pathway has been evaluated. Besides cytoplasmatic pGSK3β (Y216) and membranous β-catenin (both part of the inactive state of the Wnt signaling pathway), high tumoral PAF-AH expression was associated with prolonged OS of EOC patients in univariate analysis (Figure 1). A multivariate Cox regression model proved the independence of PAF-AH as a favorable prognostic factor (Table 5). In vitro experiments confirmed protective functional effects of PAF-AH. Silencing of its gene PLA2G7 caused activation of viability, proliferation, and migration of BRCA1 mutant ovarian cancer cells (Figure 5). Since the relevant gene and protein expression of PLA2G7/PAF-AH were detected exclusively in the BRCA1 mutant cell line UWB1.289 (Figure 4), PAF-AH can be considered a new biomarker for BRCA1 mutant ovarian cancer, indicating good prognosis. Significantly higher PAF-AH levels were detected in tumor biopsies (Figure 2) and in the serum of BRCA1 mutation carriers compared to BRCA WT patients (Figure 3). An advantage of PAF-AH as a potential biomarker is the possibility of its non-invasive determination in blood samples before surgery. Since the blood analysis conducted in this study is somewhat preliminary, we suggest further investigation of PAF-AH as a biomarker with prediction ability in BRCA mutant ovarian cancer in a large-scale prospective clinical trial.

We further show that PAF-AH expression positively correlated with cytoplasmatic pGSK3β (Y216) and membranous β-catenin expression, which suggests an interaction with the Wnt/β-catenin signaling pathway. A changed distribution pattern of β-catenin within the cellular departments in BRCA mutant ovarian cancer cells caused by PLA2G7 gene knockdown confirmed this assumption. Membrane expression of β-catenin was reduced, while nuclear expression was upregulated (Figure 6). Thus, increased activation of the Wnt signaling could be responsible for tumor progression under PLA2G7 knockdown. We assume that PAF/PTAFR and PLA2G7/PAF-AH might have a negative regulatory influence on the Wnt signaling pathway, especially in BRCA1 mutant EOC (Figure 7) [53].

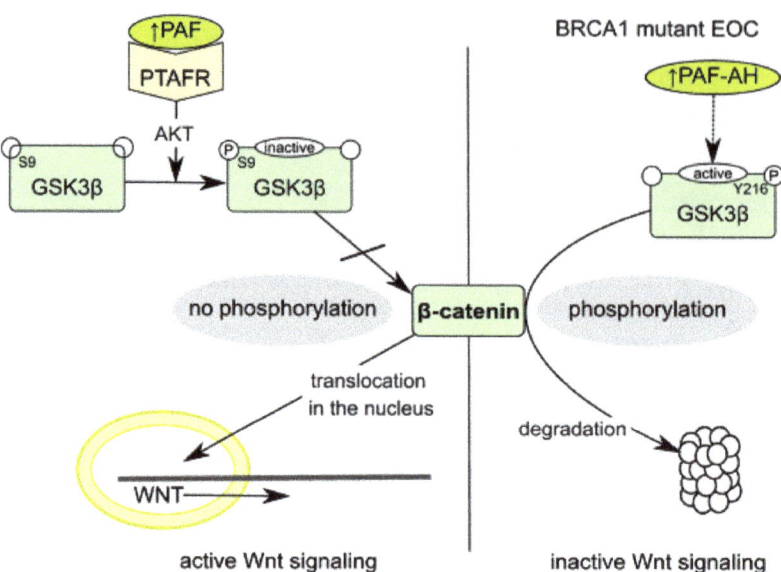

Figure 7. Activation states of canonical Wnt signaling pathway and possible regulation by PAF/PTAFR or PAF-AH. Inactivation of GSK3β by phosphorylation at S9 either in the presence of Wnt ligands or following signal transduction through PAF/PTAFR/AKT (left) led to accumulation of non-phosphorylated β-catenin and translocation in the nucleus [40,53]. There, β-catenin displaces Groucho/TLE repressors from transcription factors Tcf/Lef and activates transcription of Wnt-responsive genes [54]. In the absence of Wnt ligands or PAF signaling, e.g., through enhanced PAF degradation by PAF-AH (right), β-catenin is marked by active GSK3β for ubiquitination and proteasomal degradation [8,39].

Similarly, studies of Furihata et al. [55] and Boccellino and Camussi et al. [56] indicate a functional link between PAF/PTAFR and β-catenin. A PTAFR antagonist reduced inflammation-induced colon carcinogenesis in rats, and β-catenin was localized in the cell membrane in healthy tissue, while it was overexpressed in the nucleus in precursor lesions and colon cancer [55]. Immunofluorescence analysis of Kaposi's sarcoma cells also showed a change in β-catenin distribution from the membrane to a diffuse pattern as a reaction to PAF treatment [56].

On the basis of our findings and evidence from literature, we can consider two explanatory approaches for the protective effects of PAF-AH: (1) Influence of PAF-AH on the Wnt signaling pathway by regulating PAF levels in the tumor microenvironment. (2) PAF independent regulatory effect of PAF-AH on Wnt downstream genes. Indeed, the anti-inflammatory properties of PAF-AH further contribute to its protective character [57].

PAF induces various signaling pathways via its G-protein-coupled receptor PTAFR through the activation of phosphorylation cascades [15,58]. These phospholipid-mediated protein phosphorylation cascades often represent early responses to mitogenic induction [59]. While PAF exposure activates, e.g., Src/FAK, FAK/STAT, and AKT, leading to enhanced proliferation, invasion, and migration, respectively (Figure 8) [15,53,60,61], GSK3β is inactivated by phosphorylation at S9 [53,60]. β-Catenin is thereby stabilized and activates Wnt-responsive genes (Figure 7).

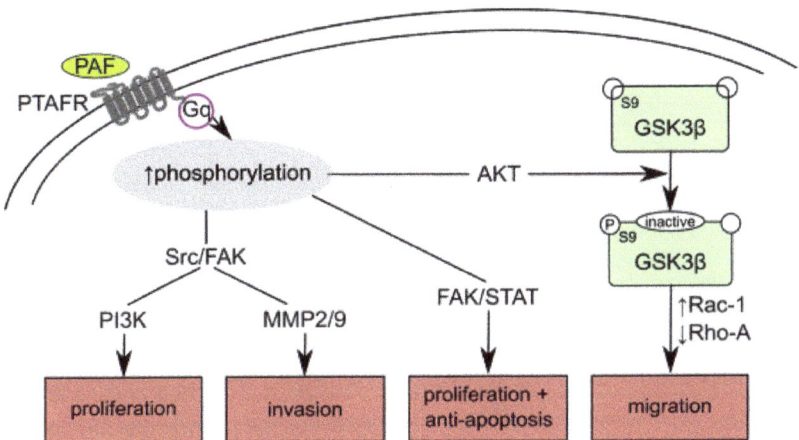

Figure 8. Functional consequences of PAF-AH silencing. By PLA2G7 silencing, PAF-mediated signaling dominated. Binding to its Gq-coupled receptor PTAFR, PAF activated phosphorylation cascades, which often lead to oncogenic transformation, tumor growth, angiogenesis, and metastasis [15,53,60,61]. Activation of Src/FAK and their downstream targets PI3K and MMP2/MMP9 resulted in cancer cell proliferation and cancer invasion, respectively [15]. Proliferation and anti-apoptosis are induced via FAK/STAT [61]. GSK-3β is inactivated by AKT, leading to enhanced migration by Rac-1 activation and Rho-A inactivation and active Wnt signaling by stabilizing β-catenin [53].

Zhang et al. reported an elevated expression of PTAFR in BRCA1 mutant cell lines and tissue of BRCA1 mutation carriers. Additionally, they showed PAF/PTAFR-mediated malignant transition of BRCA1-mutated non-malignant ovarian epithelial cells by FAK/STAT phosphorylation, thereby inducing proliferation and anti-apoptosis [61]. As we also found higher PAF-AH levels in BRCA1 mutation carriers and BRCA1 mutant ovarian cancer cells, we conclude that PAF-AH upregulation might be relevant to counteract PAF and Wnt signaling, respectively. By increased PAF degradation, GSK3β remains active, and β-catenin is marked for degradation, resulting in an inactive Wnt pathway (Figure 7) [39]. The same effect was observed for PTAFR antagonism [61].

Direct modulation of the Wnt signaling pathway by the catalytic subunits of intracellular PAF-AH isoform IB was discovered by Livnat et al. in restricted areas of the cerebral cortex [62]. In addition to PAF degradation, it is conceivable that the PAF-AH isoforms show other parallels on a regulatory level. In line with our results, Livnat et al. showed enhanced proliferation and tangential migration of GABAergic interneurons in PAF-AH knockout mice. Overexpression of each of the catalytic subunits provoked a shift of β-catenin from the nucleus to the cytoplasm and repressed Wnt gene expression [62]. However, the molecular interaction between PAF-AH and β-catenin remains unclear and needs to be defined in future studies.

For breast cancer, an interplay between BRCA1 and the Wnt signaling pathway has been previously described. Wu et al. found an inverse correlative association between Wnt signaling and BRCA1 expression in basal-like breast cancer due to epigenetic repression of BRCA1 by the Wnt effector Slug [40]. Li et al. reported that the nuclear form of β-catenin was lower or absent in most BRCA1 familial breast cancer tissues compared to sporadic breast cancer or healthy tissue [8]. For BRCA1 WT, but not mutated BRCA1, direct interaction with β-catenin on the same binding site as the ubiquitinylating enzyme was described. Consequently, the half-life of β-catenin is prolonged, and the Wnt signaling pathway is active in the presence of BRCA1 WT [8]. In BRCA mutant ovarian cancer, Wnt signaling might be repressed by PAF-AH. Nevertheless, we cannot exclude participations or crosstalk with other signaling pathways and regulatory factors resulting in the observed phenotypes.

5. Conclusions

Patients and in vitro generated data indicate that PAF/PTAFR and PLA2G7/PAF-AH signaling plays a crucial role in BRCA1 mutant ovarian cancer. While PAF and its receptor PTAFR promote malignant transformation [59,61], tumor progression [12,15,55,63], and chemoresistance [19], we were able to identify PLA2G7/PAF-AH as counterpart and protective factor. Strong positive correlations between PAF-AH and the Wnt signaling proteins pGSK3β and β-catenin and a shift of β-catenin from the membrane to the nucleus by PLA2G7 silencing suggest a negative regulatory impact of PAF-AH on the Wnt/β-catenin signaling pathway. Since PAF-AH mediates protective effects and is non-invasively detectable in blood samples, it should be considered a potential biomarker that indicates a good prognosis for patients with BRCA1 mutant ovarian cancer. Thus, further studies are needed to validate our findings.

Supplementary Materials: The following are available online at https://www.mdpi.com/article/10.3390/biomedicines9070706/s1, Table S1: Antibodies used for immunostainings. Table S2: Sequences of primers used in qPCR to determine mRNA expression levels. Figure S1: Positive and negative system controls. Figure S2: Combined survival analysis of PAF-AH, pGSK3β (cytoplasmatic), and β-catenin (membranous). Figure S3: Successful PLA2G7/PAF-AH downregulation by siRNA knockdown.

Author Contributions: Y.L., S.B. (Susann Badmann): participated in design and coordination of the study, performed the experiments, performed the statistical analysis, and wrote the manuscript. D.M., E.S.: supervised immunohistochemistry as gynecologic pathologists and participated in immunohistochemistry analysis as well as in the design and coordination of the study. T.K. (Till Kaltofen), E.D., M.M., S.L., T.K. (Thomas Kolben), A.H., S.B. (Susanne Beyer), A.B. and S.M.: revised the manuscript for important intellectual content. U.J., F.T. and B.C.: conceived of the study and participated in its design and coordination, and approved the final version of the manuscript. All authors analyzed and interpreted the results. All authors have read and agreed to the published version of the manuscript.

Funding: This work was funded by the "Brigitte & Dr. Konstanze Wegener" foundation.

Institutional Review Board Statement: This study was approved by the Ethics Committee of the Ludwig-Maximilian-University Munich (approval numbers 227-09, 17-471, 17-527, and 19-972). The ovarian cancer specimens were obtained in clinically indicated surgeries and were initially used for histopathological diagnostics. When the current study was performed, all diagnostic procedures were completed, and the patients' data were anonymized. The ethical principles adopted in the Declaration of Helsinki 1975 have been respected.

Informed Consent Statement: Before the current study was performed, all diagnostic procedures were completed, and the patients' data were fully anonymized. Due to these circumstances, our ethics committee declared that no written informed consent of the participants or permission to publish is needed.

Data Availability Statement: The datasets generated and/or analyzed during the current study are available from the corresponding author on reasonable request.

Acknowledgments: The authors thank Christina Kuhn, Martina Rahmeh, Sabine Fink, Cornelia Herbst, and Andrea Sendelhofert for her excellent technical assistance.

Conflicts of Interest: Thomas Kolben holds stock of Roche AG and his relative is employed at Roche AG. Anna Hester has received a research grant from the "Walter Schulz" foundation and advisory board, speech honoraria, and travel expenses from Roche and Pfizer. Alexander Burges has received advisory board and honoraria from AstraZeneca, Clovis, Roche, and Tesaro. Research support, advisory board, honoraria, and travel expenses from AstraZeneca, Clovis, Medac, MSD, Novartis, PharmaMar, Roche, Sensor Kinesis, Tesaro, and Teva have been received by Sven Mahner, and from AstraZeneca, Medac, PharmaMar, Roche, and Tesaro by Fabian Trillsch. All other authors declare no conflict of interest.

Abbreviations

ADP	adenosine diphosphate
AKT	protein kinase B
BRCA	breast cancer gene
BrDU	5-bromo-2-deoxyuridine
Cc	correlation coefficient
CI	confidence interval
DNA	deoxyribonucleic acid
ELISA	enzyme-linked immunosorbent assay
EMT	epithelial–mesenchymal transition
EOC	epithelial ovarian cancer
FBS	fetal bovine serum
FIGO	International Federation of Gynecology and Obstetrics
GAPDH	glycerinaldehyd-3-phosphat-dehydrogenase
GSK3β	glycogen synthase kinase-3β
ICC	immunocytochemistry
IHC	immunohistochemistry
IRScore	immunoreactive score
MMP	matrix metalloproteinase
mRNA	messenger ribonucleic acid
MTT	3-(4,5-dimethylthiazol-2-yl)-2,5-diphenyltetrazolium bromide
OS	overall survival
PAF	platelet-activating factor
PBS	phosphate-buffered saline
PI3K	phosphatidylinositol 3-kinase
PLA2G7/PAF-AH	platelet-activating factor acetylhydrolase
PTAFR	platelet-activating factor receptor
qPCR	quantitative polymerase chain reaction
Rac-1	ras-related C3 botulinum toxin substrate 1
Rho-A	ras homolog family member A
RIPA	radioimmunoprecipitation assay
ROC	receiver operating characteristic
RT	room temperature
siRNA	small interfering ribonucleic acid
Src/FAK	steroid receptor coactivator/focal adhesion kinase
STAT	signal transducer and activator of transcription
Tcf/Lef	transcription factor/lymphoid enhancer-binding factor
TLE	transducin-like enhancer
WHO	World Health Organization
WT	wildtype

References

1. Oberaigner, W.; Minicozzi, P.; Bielska-Lasota, M.; Allemani, C.; de Angelis, R.; Mangone, L.; Sant, M. Eurocare Working G: Survival for ovarian cancer in Europe: The across-country variation did not shrink in the past decade. *Acta Oncol.* **2012**, *51*, 441–453. [CrossRef]
2. Torre, L.A.; Trabert, B.; DeSantis, C.E.; Miller, K.D.; Samimi, G.; Runowicz, C.D.; Gaudet, M.M.; Jemal, A.; Siegel, R.L. Ovarian cancer statistics. 2018. *CA Cancer J. Clin.* **2018**, *68*, 284–296. [CrossRef]
3. Aletti, G.D.; Gostout, B.S.; Podratz, K.C.; Cliby, W.A. Ovarian cancer surgical resectability: Relative impact of disease, patient status, and surgeon. *Gynecol. Oncol.* **2006**, *100*, 33–37. [CrossRef]
4. Dembo, A.J.; Davy, M.; Stenwig, A.E.; Berle, E.J.; Bush, R.S.; Kjorstad, K. Prognostic factors in patients with stage I epithelial ovarian cancer. *Obstet. Gynecol.* **1990**, *75*, 263–273.
5. Vergote, I.; De Brabanter, J.; Fyles, A.; Bertelsen, K.; Einhorn, N.; Sevelda, P.; Gore, M.E.; Kaern, J.; Verrelst, H.; Sjovall, K.; et al. Prognostic importance of degree of differentiation and cyst rupture in stage I invasive epithelial ovarian carcinoma. *Lancet* **2001**, *357*, 176–182. [CrossRef]
6. Nelson, H.D.; Pappas, M.; Cantor, A.; Haney, E.; Holmes, R. Risk Assessment, Genetic Counseling, and Genetic Testing for BRCA-Related Cancer in Women: Updated Evidence Report and Systematic Review for the US Preventive Services Task Force. *JAMA* **2019**, *322*, 666–685. [CrossRef]

7. Madariaga, A.; Lheureux, S.; Oza, A.M. Tailoring Ovarian Cancer Treatment: Implications of BRCA1/2 Mutations. *Cancers* **2019**, *11*, 416. [CrossRef]
8. Li, H.; Sekine, M.; Tung, N.; Avraham, H.K. Wild-type BRCA1, but not mutated BRCA1, regulates the expression of the nuclear form of beta-catenin. *Mol. Cancer Res.* **2010**, *8*, 407–420. [CrossRef]
9. Yu, V. Caretaker Brca1: Keeping the genome in the straight and narrow. *Breast Cancer Res.* **2000**, *2*, 82–85. [CrossRef]
10. Kuchenbaecker, K.B.; Hopper, J.L.; Barnes, D.R.; Phillips, K.A.; Mooij, T.M.; Roos-Blom, M.J.; Jervis, S.; van Leeuwen, F.E.; Milne, R.L.; Andrieu, N.; et al. Risks of Breast, Ovarian, and Contralateral Breast Cancer for BRCA1 and BRCA2 Mutation Carriers. *JAMA* **2017**, *317*, 2402–2416. [CrossRef] [PubMed]
11. Tsoupras, A.B.; Iatrou, C.; Frangia, C.; Demopoulos, C.A. The implication of platelet activating factor in cancer growth and metastasis: Potent beneficial role of PAF-inhibitors and antioxidants. *Infect. Disord. Drug Targets* **2009**, *9*, 390–399. [CrossRef]
12. Melnikova, V.; Bar-Eli, M. Inflammation and melanoma growth and metastasis: The role of platelet-activating factor (PAF) and its receptor. *Cancer Metastasis Rev.* **2007**, *26*, 359–371. [CrossRef]
13. Chen, J.; Lan, T.; Zhang, W.; Dong, L.; Kang, N.; Zhang, S.; Fu, M.; Liu, B.; Liu, K.; Zhan, Q. Feed-Forward Reciprocal Activation of PAFR and STAT3 Regulates Epithelial-Mesenchymal Transition in Non-Small Cell Lung Cancer. *Cancer Res.* **2015**, *75*, 4198–4210. [CrossRef]
14. Gao, T.; Yu, Y.; Cong, Q.; Wang, Y.; Sun, M.; Yao, L.; Xu, C.; Jiang, W. Human mesenchymal stem cells in the tumour microenvironment promote ovarian cancer progression: The role of platelet-activating factor. *BMC Cancer* **2018**, *18*, 999. [CrossRef] [PubMed]
15. Aponte, M.; Jiang, W.; Lakkis, M.; Li, M.J.; Edwards, D.; Albitar, L.; Vitonis, A.; Mok, S.C.; Cramer, D.W.; Ye, B. Activation of platelet-activating factor receptor and pleiotropic effects on tyrosine phospho-EGFR/Src/FAK/paxillin in ovarian cancer. *Cancer Res.* **2008**, *68*, 5839–5848. [CrossRef]
16. Boccellino, M.; Biancone, L.; Cantaluppi, V.; Ye, R.D.; Camussi, G. Effect of platelet-activating factor receptor expression on CHO cell motility. *J. Cell. Physiol.* **2000**, *183*, 254–264. [CrossRef]
17. Holmes, C.E.; Levis, J.E.; Ornstein, D.L. Activated platelets enhance ovarian cancer cell invasion in a cellular model of metastasis. *Clin. Exp. Metastasis* **2009**, *26*, 653–661. [CrossRef]
18. Yu, Y.; Zhang, X.; Hong, S.; Zhang, M.; Cai, Q.; Jiang, W.; Xu, C. Epidermal growth factor induces platelet-activating factor production through receptors transactivation and cytosolic phospholipase A2 in ovarian cancer cells. *J. Ovarian Res.* **2014**, *7*, 39. [CrossRef]
19. Yu, Y.; Zhang, X.; Hong, S.; Zhang, M.; Cai, Q.; Jiang, W.; Xu, C. The expression of platelet-activating factor receptor modulates the cisplatin sensitivity of ovarian cancer cells: A novel target for combination therapy. *Br. J. Cancer* **2014**, *111*, 515–524. [CrossRef]
20. Stafforini, D.M. Biology of platelet-activating factor acetylhydrolase (PAF-AH, lipoprotein associated phospholipase A2). *Cardiovasc. Drugs Ther.* **2009**, *23*, 73–83. [CrossRef] [PubMed]
21. Arai, H. Platelet-activating factor acetylhydrolase. *Prostaglandins Other Lipid Mediat.* **2002**, *68–69*, 83–94. [CrossRef]
22. Bonin, F.; Ryan, S.D.; Migahed, L.; Mo, F.; Lallier, J.; Franks, D.J.; Arai, H.; Bennett, S.A. Anti-apoptotic actions of the platelet-activating factor acetylhydrolase I alpha2 catalytic subunit. *J. Biol. Chem.* **2004**, *279*, 52425–52436. [CrossRef] [PubMed]
23. Ma, C.; Guo, Y.; Zhang, Y.; Duo, A.; Jia, Y.; Liu, C.; Li, B. PAFAH1B2 is a HIF1a target gene and promotes metastasis in pancreatic cancer. *Biochem. Biophys. Res. Commun.* **2018**, *501*, 654–660. [CrossRef] [PubMed]
24. Xu, J.; Zang, Y.; Cao, S.; Lei, D.; Pan, X. Aberrant expression of PAFAH1B3 associates with poor prognosis and affects proliferation and aggressiveness in hypopharyngeal squamous cell carcinoma. *Onco Targets Ther.* **2019**, *12*, 2799–2808. [CrossRef]
25. Mulvihill, M.M.; Benjamin, D.I.; Ji, X.; Le Scolan, E.; Louie, S.M.; Shieh, A.; Green, M.; Narasimhalu, T.; Morris, P.; Luo, K.; et al. Metabolic profiling reveals PAFAH1B3 as a critical driver of breast cancer pathogenicity. *Chem. Biol.* **2014**, *21*, 831–840. [CrossRef] [PubMed]
26. Vainio, P.; Lehtinen, L.; Mirtti, T.; Hilvo, M.; Seppänen-Laakso, T.; Virtanen, J.; Sankila, A.; Nordling, S.; Lundin, J.; Rannikko, A.; et al. Phospholipase PLA2G7, associated with aggressive prostate cancer, promotes prostate cancer cell migration and invasion and is inhibited by statins. *Oncotarget* **2011**, *2*, 1176–1190. [CrossRef]
27. Lehtinen, L.; Vainio, P.; Wikman, H.; Huhtala, H.; Mueller, V.; Kallioniemi, A.; Pantel, K.; Kronqvist, P.; Kallioniemi, O.; Carpèn, O.; et al. PLA2G7 associates with hormone receptor negativity in clinical breast cancer samples and regulates epithelial-mesenchymal transition in cultured breast cancer cells. *J. Pathol. Clin. Res.* **2017**, *3*, 123–138. [CrossRef]
28. Biancone, L.; Cantaluppi, V.; Del Sorbo, L.; Russo, S.; Tjoelker, L.W.; Camussi, G. Platelet-activating factor inactivation by local expression of platelet-activating factor acetyl-hydrolase modifies tumor vascularization and growth. *Clin. Cancer Res.* **2003**, *9*, 4214–4220.
29. Arend, R.C.; Londono-Joshi, A.I.; Straughn, J.M., Jr.; Buchsbaum, D.J. The Wnt/beta-catenin pathway in ovarian cancer: A review. *Gynecol. Oncol.* **2013**, *131*, 772–779. [CrossRef]
30. Nagaraj, A.B.; Joseph, P.; Kovalenko, O.; Singh, S.; Armstrong, A.; Redline, R.; Resnick, K.; Zanotti, K.; Waggoner, S.; DiFeo, A. Critical role of Wnt/beta-catenin signaling in driving epithelial ovarian cancer platinum resistance. *Oncotarget* **2015**, *6*, 23720–23734. [CrossRef]
31. Yamamoto, T.M.; McMellen, A.; Watson, Z.L.; Aguilera, J.; Ferguson, R.; Nurmemmedov, E.; Thakar, T.; Moldovan, G.L.; Kim, H.; Cittelly, D.M.; et al. Activation of Wnt signaling promotes olaparib resistant ovarian cancer. *Mol. Carcinog.* **2019**, *58*, 1770–1782. [CrossRef]

32. Moon, R.T.; Kohn, A.D.; De Ferrari, G.V.; Kaykas, A. WNT and beta-catenin signalling: Diseases and therapies. *Nat. Rev. Genet.* **2004**, *5*, 691–701. [CrossRef] [PubMed]
33. Clevers, H. Wnt/beta-catenin signaling in development and disease. *Cell* **2006**, *127*, 469–480. [CrossRef]
34. Taketo, M.M. Shutting down Wnt signal-activated cancer. *Nat. Genet.* **2004**, *36*, 320–322. [CrossRef]
35. Giles, R.H.; van Es, J.H.; Clevers, H. Caught up in a Wnt storm: Wnt signaling in cancer. *Biochim. Biophys. Acta* **2003**, *1653*, 1–24. [CrossRef]
36. Teeuwssen, M.; Fodde, R. Wnt Signaling in Ovarian Cancer Stemness, EMT, and Therapy Resistance. *J. Clin. Med.* **2019**, *8*, 1658. [CrossRef]
37. Marchion, D.C.; Xiong, Y.; Chon, H.S.; Al Sawah, E.; Bou Zgheib, N.; Ramirez, I.J.; Abbasi, F.; Stickles, X.B.; Judson, P.L.; Hakam, A.; et al. Gene expression data reveal common pathways that characterize the unifocal nature of ovarian cancer. *Am. J. Obstet. Gynecol.* **2013**, *209*, 576.e1–576.e16. [CrossRef] [PubMed]
38. Reinartz, S.; Finkernagel, F.; Adhikary, T.; Rohnalter, V.; Schumann, T.; Schober, Y.; Nockher, W.A.; Nist, A.; Stiewe, T.; Jansen, J.M.; et al. A transcriptome-based global map of signaling pathways in the ovarian cancer microenvironment associated with clinical outcome. *Genome Biol.* **2016**, *17*, 108. [CrossRef]
39. Domoto, T.; Pyko, I.V.; Furuta, T.; Miyashita, K.; Uehara, M.; Shimasaki, T.; Nakada, M.; Minamoto, T. Glycogen synthase kinase-3beta is a pivotal mediator of cancer invasion and resistance to therapy. *Cancer Sci.* **2016**, *107*, 1363–1372. [CrossRef]
40. Wu, Z.Q.; Li, X.Y.; Hu, C.Y.; Ford, M.; Kleer, C.G.; Weiss, S.J. Canonical Wnt signaling regulates Slug activity and links epithelial-mesenchymal transition with epigenetic Breast Cancer 1, Early Onset (BRCA1) repression. *Proc. Natl. Acad. Sci. USA* **2012**, *109*, 16654–16659. [CrossRef] [PubMed]
41. Xu, C.; Reichert, E.C.; Nakano, T.; Lohse, M.; Gardner, A.A.; Revelo, M.P.; Topham, M.K.; Stafforini, D.M. Deficiency of phospholipase A2 group 7 decreases intestinal polyposis and colon tumorigenesis in Apc(Min/+) mice. *Cancer Res.* **2013**, *73*, 2806–2816. [CrossRef]
42. Scholz, C.; Heublein, S.; Lenhard, M.; Friese, K.; Mayr, D.; Jeschke, U. Glycodelin A is a prognostic marker to predict poor outcome in advanced stage ovarian cancer patients. *BMC Res. Notes* **2012**, *5*, 551. [CrossRef]
43. Remmele, W.; Stegner, H.E. Recommendation for uniform definition of an immunoreactive score (IRS) for immunohistochemical estrogen receptor detection (ER-ICA) in breast cancer tissue. *Pathologe* **1987**, *8*, 138–140. [PubMed]
44. Whitney, J. Testing for differences with the nonparametric Mann-Whitney U test. *J. Wound Ostomy Cont. Nurs.* **1997**, *24*, 12. [CrossRef]
45. Spearman, C. The proof and measurement of association between two things; By, C. Spearman, 1904. *Am. J. Psychol.* **1987**, *100*, 441–471. [CrossRef]
46. Kaplan, E.L.; Meier, P. Nonparametric Estimation from Incomplete Observations. *J. Am. Stat. Assoc.* **1958**, *53*, 457–481. [CrossRef]
47. Youden, W.J. Index for rating diagnostic tests. *Cancer* **1950**, *3*, 32–35. [CrossRef]
48. Perkins, N.J.; Schisterman, E.F. The Inconsistency of "Optimal" Cut-points Using Two ROC Based Criteria. *Am. J. Epidemiol.* **2006**, *163*, 670–675. [CrossRef]
49. Fluss, R.; Faraggi, D.; Reiser, B. Estimation of the Youden Index and its Associated Cutoff Point. *Biom. J.* **2005**, *47*, 458–472. [CrossRef]
50. Cox, D.R. Regression Models and Life-Tables. *J. R. Stat. Soc. Ser. B* **1972**, *34*, 187–220. [CrossRef]
51. Livak, K.J.; Schmittgen, T.D. Analysis of relative gene expression data using real-time quantitative PCR and the 2(-Delta Delta C(T)) Method. *Methods* **2001**, *25*, 402–408. [CrossRef] [PubMed]
52. Tremmel, E.; Hofmann, S.; Kuhn, C.; Heidegger, H.; Heublein, S.; Hermelink, K.; Wuerstlein, R.; Harbeck, N.; Mayr, D.; Mahner, S.; et al. Thyronamine regulation of TAAR1 expression in breast cancer cells and investigation of its influence on viability and migration. *Breast Cancer* **2019**, *11*, 87–97. [CrossRef] [PubMed]
53. Nandy, D.; Asmann, Y.W.; Mukhopadhyay, D.; Basu, A. Role of AKT-glycogen synthase kinase axis in monocyte activation in human beings with and without type 2 diabetes. *J. Cell. Mol. Med.* **2010**, *14*, 1396–1407. [CrossRef] [PubMed]
54. Daniels, D.L.; Weis, W.I. Beta-catenin directly displaces Groucho/TLE repressors from Tcf/Lef in Wnt-mediated transcription activation. *Nat. Struct. Mol. Biol.* **2005**, *12*, 364–371. [CrossRef]
55. Furihata, T.; Kawamata, H.; Kubota, K.; Fujimori, T. Evaluation of the malignant potential of aberrant crypt foci by immunohistochemical staining for beta-catenin in inflammation-induced rat colon carcinogenesis. *Int. J. Mol. Med.* **2002**, *9*, 353–358.
56. Boccellino, M.; Camussi, G.; Giovane, A.; Ferro, L.; Calderaro, V.; Balestrieri, C.; Quagliuolo, L. Platelet-activating factor regulates cadherin-catenin adhesion system expression and beta-catenin phosphorylation during Kaposi's sarcoma cell motility. *Am. J. Pathol.* **2005**, *166*, 1515–1522. [CrossRef]
57. Tjoelker, L.W.; Wilder, C.; Eberhardt, C.; Stafforinit, D.M.; Dietsch, G.; Schimpf, B.; Hooper, S.; Le Trong, H.; Cousens, L.S.; Zimmerman, G.A.; et al. Anti-inflammatory properties of a platelet-activating factor acetylhydrolase. *Nature* **1995**, *374*, 549–553. [CrossRef]
58. Yu, Y.; Zhang, M.; Zhang, X.; Cai, Q.; Hong, S.; Jiang, W.; Xu, C. Synergistic effects of combined platelet-activating factor receptor and epidermal growth factor receptor targeting in ovarian cancer cells. *J. Hematol. Oncol.* **2014**, *7*, 39. [CrossRef]
59. Rozengurt, E. Mitogenic signaling pathways induced by G protein-coupled receptors. *J. Cell. Physiol.* **2007**, *213*, 589–602. [CrossRef]

60. Penna, C.; Mognetti, B.; Tullio, F.; Gattullo, D.; Mancardi, D.; Moro, F.; Pagliaro, P.; Alloatti, G. Post-ischaemic activation of kinases in the pre-conditioning-like cardioprotective effect of the platelet-activating factor. *Acta Physiol.* **2009**, *197*, 175–185. [CrossRef]
61. Zhang, L.; Wang, D.; Jiang, W.; Edwards, D.; Qiu, W.; Barroilhet, L.M.; Rho, J.H.; Jin, L.; Seethappan, V.; Vitonis, A.; et al. Activated networking of platelet activating factor receptor and FAK/STAT1 induces malignant potential in BRCA1-mutant at-risk ovarian epithelium. *Reprod. Biol. Endocrinol.* **2010**, *8*, 74. [CrossRef] [PubMed]
62. Livnat, I.; Finkelshtein, D.; Ghosh, I.; Arai, H.; Reiner, O. PAF-AH Catalytic Subunits Modulate the Wnt Pathway in Developing GABAergic Neurons. *Front. Cell. Neurosci.* **2010**, *4*, 4. [CrossRef] [PubMed]
63. Axelrad, T.W.; Deo, D.D.; Ottino, P.; Van Kirk, J.; Bazan, N.G.; Bazan, H.E.; Hunt, J.D. Platelet-activating factor (PAF) induces activation of matrix metalloproteinase 2 activity and vascular endothelial cell invasion and migration. *FASEB J.* **2004**, *18*, 568–570. [CrossRef] [PubMed]

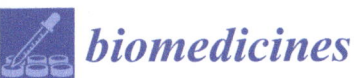

Article

Synergistic AHR Binding Pathway with EMT Effects on Serous Ovarian Tumors Recognized by Multidisciplinary Integrated Analysis

Kuo-Min Su [1,2], Hong-Wei Gao [3], Chia-Ming Chang [4,5], Kai-Hsi Lu [6], Mu-Hsien Yu [1,2], Yi-Hsin Lin [2], Li-Chun Liu [2,7], Chia-Ching Chang [2], Yao-Feng Li [3,*,†] and Cheng-Chang Chang [1,2,*,†]

[1] Graduate Institute of Medical Sciences, National Defense Medical Center, Taipei 114, Taiwan; aeolusfield@hotmail.com (K.-M.S.); hsienhui@ms15.hinet.net (M.-H.Y.)
[2] Department of Obstetrics and Gynecology, Tri-Service General Hospital, National Defense Medical Center, Taipei 114, Taiwan; m860371@gmail.com (Y.-H.L.); lvita.tw@gmail.com (L.-C.L.); t791212@gmail.com (C.-C.C.)
[3] Department of Pathology, Tri-Service General Hospital, National Defense Medical Center, Taipei 114, Taiwan; doc31796@gmail.com
[4] School of Medicine, National Yang Ming Chiao Tung University, Taipei 112, Taiwan; cm_chang@vghtpe.gov.tw
[5] Department of Obstetrics and Gynecology, Taipei Veterans General Hospital, Taipei 112, Taiwan
[6] Department of Medical Research and Education, Cheng-Hsin General Hospital, Taipei 112, Taiwan; lionel.lu@gmail.com
[7] Division of Obstetrics and Gynecology, Tri-Service General Hospital Songshan Branch, National Defense Medical Center, Taipei 105, Taiwan
* Correspondence: liyaofeng1109@gmail.com (Y.-F.L.); obsgynchang@gmail.com (C.-C.C.); Tel.: +886-2-8792-3311 (ext. 16734) (Y.-F.L.); +886-2-8792-7205 (C.-C.C.)
† Equal contribution.

Citation: Su, K.-M.; Gao, H.-W.; Chang, C.-M.; Lu, K.-H.; Yu, M.-H.; Lin, Y.-H.; Liu, L.-C.; Chang, C.-C.; Li, Y.-F.; Chang, C.-C. Synergistic AHR Binding Pathway with EMT Effects on Serous Ovarian Tumors Recognized by Multidisciplinary Integrated Analysis. *Biomedicines* **2021**, *9*, 866. https://doi.org/10.3390/biomedicines9080866

Academic Editor: Naomi Nakayama

Received: 5 June 2021
Accepted: 20 July 2021
Published: 22 July 2021

Publisher's Note: MDPI stays neutral with regard to jurisdictional claims in published maps and institutional affiliations.

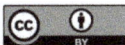

Copyright: © 2021 by the authors. Licensee MDPI, Basel, Switzerland. This article is an open access article distributed under the terms and conditions of the Creative Commons Attribution (CC BY) license (https://creativecommons.org/licenses/by/4.0/).

Abstract: Epithelial ovarian cancers (EOCs) are fatal and obstinate among gynecological malignancies in advanced stage or relapsed status, with serous carcinomas accounting for the vast majority. Unlike EOCs, borderline ovarian tumors (BOTs), including serous BOTs, maintain a semimalignant appearance. Using gene ontology (GO)-based integrative analysis, we analyzed gene set databases of serous BOTs and serous ovarian carcinomas for dysregulated GO terms and pathways and identified multiple differentially expressed genes (DEGs) in various aspects. The *SRC* (SRC proto-oncogene, non-receptor tyrosine kinase) gene and dysfunctional aryl hydrocarbon receptor (AHR) binding pathway consistently influenced progression-free survival and overall survival, and immunohistochemical staining revealed elevated expression of related biomarkers (SRC, ARNT, and TBP) in serous BOT and ovarian carcinoma samples. Epithelial–mesenchymal transition (EMT) is important during tumorigenesis, and we confirmed the *SNAI2* (Snail family transcriptional repressor 2, *SLUG*) gene showing significantly high performance by immunohistochemistry. During serous ovarian tumor formation, activated AHR in the cytoplasm could cooperate with SRC, enter cell nuclei, bind to AHR nuclear translocator (ARNT) together with TATA-Box Binding Protein (TBP), and act on DNA to initiate AHR-responsive genes to cause tumor or cancer initiation. Additionally, SNAI2 in the tumor microenvironment can facilitate EMT accompanied by tumorigenesis. Although it has not been possible to classify serous BOTs and serous ovarian carcinomas as the same EOC subtype, the key determinants of relevant DEGs (*SRC*, *ARNT*, *TBP*, and *SNAI2*) found here had a crucial role in the pathogenetic mechanism of both tumor types, implying gradual evolutionary tendencies from serous BOTs to ovarian carcinomas. In the future, targeted therapy could focus on these revealed targets together with precise detection to improve therapeutic effects and patient survival rates.

Keywords: gene ontology; epithelial ovarian cancers; borderline ovarian tumors; differentially expressed genes; aryl hydrocarbon receptor; epithelial–mesenchymal transition; integrative analysis

1. Introduction

Ovarian tumors occupy a certain place among gynecological diseases and most cases are benign in clinical and pathological features such as follicular cysts, corpus luteum cysts, serous or mucinous cystadenomas, endometriomas, and teratomas [1,2]. Comparatively, ovarian cancer is the most lethal gynecological malignancy worldwide although the proportion is relatively low [3]. Epithelial ovarian cancers (EOCs) are the leading cause of death among patients with gynecologic cancers accounting for the vast majority of all ovarian cancers [4,5]; furthermore, serous carcinoma (SC) accounts for the most common of EOCs, with a poor prognosis and a five-year survival rate of only 25% with metastases [6,7]. SC is less likely to be found in the early stages (International Federation of Gynecology and Obstetrics (FIGO) stages I and II), which have higher survival rates because they are easier to treat, whereas patients at advanced stages (FIGO stages III and IV) have poor prognosis and high recurrence rates even after complete debulking surgery combined with chemotherapy (carboplatin and paclitaxel) due to resistance to chemotherapy [6,8,9].

Borderline ovarian tumors (BOTs), a specific subtype of EOCs, consist of disparate groups of neoplasms based on histopathological features, molecular characteristics, and clinical behaviors and BOTs can generally be classified into serous, mucinous, and other subtypes according to clinical and histopathological features [10,11]. Besides, BOTs account for approximately 10–15% of EOCs and usually occur in younger women, resulting in an excellent prognosis [12]. Compared with ovarian cancer patients, who almost always require chemotherapy after a debulking operation, patients with BOTs usually have better prognoses after adequate surgery with an extremely low probability of recurrence or metastasis [13,14]. Serous BOTs, comprising approximately 65% of BOTs, occur mostly in North America, the Middle East, and most of Europe [15]. To date, surgery is still the ideal method to treat BOTs, while adjuvant chemotherapy and radiotherapy are not usually considered as standard therapies [14,16]. Recent studies have inferred several assumptions, including the incessant ovulation, gonadotropin, hormonal, and inflammation hypotheses, to explain the tumorigenesis of serous BOTs [17–19]. Serous BOTs are characterized by mutations in the *KRAS*, *BRAF*, and *ERBB2* genes and overexpression of the *p53* and *Claudin-1* genes; furthermore, the mitogen-activated protein kinase (MAPK)/extracellular signal-regulated kinase (ERK) pathway, PI3K/AKT/mTOR pathway, Hedgehog pathway, and angiogenesis pathway are frequently activated in serous BOTs [13,14,20–25].

As a complex disease, several genetic and environmental factors contribute to SC development with a complicated carcinogenesis pathway, and the carcinogenesis of SC evolves through several aberrant functions, which fluctuate with disease progression based on findings through the widely utilized FIGO system [13,26–32]. It is widely known that most serous ovarian carcinomas are associated with *TP53* mutations [30,33–36]; about half of them have undergone abnormal DNA repair processes through homologous recombination due to epigenetic or genetic alterations of *BRCA1*, *BRCA2*, or other DNA repair molecules [37,38]; and some show gene mutations, such as in BRAF and KRAS [20]. In addition to debulking surgery and subsequent adjuvant chemotherapy, targeted therapy and systemic immunotherapy can also be utilized to enhance the therapeutic effects. Poly-adenosine diphosphate (ADP) ribose polymerase inhibitors (PARPis), the first approved cancer drugs, were widely used targeted therapies for BRCA1/2-mutated breast and ovarian cancers, and they specifically target DNA damage and repair responses, especially for patients with homologous recombination deficiencies, resulting in increased survival [39–41]. However, resistance to PARPi has recently become an emerging issue and breast-related cancer antigens (BRCA) and homologous recombination deficiency (HRD) status can be considered novel predictive biomarkers of response [42–45]. Therefore, identifying potential crucial biomarkers for monitoring drug resistance and formulating new drug combination strategies are efficacious methods to resolve PARPi resistance along with precision medicine [46,47].

Furthermore, it is well known that serous ovarian carcinomas have a poor clinical prognosis because they are usually diagnosed too late, while advanced stages usually result in frequent emergence of chemoresistance [4,5,8,48,49]. Recent growing evidence suggests that epithelial–mesenchymal transition (EMT) may contribute to tumor invasion and metastasis and promote chemotherapeutic resistance, especially to cisplatin, by converting the motionless epithelial cells into mobile mesenchymal cells, escaping cell adhesion, and altering the cellular extracellular matrix [50–52]. EMT is a reversible process in which many crucial components, such as E-cadherin, EpCAM, vimentin, fibronectin, neural cadherin, matrix metalloproteinases, various integrins, and different cytokeratins, are regulated by a complex functional network of transcription factors, including the zinc-finger E-box-binding homeobox factors (Zeb1 and Zeb2), Snail (SNAI1), Slug (SNAI2), and the basic helix–loop–helix factors (Twist1 and Twist2) [53–55]. Loss of breast cancer type 1 susceptibility protein (BRCA1), a tumor suppressor that plays a role in mending double-stranded DNA breaks, is also associated with EMT and tumor initiation [50,56]. The expression of EMT signaling pathways has been correlated with poor prognosis in various epithelial cancers, including breast, pancreas, prostate, and ovarian cancer, and the role of EMT in ovarian cancer progression and therapy resistance is highlighted in current studies [57]; however, the role of EMT plasticity in serous ovarian tumors has not been comprehensively investigated.

As mentioned above, although both are named the "serous" subtype in terms of classification, serous BOTs and serous ovarian carcinomas still have decisive differences in genetic mechanisms, pathological characteristics, and clinical manifestations [13,32]. Various functions can be investigated using differentially expressed genes (DEGs) detected by microarrays. In contrast to DEGs, we established a gene set regularity (GSR) model, which reconstructed the functionomes, that is, the GSR indices of the global functions, and then investigated the dysregulated functions and dysfunctional pathways involved in the complex disease. Constructing a functionome can provide information about the dysregulated functionomes accompanied with dysfunctional pathways of complicated illness and we had conducted several gene set-based analyses by integrating microarray gene expression profiles downloaded from publicly available databases, which revealed that comprehensive methods based on functionome defined by gene ontology (GO) are useful for successfully conducting significant research on BOTs and ovarian carcinomas of different stages and subtypes [58–64]. Previously, individual studies have focused on gene set analysis of serous ovarian carcinomas and serous BOTs to uncover pathogenic mechanisms during tumorigenesis. However, there is no integrated analysis to compare and discover the genomic functionome of serous BOTs and serous ovarian carcinomas. Therefore, we first utilized GO-based integrative approaches to explore expression profile datasets of serous ovarian tumors, including serous BOTs and all stages of serous ovarian carcinomas, to identify common and meaningful dysregulated functions and dysfunctional pathways between these two groups. We then selected the featured DEGs by checking the significant biomarkers related to EMT with cross comparison. In this experiment, we aimed to excavate newly discovered pathogenetic mechanisms based on previous studies that differ from previous theories and hoped to take advantage of these new findings applied in medical detection with targeted therapy and effective avoidance of recurrence for better prognosis of serous ovarian tumors and patient survival.

2. Materials and Methods

2.1. Workflow for the Integrative Analytic Model

The workflow for this study is shown in the flowchart in Figure 1, and detailed information is explained below. First, we converted the gene expression profile of the extracted gene elements downloaded from the Gene Expression Omnibus (GEO) database with selection criteria for serous ovarian tumors and normal controls to ordered data and then transformed them into 10,192 quantified GO terms according to the sequential expression from the gene elements in each gene set. This process produced functionomes consisting of 10,192 GSR indices, which defined the relatively comprehensive biological and molecular functions to explore serous ovarian tumors, including serous BOTs and all stages of serous ovarian carcinomas. Next, we individually calculated the quantified functions and functional regularity patterns among serous ovarian tumors and 136 normal ovarian controls with GSR indices and established the GSR model for the functionome pattern. Then, we investigated the whole informativeness of genomic functionomes consisting of the GSR indices and constructed a functionome-based training model of classification and prediction using the support vector machine (SVM), a set of supervised mathematical commands from machine learning. The variation in the GSR indices between each serous ovarian tumor group and normal control group revealed that the biomolecular functions among serous ovarian tumors were significantly extensively dysregulated in contrast to the normal control group. Finally, we conducted whole-genome integrative analysis to identify meaningful dysfunctional pathways together with significant biomarkers of EMT involved in the progression of serous ovarian carcinomas to determine crucial DEGs that may be essential parts of the pathogenetic mechanisms for serous ovarian tumors by elucidating dysregulated functionomes using microarray analysis of gene expression profiles. The key biological functions and genes involved in the pathogenesis of serous BOTs and all stages of serous ovarian carcinomas were determined by identifying genome-wide and GO-defined functions and DEGs.

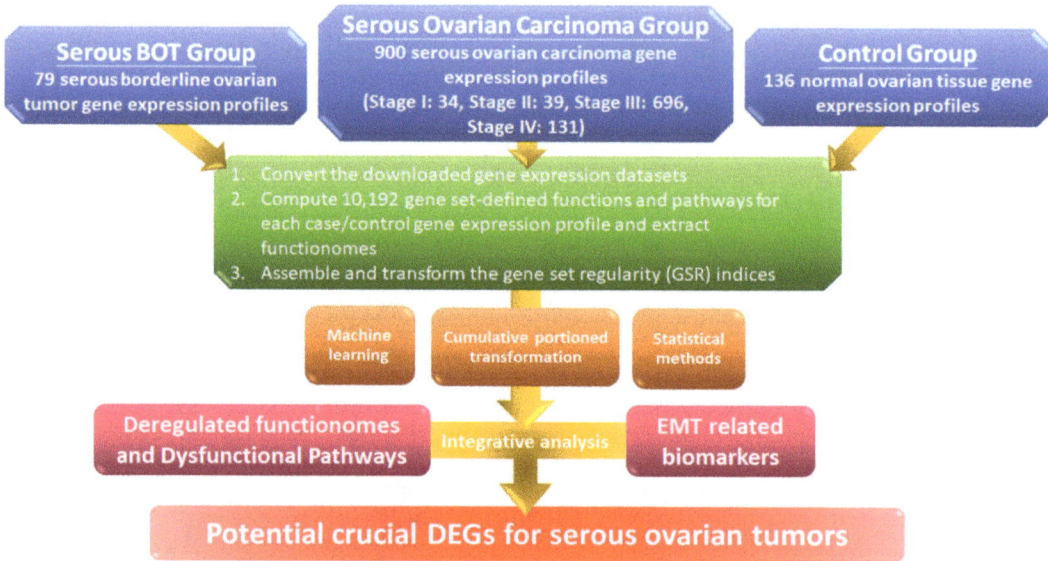

Figure 1. Workflow of this study. The DNA microarray gene expression profiles of 79 serous borderline tumor (BOT) samples, 900 serous ovarian carcinoma specimens including all stages, and 136 normal ovarian controls were downloaded from publicly available databases with gene set regularity (GSR) indices calculated by the Gene Ontology (GO) gene set. Functionomes consisting of 10,192 GO gene sets established from the polygenic models and cumulative portion transformations with machine learning and statistical methods were utilized to identify the functionome-based patterns to investigate dysregulated GO terms, dysfunctional pathways, and biomarkers of epithelial–mesenchymal transition (EMT) together with integrative analysis and to discover potential crucial differentially expressed genes (DEGs).

2.2. Microarray Dataset Collections and the Selection Criteria

The selection criteria for the microarray gene expression datasets from the GEO database were as follows: (1) samples of normal controls and serous ovarian tumor samples, including serous BOTs and serous ovarian carcinomas, should all originate from ovarian tissues of homo sapiens; (2) datasets should offer sufficient information about the diagnosis and clinical histopathological subtypes of serous ovarian tumors and normal controls should consist of tissues or cell cultures from normal ovarian surface epithelium (NOSE) judged by histology; and (3) any extracted sample that did not meet the above-mentioned conditions was discarded and any gene expression profile in a dataset was abandoned if it contained missing data.

2.3. Computing the GSR Indices and Rebuilding the Functionomes

GSR indices were calculated and extracted from the gene expression datasets by modifying the differential rank retention (DIRAC) algorithm [65] and used to measure sequential changes among the gene elements in the gene set datasets of the gene expression profiles of serous BOTs, all stages of serous ovarian carcinomas, and the most common gene expression ordering from the normal control samples. The details and calculation process of the GSR model were described in our previous studied papers [58–64]. The microarray-based gene expression profiles from serous ovarian tumors and normal ovarian samples obtained from the GEO database were produced using the corresponding gene expression levels constructed according to the genetic elements in the GO-based functionome, which were then con-verted into ordered data based on each expression level. By definition, the GSR index refers to the ratio of the gene expression sequence in a gene set between the case group and the most common gene expression sequence from the normal ovarian tissue samples, ranging from 0 to 1, where 0 represents the most dysregulated state of a gene set with oppositely ordered gene set regularities between the serous ovarian tumors and the most common gene expression orderings in the normal controls, whereas 1 indicates that the genomic regularities in a gene set remain the same between the groups of serous ovarian tumors and the normal ovarian group. All GSR indices were measured using the R programming language. A functionome was defined as the complete gene set of biological functions, and we annotated and defined the human functionome using the 10,192 GO gene set-defined functions because the definitions for comprehensive biological functions are not yet available. Therefore, the functionomes used in this study were defined as a combination of 10,192 GSR indices for all samples.

2.4. Statistical Analysis

The Mann–Whitney U-test was used to test the differences in serous BOTs, all stages of serous ovarian carcinomas, and controls, and then corrected by multiple hypotheses using the false discovery rate (Benjamini–Hochberg procedure) [66]. The p-value was set at $p < 0.05$.

2.5. Classification and Prediction by Machine Learning with Set Analysis

An R package with the function "kvsm" provided by the "kernlab" (version 0.9–27; Comprehensive R Archive Network) and kernel-based machine learning methods were used to classify and predict patterns of GSR indices. K-fold cross-validation was used to measure the accuracy of classification and prediction of SVM. The results of ten repetitive predictions were used to evaluate the performance of the binary classification. The R package "pROC" was used to calculate the area under the curve (AUC) [67]. The R package "data.table" (version 1.12.8; Comprehensive R Archive Network) was used to display all possible logical relationships among the dysregulated gene sets of serous ovarian tumors clearly and sequentially in the tables.

2.6. Verification of Clinical Samples Using Immunohistochemical (IHC) Staining Method

Fifty clinical samples of serous ovarian tumors were collected (serous BOTs, n = 9; serous ovarian carcinomas, n = 41, including 8 stage I, 2 stage II, 23 stage III, and 8 stage IV cases). All serous ovarian tumor tissues were collected from female patients undergoing surgical treatments after signing an informed consent agreement. All patients were diagnosed and treated according to the standard therapeutic guidelines, and all tissues of patients were kept in the biobank at Tri-Service General Hospital, National Defense Medical Center, Taipei, Taiwan. The Institutional Review Board of the General Hospital of the National Defense Medical Center approved the study (2-107-05-043, approved on

October 26, 2018, and 2-108-05-091, approved on 20 May 2019). Informed consent was obtained from all patients and control subjects. All clinical tissue samples were confirmed via quantitative histopathological inspections and diagnosed by professional pathologists, and IHC staining results were scored as follows: the intensity (I) was multiplied by the percentage of positive cells (P) of all biomarkers utilized in this study (the formula is shown as IHC score [Q] = I × P; maximum = 300) [68,69].

3. Results

3.1. Microarrays of Sample Groups for Gene Expression Profiles and Definition for Gene Set Analysis

We performed a comprehensive bioinformatics method based on GO to explore and analyze all relational disordered functions of serous ovarian tumors, including serous BOTs and all stages of serous ovarian carcinomas [70]. The gene expression profiles of DNA microarray of serous ovarian tumors and normal controls were downloaded from the GEO repository at the National Center for Biotechnology Information (NCBI) archives. The whole-sample data were obtained from 30 datasets containing eight heterogeneous DNA microarray platforms without any missing data. There were 79 serous BOT samples and 900 serous ovarian carcinoma samples based on histopathological classification, including 34 stage I, 39 stage II, 696 stage III, and 131 stage IV cases among the 900 serous ovarian carcinoma samples according to the FIGO staging system (Table 1). In addition, 136 normal ovarian samples were collected as a control group for comparison. Table S1 provides detailed information about all obtained samples and controls. In total, 10,192 GO-based definitions for annotating all gene set-defined functionomes were also downloaded from the Molecular Signatures Database (MSigDB), the version "c5.all.v7.1.symbols.gmt" [71].

Table 1. Number of samples and statistics for the groups of serous BOTs and all FIGO stages of serous ovarian carcinomas.

Groups	Sample	Control	Total	Sample Mean (SD [1])	Control Mean (SD [1])	p-Value
Serous BOT [2]	79	136	215	0.7036 (0.1772)	0.7732 (0.1646)	<0.05
Serous ovarian carcinoma stage I	34	136	170	0.7298 (0.1672)	0.7715 (0.1551)	<0.05
Serous ovarian carcinoma stage II	39	136	175	0.6976 (0.1838)	0.7713 (0.1552)	<0.05
Serous ovarian carcinoma stage III	696	136	832	0.6355 (0.1940)	0.7705 (0.1606)	<0.05
Serous ovarian carcinoma stage IV	131	136	267	0.6147 (0.1969)	0.7706 (0.1565)	<0.05

[1] SD, standard deviation; [2] BOT, borderline ovarian tumor.

3.2. Histograms of GSR Indices of Functionomes among Each Group with Diverse Differences

According to the divergence in ranking within a gene set between the case and control groups characterized by GO terms, GSR indices were individually calculated by quantifying alterations in the ranking of gene expression in a gene set or functionome. As displayed in Figure 2, all averages of GSR indices for the functions of serous ovarian tumors were computed and then rectified by the mean values of the control group. Divergences in GSR indices between serous ovarian tumor and normal control groups were statistically significant ($p < 0.05$). We found that in the serous ovarian carcinoma group, as the FIGO stage progressed from early stages (I and II, yellow-green grids in Figure 2B,C, respectively) to advanced stages (III and IV, yellow-green grids in Figure 2D,E, respectively), the differences from corresponding normal controls (blue grids in Figure 2) became increasingly distinct. Furthermore, differences in mutations among serous BOTs (yellow-green grids in Figure 2A) and normal controls seemed to be more irregular than those at the early stages (FIGO stage I and II) but less aberrant than at the late stages (FIGO stage III and IV) of serous ovarian carcinomas. The modulation of dysregulated functionomes was quantified using the means of the total GSR indices of each functionome of serous ovarian tumors and control groups with adjustments compared to the control group. The average corrected GSR indices for serous BOTs and serous ovarian carcinomas from stage I to IV were 0.7036, 0.7230, 0.6976, 0.6355, and 0.6147, respectively.

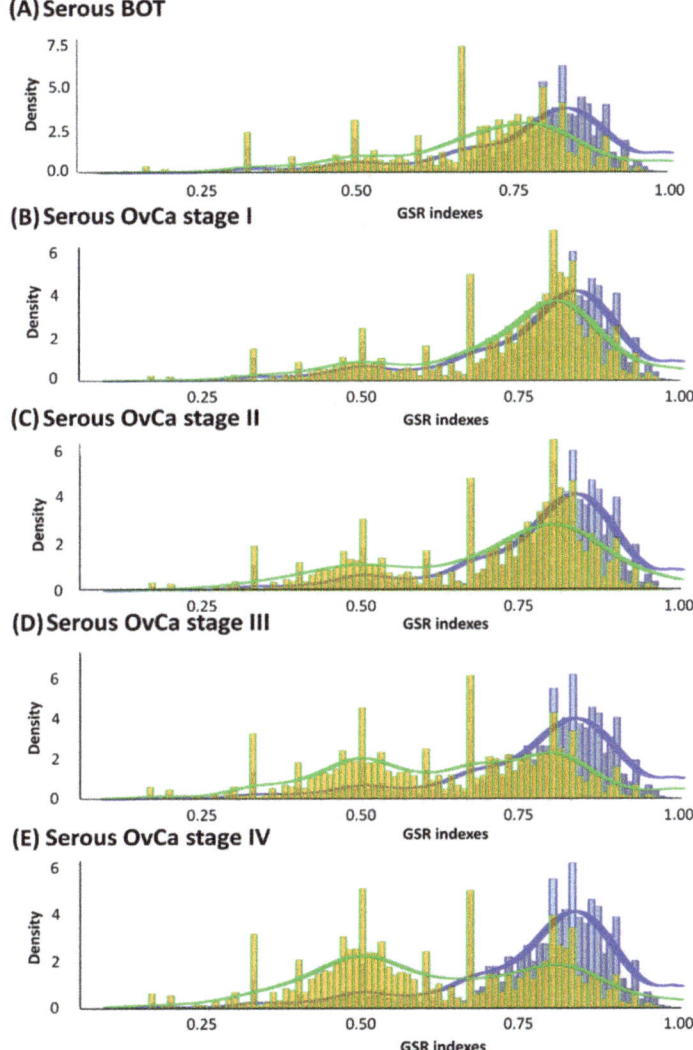

Figure 2. Histograms of global GSR indices of functionomes for serous BOTs, all stages of serous ovarian carcinomas (yellow green), and control groups (blue). Different distributions of the functionomes among five case sample groups and control groups are shown with statistical significance ($p < 0.05$). The normal control group (blue, right) was used as the control and is the same in all panels. Peaks in distribution were observed (yellow green), indicating dysregulated biomolecular functionomes of serous BOTs and all stages of serous ovarian carcinomas. (**A–E**) Corrected GSR indices of serous BOTs: 0.7036 (**A**); FIGO stage I: 0.7230 (**B**); FIGO stage II: 0.6976 (**C**); FIGO stage III: 0.6355 (**D**); and FIGO stage IV: 0.6147 (**E**).

3.3. Regularity Patterns of Functionomes Classified and Predicted by Supervised Machine Learning with High Sensitivity, Specificity, and Accuracy

As displayed in Figure 2, the regularity patterns of functionomes among the five serous ovarian tumor groups were compared with those of the normal control group, and the functional regularity patterns of the five case groups (serous BOTs and all four stages of serous ovarian carcinomas) showed significant divergence. We then identified, classified, and predicted different functions of various gene sets defined by GO using SVM, a powerful technological algorithm for supervised machine learning. The accumulated data of assessed performances were operated with ten consecutive binary classifications and checked with forecasting approaches by five-fold cross-validation; all the calculated results with high sensitivity, specificity, and accuracy are listed in Table S2. The sensitivity, specificity, and accuracy of binary classification for gene set databases among serous ovarian tumor and control groups were approximately 95.13–100.00%, 99.85–100.00%, and 98.97–100.00%, respectively. The AUCs for the performance of each case group ranged from 0.9771 to 1.0000. The evaluated performances by binary classifications between serous ovarian carcinoma, FIGO stage IV, and normal control groups had the best overall effects. The results revealed that the quantified functional regularity patterns with the GSR indices transformed from the DNA microarray gene expression profiles could offer sufficient and credible information to the SVM for accurate identification and classification. These results also indicated that all the functional regularity patterns of serous ovarian tumors were demarcated and suitable for integrated genetic and molecular classifications interpreted in this study.

3.4. The Most Dysregulated and Common GO Terms among Serous Ovarian Tumors

We used the cluster weight index (CWI) with SVM to uncover 655, 662, 643, 828, and 841 GO terms among serous BOTs and serous ovarian carcinomas at FIGO stages I–IV, respectively. CWI, a calculated exponent based on the p-values with statistical significance, is defined as the weighted ratio of the single weight of each clustered GO term divided by the total weights of the whole clusters, and it is used to measure the representative weight and express the mutual correlation for every cluster in the GO trees. All identified GO terms were meaningful and could represent dysregulated functionomes in each group of serous ovarian tumors. We used the calculated CWI to quantify and judge the value of each dysregulated GO cluster among the pathogenetic mechanisms of serous ovarian tumors. We ranked the 50 most dysregulated GO terms judged by CWI for serous ovarian tumors, as shown in Table 2. The first dysregulated GO terms for each group were "regulation of immune system process (GO:0002682)" for serous BOT; "transporter activity (GO:0005215)" for serous ovarian carcinoma, FIGO stage I; "small molecule metabolic process (GO:0044281)" for serous ovarian carcinoma, FIGO stage II; "regulation of immune system process (GO:0002682)" for serous ovarian carcinoma, FIGO stage III; and "small molecule metabolic process (GO:0044281)" for serous ovarian carcinoma, FIGO stage IV. Details on dysregulated GO terms for all disease groups of serous ovarian tumors are listed in Table S3. We then selected and reorganized the top 25 from the 50 most dysregulated GO terms among the five groups by comprehensively comparing weighted CWIs with their original rankings in each group, as listed in Table S4. Next, we summarized the 25 most common dysregulated GO terms among the five disease groups of serous ovarian tumors with representative biological and molecular effects and reclassified them into three major categories: cellular cycle and signaling-related effects, membrane and transport-related effects, and metabolic, immunological, and other effects.

Table 2. The 50 most dysregulated GO terms for serous BOT and all stages of serous ovarian carcinoma ranked by cluster weight index (CWI).

Groups	Serous BOT		Serous Ovarian Carcinoma Stage I		Serous Ovarian Carcinoma Stage II		Serous Ovarian Carcinoma Stage III		Serous Ovarian Carcinoma Stage IV	
Ranking	GO ID	GO Term	GO ID	GO Term	GO ID	GO Term	GO ID	GO Term	GO ID	GO Term
1	GO:0002682	Regulation of immune system process	GO:0005215	Transporter activity	GO:0044281	Small molecule metabolic process	GO:0002682	Regulation of immune system process	GO:0044281	Small molecule metabolic process
2	GO:0005215	Transporter activity	GO:0044281	Small molecule metabolic process	GO:0005215	Transporter activity	GO:0044281	Small molecule metabolic process	GO:0002682	Regulation of immune system process
3	GO:0001775	Cell activation	GO:0006811	Ion transport	GO:0002682	Regulation of immune system process	GO:0005215	Transporter activity	GO:0005215	Transporter activity
4	GO:0006811	Ion transport	GO:0006629	Lipid metabolic process	GO:0006811	Ion transport	GO:0001775	Cell activation	GO:0051049	Regulation of transport
5	GO:0044281	Small molecule metabolic process	GO:0051049	Regulation of transport	GO:0006629	Lipid metabolic process	GO:0051049	Regulation of transport	GO:0006811	Ion transport
6	GO:0051049	Regulation of transport	GO:0007267	Cell-cell signaling	GO:0051049	Regulation of transport	GO:0006811	Ion transport	GO:0006629	Lipid metabolic process
7	GO:0002252	Immune effector process	GO:0046649	Lymphocyte activation	GO:0001775	Cell activation	GO:0016070	RNA metabolic process	GO:0001775	Cell activation
8	GO:0002520	Immune system development	GO:0040011	Locomotion	GO:0007267	Cell-cell signaling	GO:0045595	Regulation of cell differentiation	GO:0016070	RNA metabolic process
9	GO:0001816	Cytokine production	GO:0055085	Transmembrane transport	GO:0016070	RNA metabolic process	GO:0006629	Lipid metabolic process	GO:0045595	Regulation of cell differentiation
10	GO:0045595	Regulation of cell differentiation	GO:0042592	Homeostatic process	GO:0045595	Regulation of cell differentiation	GO:0040011	Locomotion	GO:0007267	Cell-cell signaling
11	GO:0031399	Regulation of protein modification process	GO:0045595	Regulation of cell differentiation	GO:0046903	Secretion	GO:0001816	Cytokine production	GO:0022008	Neurogenesis
12	GO:0006629	Lipid metabolic process	GO:0051174	Regulation of phosphorus metabolic process	GO:0040011	Locomotion	GO:0002252	Immune effector process	GO:0046903	Secretion
13	GO:0048585	Negative regulation of response to stimulus	GO:0016491	Oxidoreductase activity	GO:0042592	Homeostatic process	GO:0022008	Neurogenesis	GO:0040011	Locomotion
14	GO:0042592	Homeostatic process	GO:0022008	Neurogenesis	GO:0022008	Neurogenesis	GO:0007267	Cell-cell signaling	GO:0042592	Homeostatic process
15	GO:0022610	Biological adhesion	GO:0098772	Molecular function regulator	GO:0007049	Cell cycle	GO:0046903	Secretion	GO:0019219	Regulation of nucleobase-containing compound metabolic process
16	GO:0055085	Transmembrane transport	GO:0031399	Regulation of protein modification process	GO:0060429	Epithelium development	GO:0070727	Cellular macromolecule localization	GO:0002520	Immune system development
17	GO:0051240	Positive regulation of multicellular organismal process	GO:0048585	Negative regulation of response to stimulus	GO:0048585	Negative regulation of response to stimulus	GO:0002520	Immune system development	GO:0051276	Chromosome organization
18	GO:0006915	Apoptotic process	GO:0050865	Regulation of cell activation	GO:0051174	Regulation of phosphorus metabolic process	GO:0051276	Chromosome organization	GO:0060429	Epithelium development
19	GO:0046903	Secretion	GO:0070727	Cellular macromolecule localization	GO:0033043	Regulation of organelle organization	GO:0042592	Homeostatic process	GO:0007049	Cell cycle
20	GO:0060429	Epithelium development	GO:0010817	Regulation of hormone levels	GO:0019219	Regulation of nucleobase-containing compound metabolic process	GO:0007049	Cell cycle	GO:0001816	Cytokine production

Table 2. Cont.

Groups	Serous BOT		Serous Ovarian Carcinoma Stage I		Serous Ovarian Carcinoma Stage II		Serous Ovarian Carcinoma Stage III		Serous Ovarian Carcinoma Stage IV	
Ranking	GO ID	GO Term	GO ID	GO Term	GO ID	GO Term	GO ID	GO Term	GO ID	GO Term
21	GO:0051174	Regulation of phosphorus metabolic process	GO:0023056	Positive regulation of signaling	GO:0055085	Transmembrane transport	GO:0051240	Positive regulation of multicellular organismal process	GO:0048585	Negative regulation of response to stimulus
22	GO:0051276	Chromosome organization	GO:0007049	Cell cycle	GO:0002520	Immune system development	GO:0019219	Regulation of nucleobase-containing compound metabolic process	GO:0002252	Immune effector process
23	GO:0007267	Cell-cell signaling	GO:0002520	Immune system development	GO:0051276	Chromosome organization	GO:0033043	Regulation of organelle organization	GO:0051174	Regulation of phosphorus metabolic process
24	GO:0007049	Cell cycle	GO:0015849	Organic acid transport	GO:0031399	Regulation of protein modification process	GO:0031399	Regulation of protein modification process	GO:0031399	Regulation of protein modification process
25	GO:0070727	Cellular macromolecule localization	GO:0007017	Microtubule-based process	GO:0002252	Immune effector process	GO:0060429	Epithelium development	GO:0033043	Regulation of organelle organization
26	GO:0016070	RNA metabolic process	GO:0000003	Reproduction	GO:0070727	Cellular macromolecule localization	GO:0048585	Negative regulation of response to stimulus	GO:0009719	Response to endogenous stimulus
27	GO:0040011	Locomotion	GO:0060089	Molecular transducer activity	GO:0023056	Positive regulation of signaling	GO:0046907	Intracellular transport	GO:0019637	Organophosphate metabolic process
28	GO:0033043	Regulation of organelle organization	GO:0033043	Regulation of organelle organization	GO:0010817	Regulation of hormone levels	GO:0006915	Apoptotic process	GO:0051240	Positive regulation of multicellular organismal process
29	GO:0046907	Intracellular transport	GO:0019219	Regulation of nucleobase-containing compound metabolic process	GO:0016491	Oxidoreductase activity	GO:0051174	Regulation of phosphorus metabolic process	GO:0070727	Cellular macromolecule localization
30	GO:0023056	Positive regulation of signaling	GO:0051240	Positive regulation of multicellular organismal process	GO:0009719	Response to endogenous stimulus	GO:0023056	Positive regulation of signaling	GO:0000003	Reproduction
31	GO:0019219	Regulation of nucleobase-containing compound metabolic process	GO:0046907	Intracellular transport	GO:0098772	Molecular function regulator	GO:0006259	DNA metabolic process	GO:0006915	Apoptotic process
32	GO:0006468	Protein phosphorylation	GO:0022610	Biological adhesion	GO:0006915	Apoptotic process	GO:0055085	Transmembrane transport	GO:0006259	DNA metabolic process
33	GO:0051241	Negative regulation of multicellular organismal process	GO:0050877	Nervous system process	GO:0007010	Cytoskeleton organization	GO:0000003	Reproduction	GO:0007417	Central nervous system development
34	GO:0006259	DNA metabolic process	GO:0030054	Cell junction	GO:0001816	Cytokine production	GO:0044419	Interspecies interaction between organisms	GO:0055085	Transmembrane transport
35	GO:0005102	Signaling receptor binding	GO:0002683	Negative regulation of immune system process	GO:0051240	Positive regulation of multicellular organismal process	GO:0007417	Central nervous system development	GO:0023056	Positive regulation of signaling

Table 2. Cont.

Groups	Serous BOT		Serous Ovarian Carcinoma Stage I		Serous Ovarian Carcinoma Stage II		Serous Ovarian Carcinoma Stage III		Serous Ovarian Carcinoma Stage IV	
Ranking	GO ID	GO Term	GO ID	GO Term	GO ID	GO Term	GO ID	GO Term	GO ID	GO Term
36	GO:0098772	Molecular function regulator	GO:0030030	Cell projection organization	GO:0019637	Organophosphate metabolic process	GO:0030030	Cell projection organization	GO:0051241	Negative regulation of multicellular organismal process
37	GO:0080134	Regulation of response to stress	GO:0042127	Regulation of cell proliferation	GO:0046907	Intracellular transport	GO:0065003	Protein-containing complex assembly	GO:0046907	Intracellular transport
38	GO:0022008	Neurogenesis	GO:0042493	Response to drug	GO:0022610	Biological adhesion	GO:0022610	Biological adhesion	GO:0030030	Cell projection organization
39	GO:0015849	Organic acid transport	GO:0023057	Negative regulation of signaling	GO:0000003	Reproduction	GO:0009607	Response to biotic stimulus	GO:0007010	Cytoskeleton organization
40	GO:0044419	Interspecies interaction between organisms	GO:0071495	Cellular response to endogenous stimulus	GO:0030030	Cell projection organization	GO:0007010	Cytoskeleton organization	GO:0098772	Molecular function regulator
41	GO:0023057	Negative regulation of signaling	GO:0051270	Regulation of cellular component movement	GO:0051241	Negative regulation of multicellular organismal process	GO:0009719	Response to endogenous stimulus	GO:0065003	Protein-containing complex assembly
42	GO:0010941	Regulation of cell death	GO:0051338	Regulation of transferase activity	GO:0007417	Central nervous system development	GO:0080134	Regulation of response to stress	GO:0022610	Biological adhesion
43	GO:0042127	Regulation of cell population proliferation	GO:0022603	Regulation of anatomical structure morphogenesis	GO:0007017	Microtubule-based process	GO:0006468	Protein phosphorylation	GO:0009790	Embryo development
44	GO:0009790	Embryo development	GO:0009057	Macromolecule catabolic process	GO:0014070	Response to organic cyclic compound	GO:0032101	Regulation of response to external stimulus	GO:0006468	Protein phosphorylation
45	GO:0002250	Adaptive immune response	GO:0009790	Embryo development	GO:0023057	Negative regulation of signaling	GO:0098772	Molecular function regulator	GO:0016491	Oxidoreductase activity
46	GO:0019637	Organophosphate metabolic process	GO:0051093	Negative regulation of developmental process	GO:0006259	DNA metabolic process	GO:0018193	Peptidyl-amino acid modification	GO:0018193	Peptidyl-amino acid modification
47	GO:0018193	Peptidyl amino acid modification	GO:0043603	Cellular amide metabolic process	GO:0098796	Membrane protein complex	GO:0006952	Defense response	GO:0010817	Regulation of hormone levels
48	GO:0009628	Response to abiotic stimulus	GO:0030855	Epithelial cell differentiation	GO:0042493	Response to drug	GO:0051241	Negative regulation of multicellular organismal process	GO:0080134	Regulation of response to stress
49	GO:0000003	Reproduction	GO:0010876	Lipid localization	GO:0015849	Organic acid transport	GO:0019637	Organophosphate metabolic process	GO:0014070	Response to organic cyclic compound
50	GO:0009719	Response to endogenous stimulus	GO:0051094	Positive regulation of developmental process	GO:0006468	Protein phosphorylation	GO:0044093	Positive regulation of molecular function	GO:0023057	Negative regulation of signaling

3.5. Three Reclassified Categories of the Top 25 Common Dysregulated GO Terms and the Most Relevant Corresponding DEGs

As displayed in Table 3, we reclassified the top 25 most common dysregulated GO terms among serous ovarian tumors into three major categories based on each representative function. There were 9, 8, and 8 GO terms belonging to "cellular cycle and signaling-related effects", "membrane and transport-related effects", and "metabolic, immunological, and other effects", respectively. We sorted the potential genes annotated for all regrouped GO terms among each category with definitions (http://geneontology.org/, accessed on 5 June 2021) and selected the most relevant DEGs with the highest repetitive frequencies determined statistically with cross comparisons. Nine GO terms were reclassified to cellular cycle- and signaling-related effects and four most relevant DEGs were identified with the highest repetition: *EDN1* (endothelin 1), *AKT1* (AKT serine/threonine kinase 1), *IL1B* (interleukin 1 beta), and *INS* (insulin). Eight GO terms were reclassified to membrane- and transport-related effects and the two most relevant DEGs were identified with the highest repetition: *CDK5* (cyclin dependent kinase 5) and *ATP1B1* (sodium/potassium-transporting ATPase subunit beta-1). Eight GO terms were reclassified to metabolic, immunological, and other effects and the seven most relevant DEGs were identified with the highest repetition: *PTK2B* (protein tyrosine kinase 2 beta), *MTOR* (mechanistic target of rapamycin kinase), *APP* (amyloid beta precursor protein), *KIT* (tyrosine-protein kinase KIT), *LEP* (leptin), *MAPK3* (mitogen-activated protein kinase 3), and *SRC* (proto-oncogene tyrosine-protein kinase Src).

3.6. The Significant Common Dysfunctional GO-Defined Pathways and Corresponding DEGs

We firstly discovered that there were 5346, 4047, 6779, 7985, and 8251 dysfunctional pathways defined with GO terms in the serous BOT and serous ovarian carcinoma stage I–IV groups, respectively. Then, we placed these pathways in order of correlation for each group according to statistically significant *p*-values. Next, we selected the top 50 most dysfunctional pathways ranked by *p*-value for each disease group to investigate meaningful correlations, as listed in Table 4 and the detailed GO-defined pathways for serous ovarian tumors are listed in Table S5. "Negative regulation of isotype switching (GO:0045829)" ranked first in the serous BOT group; "modified amino acid transmembrane transporter activity (GO:0072349)" ranked first in serous ovarian carcinoma, FIGO stage I; "DNA double-strand break processing involved in repair via single-strand annealing (GO:0010792)" ranked first in serous ovarian carcinoma, FIGO stage II; "DNA double-strand break processing involved in repair via single-strand annealing (GO:0010792)" ranked first in serous ovarian carcinoma, FIGO stage III; and "aryl hydrocarbon receptor binding (GO:0017162)" ranked first in serous ovarian carcinoma, FIGO stage IV. Moreover, we found only one common dysfunctional pathway among the five disease groups of serous ovarian tumors: "aryl hydrocarbon receptor binding (GO:0017162)," which is ranked at 42, 2, 2, 29, and 1 in the groups of serous BOTs and serous ovarian carcinomas of stages I–IV, respectively. Meanwhile, we also found ten corresponding genes, *AHR* (aryl-hydrocarbon receptor), *AIP* (aryl-hydrocarbon receptor-interacting protein), *ARNT* (aryl hydrocarbon receptor nuclear translocator), *ARNT2* (aryl hydrocarbon receptor nuclear translocator 2), ARNTL (aryl hydrocarbon receptor nuclear translocator-like), *NCOA1* (nuclear receptor coactivator 1), *NCOA2* (nuclear receptor coactivator 2), *TAF4* (TATA-box binding protein associated factor 4), *TAF6* (TATA-box binding protein associated factor 6), and *TBP* (TATA box binding protein), with their representative proteins annotated for these GO term-defined dysfunctional pathways acquired from the GO gene set database (http://geneontology.org/, accessed on 5 June 2021).

Table 3. Categorized lists of the top 25 common dysregulated GO terms among serous ovarian tumors reclassified by biological functions and the most relevant corresponding DEGs in each group.

	Cellular Cycle and Signaling Related Effects	
GO ID	**GO Term**	**Most Relevant DEGs**
GO:0045595	Regulation of cell differentiation	
GO:0007267	Cell-cell signaling	
GO:0042592	Homeostatic process	
GO:0048585	Negative regulation of response to stimulus	
GO:0007049	Cell cycle	EDN1, AKT1, IL1B, INS
GO:0033043	Regulation of organelle organization	
GO:0051240	Positive regulation of multicellular organismal process	
GO:0023056	Positive regulation of signaling	
GO:0098772	Molecular function regulator	
	Membrane and Transport Related Effects	
GO ID	**GO Term**	**Most Relevant DEGs**
GO:0005215	Transporter activity	
GO:0006811	Ion transport	
GO:0051049	Regulation of transport	
GO:0040011	Locomotion	
GO:0055085	Transmembrane transport	CDK5, ATP1B1
GO:0070727	Cellular macromolecule localization	
GO:0046907	Intracellular transport	
GO:0022610	Biological adhesion	
	Metabolic, Immunological, and Other Effects	
GO ID	**GO Term**	**Most Relevant DEGs**
GO:0044281	Small molecule metabolic process	
GO:0006629	Lipid metabolic process	
GO:0031399	Regulation of protein modification process	
GO:0051174	Regulation of phosphorus metabolic process	PTK2B, MTOR, APP, KIT, LEP, MAPK3, SRC
GO:0019219	Regulation of nucleobase containing compound metabolic process	
GO:0002520	Immune system development	
GO:0022008	Neurogenesis	
GO:0000003	Reproduction	

Table 4. The top 50 most dysfunctional GO-defined pathways among serous BOT and all stages of serous ovarian carcinoma ranked by *p*-values.

Groups	Serous BOT		Serous Ovarian Carcinoma Stage I		Serous Ovarian Carcinoma Stage II		Serous Ovarian Carcinoma Stage III		Serous Ovarian Carcinoma Stage IV	
Ranking	GO ID	GO Term	GO ID	GO Term	GO ID	GO Term	GO ID	GO Term	GO ID	GO Term
1	GO:0045829	Negative regulation of isotype switching	GO:0072349	Modified amino acid transmembrane transporter activity	GO:0010792	DNA double-strand break processing involved in repair via single-strand annealing	GO:2001269	Positive regulation of cysteine-type endopeptidase activity involved in apoptotic signaling pathway	GO:0017162	Aryl hydrocarbon receptor binding
2	GO:0008395	Steroid hydroxylase activity	GO:0017162	Aryl hydrocarbon receptor binding	GO:0017162	Aryl hydrocarbon receptor binding	GO:0042908	Xenobiotic transport	GO:0072349	Modified amino acid transmembrane transporter activity
3	GO:0016578	Histone deubiquitination	GO:0097501	Stress response to metal ion	GO:0045002	Double-strand break repair via single-strand annealing	GO:2001267	Regulation of cysteine-type endopeptidase activity involved in apoptotic signaling pathway	GO:0036507	Protein demannosylation
4	GO:0090482	Vitamin transmembrane transporter activity	GO:0016589	NURF complex	GO:0070162	Adiponectin secretion	GO:0015701	Bicarbonate transport	GO:0045618	Positive regulation of keratinocyte differentiation
5	GO:0033499	Galactose catabolic process via UDP-galactose	GO:0055059	Asymmetric neuroblast division	GO:0046643	Regulation of gamma-delta T cell activation	GO:0046007	Negative regulation of activated T cell proliferation	GO:0015106	Bicarbonate transmembrane transporter activity
6	GO:0005347	ATP transmembrane transporter activity	GO:0004865	Protein serine/threonine phosphatase inhibitor activity	GO:0010957	Negative regulation of vitamin D biosynthetic process	GO:0010957	Negative regulation of vitamin D biosynthetic process	GO:0045002	Double-strand break repair via single-strand annealing
7	GO:0015867	ATP transport	GO:0008628	Hormone-mediated apoptotic signaling pathway	GO:0036507	Protein demannosylation	GO:0072608	Interleukin-10 secretion	GO:0045793	Positive regulation of cell size
8	GO:0006825	Copper ion transport	GO:0036507	Protein demannosylation	GO:0046137	Negative regulation of vitamin metabolic process	GO:0090482	Vitamin transmembrane transporter activity	GO:0004016	Adenylate cyclase activity
9	GO:0046007	Negative regulation of activated T cell proliferation	GO:0015106	Bicarbonate transmembrane transporter activity	GO:1990239	Steroid hormone binding	GO:0072350	Tricarboxylic acid metabolic process	GO:0006171	cAMP biosynthetic process
10	GO:0044743	Protein transmembrane import into intracellular organelle	GO:0046643	Regulation of gamma-delta T cell activation	GO:0071360	Cellular response to exogenous dsRNA	GO:0033617	Mitochondrial respiratory chain complex IV assembly	GO:0006517	Protein deglycosylation
11	GO:0050859	Negative regulation of B cell receptor signaling pathway	GO:0005078	MAP-kinase scaffold activity	GO:0044854	Plasma membrane raft assembly	GO:0016409	Palmitoyltransferase activity	GO:0010957	Negative regulation of vitamin D biosynthetic process
12	GO:0099132	ATP hydrolysis coupled cation transmembrane transport	GO:0045618	Positive regulation of keratinocyte differentiation	GO:0016589	NURF complex	GO:0005451	Monovalent cation:proton antiporter activity	GO:0015701	Bicarbonate transport
13	GO:0000244	Spliceosomal tri-snRNP complex assembly	GO:0045793	Positive regulation of cell size	GO:0097501	Stress response to metal ion	GO:0018345	Protein palmitoylation	GO:0036065	Fucosylation
14	GO:0045623	Negative regulation of T-helper cell differentiation	GO:0015116	Sulfate transmembrane transporter activity	GO:0072349	Modified amino acid transmembrane transporter activity	GO:0016417	S-acyltransferase activity	GO:0072497	Mesenchymal stem cell differentiation

Table 4. Cont.

Groups	Serous BOT		Serous Ovarian Carcinoma Stage I		Serous Ovarian Carcinoma Stage II		Serous Ovarian Carcinoma Stage III		Serous Ovarian Carcinoma Stage IV	
Ranking	GO ID	GO Term	GO ID	GO Term	GO ID	GO Term	GO ID	GO Term	GO ID	GO Term
15	GO:0004089	Carbonate dehydratase activity	GO:0008271	Secondary active sulfate transmembrane transporter activity	GO:0015106	Bicarbonate transmembrane transporter activity	GO:0046137	Negative regulation of vitamin metabolic process	GO:0050859	Negative regulation of B cell receptor signaling pathway
16	GO:0033270	Paranode region of axon	GO:0004016	Adenylate cyclase activity	GO:0050428	3′-phosphoadenosine 5′-phosphosulfate biosynthetic process	GO:0002370	Natural killer cell cytokine production	GO:0019870	Potassium channel inhibitor activity
17	GO:0050686	Negative regulation of mRNA processing	GO:0006171	cAMP biosynthetic process	GO:0001765	Membrane raft assembly	GO:0045618	Positive regulation of keratinocyte differentiation	GO:0036066	Protein O-linked fucosylation
18	GO:0044183	Protein binding involved in protein folding	GO:0008272	Sulfate transport	GO:0019531	Oxalate transmembrane transporter activity	GO:0016589	NURF complex	GO:0046137	Negative regulation of vitamin metabolic process
19	GO:0061082	Myeloid leukocyte cytokine production	GO:0022821	Potassium ion antiporter activity	GO:0045618	Positive regulation of keratinocyte differentiation	GO:0015924	Mannosyl-oligosaccharide mannosidase activity	GO:0044322	Endoplasmic reticulum quality control compartment
20	GO:0000002	Mitochondrial genome maintenance	GO:0015924	Mannosyl-oligosaccharide mannosidase activity	GO:0008271	Secondary active sulfate transmembrane transporter activity	GO:0045616	Regulation of keratinocyte differentiation	GO:0004865	Protein serine/threonine phosphatase inhibitor activity
21	GO:0045591	Positive regulation of regulatory T cell differentiation	GO:0019373	Epoxygenase P450 pathway	GO:0015116	Sulfate transmembrane transporter activity	GO:0070162	Adiponectin secretion	GO:0007175	Negative regulation of epidermal growth factor-activated receptor activity
22	GO:2001182	Regulation of interleukin-12 secretion	GO:0019532	Oxalate transport	GO:0032184	SUMO polymer binding	GO:0022821	Potassium ion antiporter activity	GO:0042359	Vitamin D metabolic process
23	GO:0097503	Sialylation	GO:0099509	Regulation of presynaptic cytosolic calcium ion concentration	GO:0045586	Regulation of gamma-delta T cell differentiation	GO:0015377	Cation: chloride symporter activity	GO:0009975	Cyclase activity
24	GO:0008373	Sialyltransferase activity	GO:0019531	Oxalate transmembrane transporter activity	GO:0019532	Oxalate transport	GO:0015379	Potassium: chloride symporter activity	GO:0045616	Regulation of keratinocyte differentiation
25	GO:0008385	Ikappab kinase complex	GO:0050428	3′-phosphoadenosine 5′-phosphosulfate biosynthetic process	GO:0071447	Cellular response to hydroperoxide	GO:0098719	Sodium ion import across plasma membrane	GO:0016849	Phosphorus-oxygen lyase activity
26	GO:0072643	Interferon-gamma secretion	GO:0008391	Arachidonic acid monooxygenase activity	GO:0042363	Fat-soluble vitamin catabolic process	GO:0072643	Interferon-gamma secretion	GO:1990239	Steroid hormone binding
27	GO:0031248	Protein acetyltransferase complex	GO:0097267	Omega-hydroxylase P450 pathway	GO:0072497	Mesenchymal stem cell differentiation	GO:0097503	Sialylation	GO:0071305	Cellular response to vitamin D
28	GO:0000188	Inactivation of MAPK activity	GO:0010792	DNA double-strand break processing involved in repair via single-strand annealing	GO:0005337	Nucleoside transmembrane transporter activity	GO:0008373	Sialyltransferase activity	GO:0070162	Adiponectin secretion
29	GO:0002634	Regulation of germinal center formation	GO:0031010	ISWI-type complex	GO:0008272	Sulfate transport	GO:0017162	Aryl hydrocarbon receptor binding	GO:0006895	Golgi to endosome transport

Table 4. Cont.

Groups	Serous BOT		Serous Ovarian Carcinoma Stage I		Serous Ovarian Carcinoma Stage II		Serous Ovarian Carcinoma Stage III		Serous Ovarian Carcinoma Stage IV	
Ranking	GO ID	GO Term	GO ID	GO Term	GO ID	GO Term	GO ID	GO Term	GO ID	GO Term
30	GO:2000515	Negative regulation of CD4-positive, alpha-beta T cell activation	GO:0071360	Cellular response to exogenous dsRNA	GO:0002175	Protein localization to paranode region of axon	GO:0032689	Negative regulation of interferon-gamma production	GO:0097225	Sperm midpiece
31	GO:2000320	Negative regulation of T-helper 17 cell differentiation	GO:0006685	Sphingomyelin catabolic process	GO:0019373	Epoxygenase P450 pathway	GO:0015296	Anion:cation symporter activity	GO:2000535	Regulation of entry of bacterium into host cell
32	GO:0060907	Positive regulation of macrophage cytokine production	GO:0071577	Zinc ion transmembrane transport	GO:2001182	Regulation of interleukin-12 secretion	GO:0046643	Regulation of gamma-delta T cell activation	GO:0004198	Calcium-dependent cysteine-type endopeptidase activity
33	GO:0032426	Stereocilium tip	GO:0005385	Zinc ion transmembrane transporter activity	GO:0090177	Establishment of planar polarity involved in neural tube closure	GO:0042788	Polysomal ribosome	GO:0019373	Epoxygenase P450 pathway
34	GO:0046915	Transition metal ion transmembrane transporter activity	GO:0044854	Plasma membrane raft assembly	GO:0015858	Nucleoside transport	GO:0045503	Dynein light chain binding	GO:1905276	Regulation of epithelial tube formation
35	GO:0033549	MAP kinase phosphatase activity	GO:0099516	Ion antiporter activity	GO:0031095	Platelet dense tubular network membrane	GO:2000773	Negative regulation of cellular senescence	GO:0071313	Cellular response to caffeine
36	GO:0016854	Racemase and epimerase activity	GO:0038044	Transforming growth factor-beta secretion	GO:0019870	Potassium channel inhibitor activity	GO:0002707	Negative regulation of lymphocyte mediated immunity	GO:0045671	Negative regulation of osteoclast differentiation
37	GO:0043371	Negative regulation of CD4-positive, alpha-beta T cell differentiation	GO:0097264	Self-proteolysis	GO:0034139	Regulation of toll-like receptor 3 signaling pathway	GO:0070234	Positive regulation of T cell apoptotic process	GO:0099516	Ion antiporter activity
38	GO:0030890	Positive regulation of B cell proliferation	GO:0045852	pH elevation	GO:0101020	Estrogen 16-alpha-hydroxylase activity	GO:0071447	Cellular response to hydroperoxide	GO:0019532	Oxalate transport
39	GO:0050798	Activated T cell proliferation	GO:0009698	Phenylpropanoid metabolic process	GO:0002933	Lipid hydroxylation	GO:0099587	Inorganic ion import across plasma membrane	GO:2001222	Regulation of neuron migration
40	GO:0015662	ATPase activity, coupled to transmembrane movement of ions, phosphorylative mechanism	GO:2001182	Regulation of interleukin-12 secretion	GO:0060353	Regulation of cell adhesion molecule production	GO:0071636	Positive regulation of transforming growth factor beta production	GO:0016712	Oxidoreductase activity, acting on paired donors, with incorporation or reduction of molecular oxygen, reduced flavin or flavoprotein as one donor, and incorporation of one atom of oxygen
41	GO:0048291	Isotype switching to IgG isotypes	GO:0015491	Cation: cation antiporter activity	GO:0008391	Arachidonic acid monooxygenase activity	GO:0033962	Cytoplasmic mRNA processing body assembly	GO:2000833	Positive regulation of steroid hormone secretion
42	GO:0017162	Aryl hydrocarbon receptor binding	GO:0071313	Cellular response to caffeine	GO:1905276	Regulation of epithelial tube formation	GO:0043189	H4/H2A histone acetyltransferase complex	GO:0007077	Mitotic nuclear envelope disassembly

Table 4. Cont.

Groups	Serous BOT		Serous Ovarian Carcinoma Stage I		Serous Ovarian Carcinoma Stage II		Serous Ovarian Carcinoma Stage III		Serous Ovarian Carcinoma Stage IV	
Ranking	GO ID	GO Term	GO ID	GO Term	GO ID	GO Term	GO ID	GO Term	GO ID	GO Term
43	GO:0061081	Positive regulation of myeloid leukocyte cytokine production involved in immune response	GO:2000833	Positive regulation of steroid hormone secretion	GO:0031010	ISWI-type complex	GO:0043968	Histone H2A acetylation	GO:0015924	Mannosyl-oligosaccharide mannosidase activity
44	GO:0016226	Iron-sulfur cluster assembly	GO:0070162	Adiponectin secretion	GO:0045671	Negative regulation of osteoclast differentiation	GO:2001222	Regulation of neuron migration	GO:2001182	Regulation of interleukin-12 secretion
45	GO:0030007	Cellular potassium ion homeostasis	GO:0031995	Insulin-like growth factor II binding	GO:0031995	Insulin-like growth factor II binding	GO:0070670	Response to interleukin-4	GO:0015373	Anion: sodium symporter activity
46	GO:0015701	Bicarbonate transport	GO:0005451	Monovalent cation: proton antiporter activity	GO:0008541	Proteasome regulatory particle, lid subcomplex	GO:0018230	Peptidyl-L-cysteine S-palmitoylation	GO:0090177	Establishment of planar polarity involved in neural tube closure
47	GO:0071850	Mitotic cell cycle arrest	GO:0008541	Proteasome regulatory particle, lid subcomplex	GO:0052173	Response to defenses of other organism involved in symbiotic interaction	GO:0005416	Amino acid: cation symporter activity	GO:0016725	Oxidoreductase activity, acting on CH or CH2 groups
48	GO:0071014	Post-mRNA release spliceosomal complex	GO:0031095	Platelet dense tubular network membrane	GO:0038085	Vascular endothelial growth factor binding	GO:0006825	Copper ion transport	GO:0002335	Mature B cell differentiation
49	GO:0008242	Omega peptidase activity	GO:0016712	Oxidoreductase activity, acting on paired donors, with incorporation or reduction of molecular oxygen, reduced flavin or flavoprotein as one donor, and incorporation of one atom of oxygen	GO:0005310	Dicarboxylic acid transmembrane transporter activity	GO:0002857	Positive regulation of natural killer cell-mediated immune response to tumor cell	GO:0009111	Vitamin catabolic process
50	GO:0043966	histone H3 acetylation	GO:0050859	Negative regulation of B cell receptor signaling pathway	GO:2000270	Negative regulation of fibroblast apoptotic process	GO:0000185	Activation of MAPKKK activity	GO:0019843	rRNA binding

3.7. The Influences of Distinct Valuable DEGs with Corresponding Biomarkers Expressed in Serous Ovarian Tumors

So far, we have performed GO-based integrative methods to analyze, discover, and reclassify the 25 most important common dysregulated functions among the serous ovarian tumor groups into distinct effective categories and obtained 13 corresponding DEGs in total. We also found one common dysfunctional pathway among the five disease groups and the corresponding ten DEGs. Next, we searched several important biomarkers and relevant genes with close relationships with EMT among ovarian cancers from previous research [50,57,72] and compared them with the DEGs of the top 25 meaningful dysregulated functionomes in this experiment by checking for repetitions and cross comparisons. Five featured DEGs were selected: *CDH1* (cadherin 1), *CTNNB1* (catenin beta 1), *SNAI1* (snail family transcriptional repressor 1, *SNAIL*), *SNAI2* (snail family transcriptional repressor 2, *SLUG*), and *TWIST1* (twist-related protein 1). In addition, we have individually established three functional protein–protein interaction networks using the STRING database (https://string-db.org, accessed on 5 June 2021) based on the relevant DEGs and their corresponding proteins as biomarkers. These networks comprised the following: one, all relevant DEGs sorted from the top 25 common dysregulated functionomes (Figure 3A); two, the 10 DEGs involved in the dysfunctional AHR binding pathway (Figure 3B); and three, the featured DEGs among relevant biomarkers associated with EMT (Figure 3C). All these biomarkers revealed intensive interactions with regulatory cross effects in each network. Simultaneously, we searched the GEO (http://www.ncbi.nlm.nih.gov/geo/, accessed on 5 June 2021) and The Cancer Genome Atlas (TCGA; http://cancergenome.nih.gov, accessed on 5 June 2021) repositories, including datasets downloaded from three major microarray platforms, GPL96 (Affymetrix HG-U133A), GPL570 (Affymetrix HG-U133 Plus 2.0), and GPL571/GPL3921 (Affymetrix HG-U133A 2.0), which contained extracted and corrected raw data of 1232 patients with serous ovarian carcinoma. We entered these datasets with gene expression into the PostgreSQL relational database and compared 28 meaningful DEGs (*EDN1, AKT1, IL1B, INS, CDK5, ATP1B1, PTK2B, MTOR, APP, KIT, LEP, MAPK3, SRC, AHR, AIP, ARNT, ARNT2, ARNTL, NCOA1, NCOA2, TAF4, TAF6, TBP, CDH1, CTNNB1, SNAI1, SNAI2,* and *TWIST1*) selected from the above steps. Then, we calculated and investigated the DEG expression levels, progression-free survival (PFS), and overall survival (OS) among serous ovarian carcinoma patients using the Mann–Whitney test and the receiver operating characteristic test in the R statistical environment (http://www.r-project.org, accessed on 5 June 2021) with Bioconductor libraries (http://www.bioconductor.org, accessed on 5 June 2021) followed by a second normalization to set the average expression of the 22,277 identical probes (http://kmplot.com/analysis/index.php?p=service&cancer=ovar, accessed on 5 June 2021) [73]. Combining all the methods mentioned above, we found that only four DEGs (*SRC, ARNT, TBP,* and *SNAI2*) showed stronger and closer relationships than the other biomarkers in each functional protein–protein interaction network (Figure 3A–C) and had consistent synchronous poor effects on PFS and OS among patients with serous ovarian carcinomas with statistical significance (Figure 3D–K). The high expression levels of the four potentially crucial genes (*SRC, ARNT, TBP,* and *SNAI2*) were significantly correlated with poor prognosis and survival, and the hazard ratios of PFS and OS are shown in each graph below (Figure 3D–K).

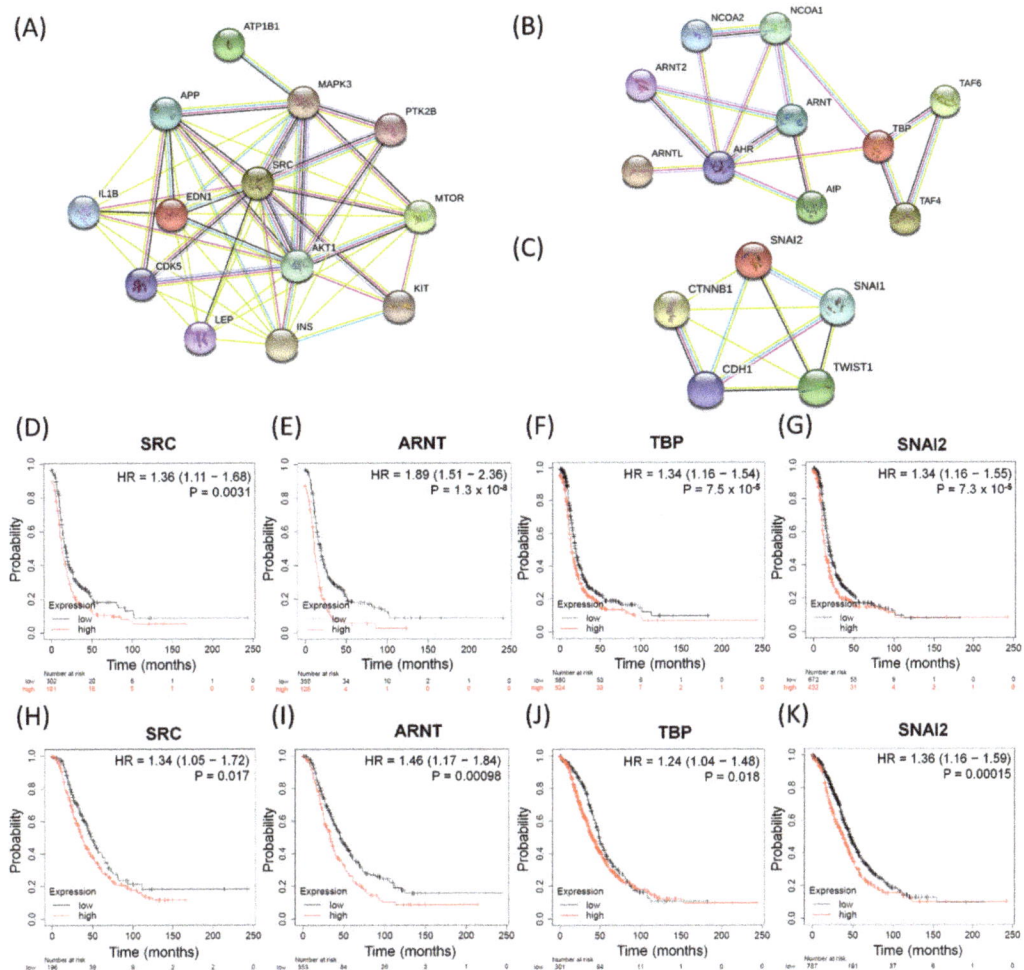

Figure 3. The significant biomarkers influencing serous ovarian tumors. (**A–C**) Panels display identified potential involving DEGs subjected to protein–protein interaction (PPI) analysis with interactive network from the STRING database (https://string-db.org (accessed on 21 July 2021)) with intensive interactions. (**A**) All 13 relevant DEGs sorted from the top 25 common dysregulated GO terms, (**B**) all ten DEGs in-volved in dysfunctional aryl hydrocarbon receptor (AHR) binding pathway, and (**C**) five featured DEGs among relevant biomarkers associated with EMT. (**D–K**) The four meaningful DEGs (SRC, ARNT, TBP and SNAI2) associated with poor survival outcomes. PFS: (**D**) SRC, (**E**) ARNT, (**F**) TBP, (**G**) SNAI2; OS: (**H**) SRC, (**I**) ARNT, (**J**) TBP, and (**K**) SNAI2 in serous ovarian carcinomas. The hazard ratios of the PFS of SRC, ARNT, TBP, and SNAI2 were 1.36 (1.11–1.68), $p = 0.0031$), 1.89 (1.51–2.36, $p = 1.3 \times 10^{-8}$), 1.34 (1.16–1.54, $p = 7.5 \times 10^{-5}$), and 1.34 (1.16–1.55, $p = 7.3 \times 10^{-5}$), respectively. The hazard ratios of the OS of SRC, ARNT, TBP, and SNAI2 were 1.34 (1.05–1.72, $p = 0.017$), 1.46 (1.17–1.84, $p = 0.00098$), 1.24 (1.04–1.48, $p = 0.018$), 1.36 (1.16–1.59, $p = 0.00015$), respectively.

3.8. Immunohistochemical Validation of Expression Levels for SRC, ARNT, TBP, and SNAI2 among Serous Ovarian Tumors

Since the inferred biomarkers including SRC, ARNT, TBP, and SNAI2 from the previous analysis were assumed to be influential in the tumorigenesis of serous ovarian tumors, we gathered relevant clinical samples from a cohort of patients (serous BOT, n = 9; serous ovarian carcinoma, n = 41, including n = 8, 2, 23, and 8 for FIGO stages I–IV, respectively) to explore the clinical characteristics and verify the specific manifestations of the four abovementioned selected DEGs that were determined to participate in the pathogenetic mechanisms of serous ovarian tumors. Because the number of samples in each group was inconsistent, we combined groups as follows to facilitate verification and comparison: serous BOTs, early-stage serous ovarian carcinomas (FIGO stages I and II), and late-stage serous ovarian carcinomas (FIGO stages III and IV). We then performed IHC staining of anti-SRC, anti-ARNT, anti-TBP, and anti-SNAI2 antibodies separately among the three modified disease groups to clinically assess the significant manifestation of SRC, ARNT, TBP, and SNAI2. Professional pathologists verified and interpreted the results evenly and repeatedly throughout the whole diagnostic process using SPSS software (IBM SPSS Statistics version 22.0 for Windows, IBM Corp., Armonk, NY, USA) to quantify the immunoscores of SRC, ARNT, TBP, and SNAI2. The organized results clearly showed that the highest biomarker expression levels tended to occur in the group of late-stage serous ovarian carcinoma, followed by the early-stage group, and lastly the serous BOT group (Figure 4A). We also found that the highest mean values of expression levels for all these biomarkers (SRC, ARNT, TBP, and SNAI2) belonged to the late-stage serous ovarian carcinoma group, with clear increasing trends from the serous BOT group to the late-stage group, and the calculated mean values of the relevant biomarkers were statistically significant (Figure 4B). The detailed results of all scores for relevant featured biomarkers of clinical samples and detailed clinical characteristics of the patients (grade, menopausal status, the presence of BRCA1, BRCA2 mutation, overall survival, and Ca125 level) are listed in Table S6. These results were in accordance with our inferences, implying that many dysregulated functionomes deduced from the integrative GO-based enrichment analysis are dedicated to the pathogenetic mechanisms of serous ovarian tumors. Similarly, these validated results also demonstrated that the dysfunctional AHR binding pathway played a role in the tumorigenesis of serous ovarian tumors. Furthermore, this verification supported the association between EMT and tumor progression. All these significant results confirmed the importance of the previously proposed DEGs and related pathogenic tumorigenesis for serous ovarian tumors.

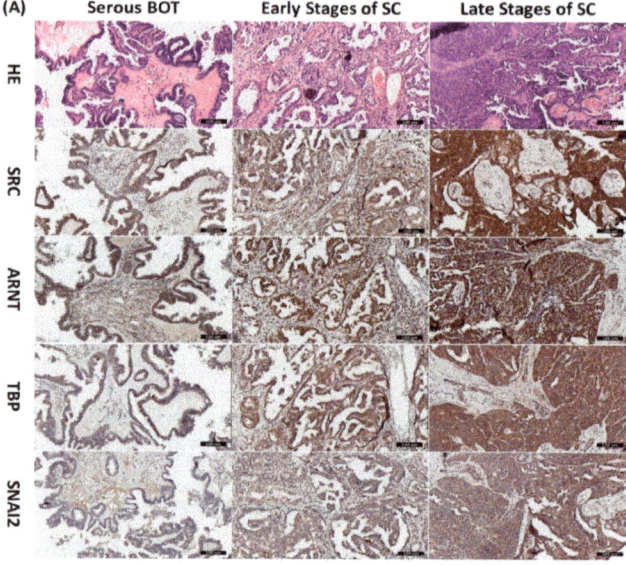

Figure 4. *Cont.*

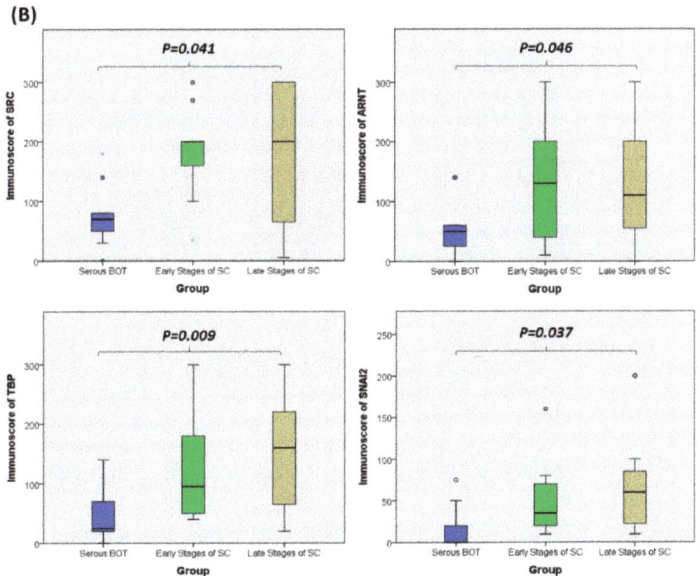

Figure 4. Verified analysis of biomarkers among serous ovarian tumors by IHC staining. (**A**) Clinical samples from patients with serous BOTs (n = 9, left column), early stages of serous ovarian carcinomas (n = 10, middle column), and late stages of serous ovarian carcinomas (n = 31, right column) were immunostained with hematoxylin and eosin (first row), anti-SRC antibody (second row), anti-ARNT antibody (third row), anti-TBP antibody (fourth row), and anti-SNAI2 antibody (fifth row). (**B**) Box plots for expressed biomarkers including SRC, ARNT, TBP, and SNAI2 among groups of serous BOTs (blue), early stages of serous ovarian carcinomas (green), and late stages of serous ovarian carcinomas (light brown). All the expression levels of these meaningful biomarkers were quantified and clearly revealed an increasing trend of mean values from serous BOTs to late stages of serous ovarian carcinomas with statistical significance.

4. Discussion

In this study, we implemented a comprehensive GO-based multi-genome interpretative model using gene set defined functionomes and GSR indices calculated based on gene expression profiles and levels downloaded from public gene set databases to further investigate the complicated and divergent molecular and genetic events of serous ovarian tumors, including serous BOTs and serous ovarian carcinomas at all stages. All results obtained using SVM were statistically significant with high sensitivity, specificity, and accuracy. The GSR indices of all groups of serous ovarian tumors compared to the control groups revealed obvious deviations. The most apparent divergence detected was in the group of serous ovarian carcinoma, FIGO stage IV, and the deviation of serous BOT was just between the early and late stages of serous ovarian carcinomas. Among all groups of serous ovarian tumors, we first identified the top 25 significant common dysregulated functionomes with 13 relevant DEGs, then found one common dysfunctional pathway, AHR binding (GO:0017162), containing 10 corresponding DEGs and excavated five applicable EMT-related DEGs that were related with ovarian neoplasms. Recently, EMT, a reversible process in which epithelial cells acquire mesenchymal cell characteristics due to the loss of cellular polarity and adhesion with increasing cellular migration, has become an important concept in research on tumorigenesis, progression, and chemoresistance of ovarian neoplasms; thus, we included biomarkers of EMT for ovarian tumors in this research. After integrative analysis, including comparison of functional protein–protein interactions and patient survival (PFS and OS) of serous ovarian carcinomas, we obtained four potentially important DEGs: *SRC*, *ARNT*, *TBP*, and *SNAI2*. Finally, IHC validation of these four biomarkers revealed that they significantly increased in samples incrementally from serous BOT to early stages and then to late stages of serous ovarian carcinomas. Since the results obtained in this study are extraordinarily rich and complex, we mainly explained and discussed the crucial dysfunctional AHR binding pathways accompanied by four consequential DEGs that were statistically verified. However, other related meaningful results deserve further exploration and investigation.

Among the preliminary results of GO-based analysis for each group of serous ovarian tumors, we noticed significant differences between serous BOT and serous ovarian carcinomas, that is similar to the divergences of clinical manifestations and histopathological characteristics between the two groups; furthermore, there were also discrepancies even in the four stages of serous ovarian carcinomas. This experiment thus revealed that serous BOTs and serous ovarian carcinomas are basically inconsistent, although all histopathological classifications are confirmed as "serous". Even so, we identified the top 25 dysregulated functionomes from the first 50 GO-defined terms among the five groups and reclassified them into three categories according to their representative functions. After statistical comparison, we noticed that the category of metabolic and immunological effects had the greatest influence on serous ovarian tumors, followed by membrane and transport-related effects, and lastly, cellular cycle and signaling-related effects. Therefore, we can reasonably infer the importance of the metabolome and immunome in the tumorigenesis of serous ovarian tumors, which require investigation in the future together with the other two effects. In our experiments, we also identified 13 highly relevant DEGs. Many related studies have examined how these DEGs affected the formation of serous ovarian tumors, such as tyrosine kinase related DEGs (*PTK2B*, *KIT*, and *SRC*) [74–76], crucial factors known to be related to tumorigenesis (*AKT1*, *MTOR*, *MAPK3*) [64,77–80], DEGs related to cellular metabolism and immunity (*EDN1*, *IL1B*, *INS*, *APP*, *LEP*) [29,56,60,81–86], and agents for signal transmission and channels of cell membranes (*CDK5* and *ATP1B1*) [59,87,88]. Among these DEGs, we found that SRC has consistently poor effects on the survival of serous ovarian carcinoma patients with a poor prognosis of PFS and OS. SRC, a non-receptor protein tyrosine kinase known as a proto-oncogene, participates in the regulation of embryonic development and cell growth [89]. SRC has been found to be activated and overexpressed in association with HER-2/neu overexpression in a high percentage of ovarian cancers, especially in the late stage, and to increase proliferation, angiogenesis, and invasion during tumor development [90]. Silencing of SRC could enhance the cytotoxicity of taxol in ovarian cancer cells to improve the efficacy of chemotherapy [91].

Of the top 50 GO-defined dysfunctional pathways, we found only one meaningful common pathway (AHR binding, GO:0017162) among the five disease groups. We conducted integrated analysis to comprehensively discover the pivotal role of the AHR binding pathway in the tumorigenesis of serous ovarian tumors for the first time. However, in addition to the dysfunctional AHR binding pathway, we also found two common disordered pathways, including positive regulation of keratinocyte differentiation (GO:0045618) and adiponectin secretion (GO:0070162), in all stages of serous ovarian carcinomas. Although not in the top 50 pathways of serous BOTs, these two disordered pathways may be potential problems to be investigated further for the pathogenesis of serous ovarian carcinoma. Through comprehensive analysis, it was revealed that ARNT and TBP have consistently poor effects on PFS and OS. AHR, a ligand-activated transcription factor, is notable for its role in environmental chemical toxicity [92–94]; however, in recent studies, AHR was also recognized to play a critical role in tumorigenesis through complex epigenetic and pathogenetic mechanisms encompassing both pro- and anti-tumorigenic activities [95,96]. AHR exists in the cytoplasm and is induced and activated by linking with a group of environmental pollutants as well as other AHR ligands from microbes and diet, and it undergoes certain conformational transformations together with SRC and other cofactors in the cytoplasm to translocate to the nucleus in a dissociated form [95,97–99]. AHR can heterodimerize with ARNT, a nuclear translocator, to compose the AhR-ARNT complex, which subsequently binds with specific DNA sequences and xenobiotic response element (XRE) in the enhancer region of certain genes associated with TBP, leading to transcriptional activation of enzymes, such as the cytochrome P450 (CYP) enzymes 1A1 (CYP1A1), CYP1A2, and CYP1B1, for xenobiotic metabolism to induce carcinogenicity of cancer stem cells as tumors or initiate cancer (Figure 5) [100–103]. Although the current research on the AHR binding pathway and serous ovarian tumors is still limited, it can be roughly understood that the AHR binding pathway influences the formation and occurrence of serous ovarian malignancy through the deep deletion and amplification of AHR transcription factors [95,96,104,105]. Moreover, localization of AHR in the nucleus of tumor cells has been associated with a worse outcome in patients with ovarian cancer, and the role of the AHR/ARNT/CYP-enzyme pathway [106,107] and AHR-driven TBP gene expression in carcinogenesis and cancer initiation, as well as its potential use, have been considered as therapeutic targets for better outcomes [108]. In addition, AHR and NCOA1 discovered in this experiment may also be targets warranting further discussion [98].

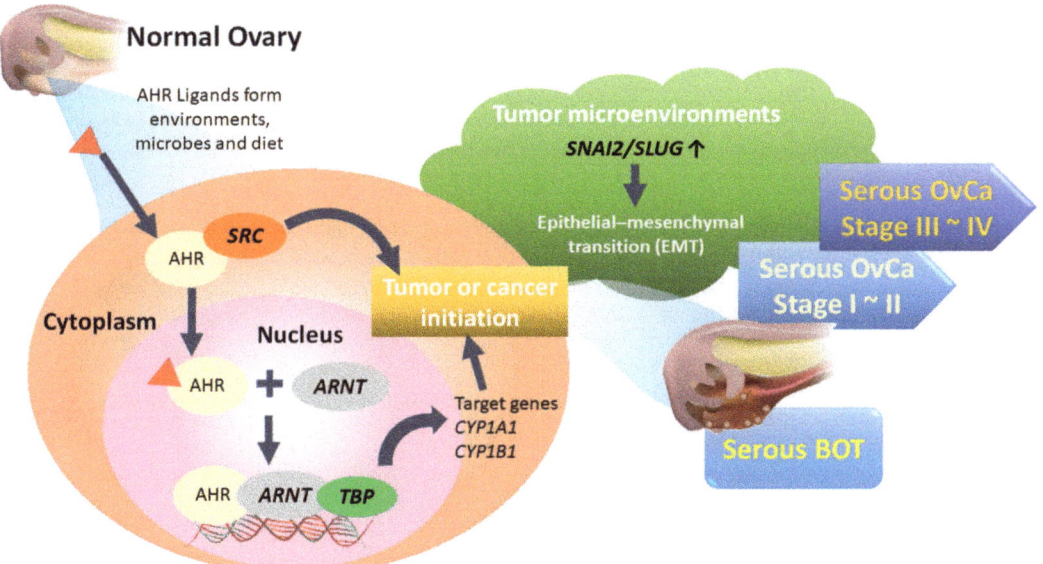

Figure 5. Proposed pathogenetic mechanism of the AHR binding pathway combined with EMT-related factors for tumorigenesis of serous ovarian tumors. BOT: borderline ovarian tumor; OvCa: ovarian carcinoma.

Approximately 80% of patients with ovarian cancer suffer from recurrence of metastasis within five years after the initial therapy with debulking operation and chemotherapy due to the development of resistance [109,110]. Accumulating findings have recently demonstrated that EMT may induce chemotherapy resistance and cancer cell stemness by regulating EMT transcription factors, such as Zeb1, Zeb2, Snail, Slug, and Twist1, in a complicated network, and all functional EMT in the tumor microenvironment could exchange tumor cell morphology to upgrade metastatic abilities via migration and invasion [72,111–113]. Because avoidance of EMT may be crucial for evaluating and managing tumor metastasis and recurrence [114], we selected five featured DEGs by proofreading and collation with all meaningful DEGs from the top 25 common functionomes of all groups of serous ovarian tumors, and we found that SNAI2 was the most influential DEG due to the concordant results of patient survival. IHC analysis showed an increasing trend from borderline tumors to the late stage of ovarian malignancy. The transcriptional factor SNAI2, also known as SLUG, is considered important for cell migration, differentiation, and metastasis [115,116]. Our study identified the expression and role of SNAI2 in serous ovarian tumors, indicating the progression of serous ovarian tumors possibly through EMT. So far, the association between the AHR binding pathway and EMT among serous ovarian tumors remains unexplored thoroughly, and this experiment provides the opportunity to solve this problem. Aromatic hydrocarbon substances, such as phthalates, di(2-ethylhexyl)phthalate (DEHP), or bisphenol A, are recognized as aggravators, as they upregulate and promote cell proliferation and tumor progression [117–119]. In contrast, dietary phytoestrogen and kaempferol could exert anti-carcinogenic and anti-proliferative effects through AHR-related pathways to inhibit the EMT process [120]. Our results showed that there is indeed a tight correlation between AHR and EMT as the degree of malignancy develops in serous ovarian tumors, just like other malignancy [121]. However, how the AHR binding pathway and EMT interact and influence each other in tumor progression and resistance to chemotherapy warrants further research.

This study had several limitations. First, we noticed some limitations in the integrative analytic methods utilized in this study, because the gene set databases of GO terms and related biomolecular pathways did not completely contain or fully define all functionomes of humans. False positivity was attributed to the heterogenicity of disparate cellular histopathological compositions and the indistinguishable elements of different gene sets among the chosen tumor and control samples, and detection by the GSR model was uncertain due to missed errors and untransformed GSR indices if the expression levels were undetectable when converting levels for ordering gene expression. However, these disadvantages may not be obvious in the overall results coupled with the statistically significant high sensitivity, specificity, and accuracy of this experiment. To eliminate these problems in the future, a more precise programming syntax design and more specified sample screening are required. The second limitation is the uneven distribution of case groups. The numbers of serous BOTs, serous ovarian carcinomas, and normal control samples are quite different, and even in the largest population of serous ovarian carcinomas, the numbers of tumors in each stage are quite different. According to the known proportions of serous ovarian tumors, serous ovarian carcinomas account for more EOCs than BOTs, and early stages of serous ovarian carcinomas are usually difficult to diagnose, resulting in fewer diagnoses than at advanced stages. The number of specimens collected for subsequent clinical verification also fits this situation. Although the number of clinical samples is small, with the support of the support vector machine (SVM) used in this study, the preliminary results of this multidisciplinary comprehensive analysis are reliable with high sensitivity, specificity, and accuracy. Even a relatively small number could obtain statistically significant results through IHC verification. Perhaps a more intact gene expression profile database could be constructed to decrease individual discrepancies among ethnic groups in retrospective or prospective cohort studies conducted on a larger scale globally. Third, this study only investigated the common pathogenetic mechanisms of serous ovarian tumors. However, due to the current lack of research, the small number of clinical specimens, and limited funds, data gathered from the GO term database are somewhat obstructed, especially data of serous BOT. Nevertheless, the results are clear and statistically significant, as determined by clinical verification with the immunostaining method. In the future, it may be necessary to gather more specimens, examine more global academic research, and utilize databases of various subtypes to compare and investigate more profoundly and comprehensively the pathogenetic mechanisms with the aid of large-scale experimental tests and funding.

In summary, to investigate potential crucial pathogenetic mechanisms, we performed an integrated GO-based analysis to obtain global genome-wide expression profiles individually and explore meaningful dysregulated functionomes, dysfunctional pathways, and relevant biomarkers of EMT among assorted groups of serous ovarian tumors with the support of elementary machine learning. Based on the above conclusions, we proposed the inferred hypothesis for the formative process of serous ovarian tumor that activated AHR could cooperate with SRC in the cytoplasm to enter cell nuclei and then bind to ARNT together with TBP to act on DNA for initiating targeted AHR-responsive genes to cause tumor or cancer initiation. Besides, biomarker of EMT such as SNAI2 in the tumor microenvironment could also facilitate EMT process accompanied with tumorigenesis (Figure 5). These results provided new directions for understanding the tumorigenesis of serous ovarian tumors and more potential crucial targets for the identification, treatment, monitoring, and even prevention of recurrence combined with targeted therapies as precision medicine in the future.

5. Conclusions

Serous ovarian tumors, consisting mainly of serous ovarian carcinoma and serous BOT, are epithelial tumors of the ovary with distinctive characteristics for each subtype. In this study, we made use of integrative analytic methods to select the top 25 significant common GO terms as dysregulated functionomes reclassified into three crucial categories (metabolic, immunological, and other effects; membrane and transport-related effects; and cellular cycle and signaling-related effects) and acquired 13 corresponding DEGs with high probability through cross comparison. For the first time, the dysfunctional AHR binding pathway accompanied with 10 corresponding DEGs was found significantly to be participated in tumorigenesis of both serous BOT and serous ovarian carcinoma and five vital biomarkers related to EMT were searched and gathered for this analytic study. Finally, four important DEGs (SRC, ARNT, TBP, and SNAI2) were compiled to have distinct effects on the survivals of serous ovarian tumor patients with the help of IHC staining for verification showing elevated expression among all clinical samples with increasing malignancy from serous BOT to early stages and to late stages of serous ovarian carcinomas. All acquired results initially supported the inference that dysregulated functionomes with active DEGs and relevant biomarkers could cooperate with the dysfunctional AHR binding pathway together with increased EMT effects in the tumor microenvironment to synergistically influence tumor initiation. These findings considerably contributed to elucidating the pathogenesis of serous ovarian tumors.

Supplementary Materials: The following are available online at https://www.mdpi.com/article/10.3390/biomedicines9080866/s1, Table S1, Detailed informative data of all collected samples. Table S2, Sensitivity, specificity, and accuracy of binary classification and prediction by supervised machine learning. Table S3, The whole deregulated GO terms of serous ovarian tumors. Table S4, The top 25 common dysregulated GO terms among the five case groups (serous BOT and all stages of serous ovarian carcinoma). Table S5, The whole dysfunctional GO pathways for serous ovarian tumors. Table S6, All IHC scores for relevant biomarkers of clinical samples and detailed clinical characteristics of the patients.

Author Contributions: Conceptualization, K.-M.S. and C.-M.C.; methodology, K.-M.S. and Y.-F.L.; software, C.-M.C. and Y.-F.L.; validation, H.-W.G., Y.-F.L., and K.-M.S.; formal analysis, L.-C.L. and C.-C.C. (Chia-Ching Chang); investigation, K.-H.L., Y.-H.L., and L.-C.L.; resources, M.-H.Y., Y.-H.L., and C.-C.C. (Chia-Ching Chang); data curation, H.-W.G., C.-M.C., and K.-H.L.; writing—original draft preparation, K.-M.S. and Y.-F.L.; writing—review and editing, K.-M.S. and C.-C.C. (Cheng-Chang Chang); visualization, K.-M.S. and H.-W.G.; supervision, M.-H.Y. and C.-C.C. (Cheng-Chang Chang); funding acquisition, K.-M.S., Y.-F.L., and C.-C.C. (Cheng-Chang Chang). All authors have read and agreed to the published version of the manuscript.

Funding: This research was supported in part and funded individually by the following grants from the Ministry of Science and Technology, R.O.C. (MOST 110-2321-B-016-002); the Tri-Service General Hospital (TSGH-D-109189, TSGH-D-109203, TSGH-D-110136, TSGH-D-110172, and TSGH-E-110230), the Teh-Tzer Study Group for Human Medical Research Foundation, the Veterans General Hospital, Tri-Service General Hospital and Academia Sinica Joint Research Programs (VTA110-T-4-1).

Institutional Review Board Statement: The study was conducted according to the guidelines of the Declaration of Helsinki and approved by the Institutional Review Board of the Tri-Service General Hospital, National Defense Medical Center for agreement of the study (2-107-05-043, approved on 26 October 2018; 2-108-05-091, approved on 20 May 2019).

Informed Consent Statement: Informed consent was obtained from all subjects involved in the study.

Data Availability Statement: The gene set databases of microarrays expression profiles are publicly available and downloaded from the National Center for Biotechnology Information (NCBI) Gene Expression Omnibus (GEO) repository (https://www.ncbi.nlm.nih.gov/geo/, accessed on 5 June 2021).

Acknowledgments: We would like to thank Kuo-Chih Su and Hui-Yin Su for figure editing.

Conflicts of Interest: The authors declare no conflict of interest.

References

1. Russell, P. The pathological assessment of ovarian neoplasms. I: Introduction to the common 'epithelial'tumours and analysis of benign 'epithelial'tumours. *Pathology* **1979**, *11*, 5–26. [CrossRef] [PubMed]
2. Iwabuchi, H.; Sakamoto, M.; Sakunaga, H.; Ma, Y.-Y.; Carcangiu, M.L.; Pinkel, D.; Yang-Feng, T.L.; Gray, J.W. Genetic analysis of benign, low-grade, and high-grade ovarian tumors. *Cancer Res.* **1995**, *55*, 6172–6180.
3. Allemani, C.; Weir, H.K.; Carreira, H.; Harewood, R.; Spika, D.; Wang, X.-S.; Bannon, F.; Ahn, J.V.; Johnson, C.J. Bonaventure, A. Global surveillance of cancer survival 1995–2009: Analysis of individual data for 25,676,887 patients from 279 population-based registries in 67 countries (CONCORD-2). *Lancet* **2015**, *385*, 977–1010. [CrossRef]
4. Runnebaum, I.B.; Stickeler, E. Epidemiological and molecular aspects of ovarian cancer risk. *J. Cancer Res. Clin. Oncol.* **2001**, *127*, 73–79. [CrossRef]
5. Karnezis, A.N.; Cho, K.R.; Gilks, C.B.; Pearce, C.L.; Huntsman, D.G. The disparate origins of ovarian cancers: Pathogenesis and prevention strategies. *Nat. Rev. Cancer* **2017**, *17*, 65. [CrossRef] [PubMed]
6. Jayson, G.C.; Kohn, E.C.; Kitchener, H.C.; Ledermann, J.A. Ovarian cancer. *Lancet* **2014**, *384*, 1376–1388. [CrossRef]
7. Vargas, A.N. Natural history of ovarian cancer. *Ecancermedicalscience* **2014**, *8*, 1–10.
8. Chien, J.; Poole, E.M. Ovarian cancer prevention, screening, and early detection: Report from the 11th biennial ovarian cancer research symposium. *Int. J. Gynecol. Cancer* **2017**, *27*. [CrossRef]
9. Santillan, A.; Kim, Y.; Zahurak, M.; Gardner, G.; Giuntoli, R.; Shih, I.; Bristow, R. Differences of chemoresistance assay between invasive micropapillary/low-grade serous ovarian carcinoma and high-grade serous ovarian carcinoma. *Int. J. Gynecol. Cancer* **2007**, *17*, 601–606. [CrossRef]
10. Song, T.; Lee, Y.-Y.; Choi, C.H.; Kim, T.-J.; Lee, J.-W.; Bae, D.-S.; Kim, B.-G. Histologic distribution of borderline ovarian tumors worldwide: A systematic review. *J. Gynecol. Oncol.* **2013**, *24*, 44–51. [CrossRef]
11. Yasmeen, S.; Hannan, A.; Sheikh, F.; Syed, A.A.; Siddiqui, N. Borderline tumors of the ovary: A clinicopathological study. *Pak. J. Med Sci.* **2017**, *33*, 369. [CrossRef]
12. Silverberg, S.G.; Bell, D.A.; Kurman, R.J.; Seidman, J.D.; Prat, J.; Ronnett, B.M.; Copeland, L.; Silva, E.; Gorstein, F.; Young, R.H. Borderline ovarian tumors: Key points and workshop summary. *Hum. Pathol.* **2004**, *35*, 910–917. [CrossRef]
13. Hauptmann, S.; Friedrich, K.; Redline, R.; Avril, S. Ovarian borderline tumors in the 2014 WHO classification: Evolving concepts and diagnostic criteria. *Virchows Arch.* **2017**, *470*, 125–142. [CrossRef] [PubMed]
14. Sun, Y.; Xu, J.; Jia, X. The Diagnosis, Treatment, Prognosis and Molecular Pathology of Borderline Ovarian Tumors: Current Status and Perspectives. *Cancer Manag. Res.* **2020**, *12*, 3651–3659. [CrossRef] [PubMed]
15. Lalwani, N.; Shanbhogue, A.K.; Vikram, R.; Nagar, A.; Jagirdar, J.; Prasad, S.R. Current update on borderline ovarian neoplasms. *Am. J. Roentgenol.* **2010**, *194*, 330–336. [CrossRef] [PubMed]
16. Trillsch, F.; Mahner, S.; Ruetzel, J.; Harter, P.; Ewald-Riegler, N.; Jaenicke, F.; Du Bois, A. Clinical management of borderline ovarian tumors. *Expert Rev. Anticancer Ther.* **2010**, *10*, 1115–1124. [CrossRef] [PubMed]
17. Fathalla, M. Incessant ovulation—A factor in ovarian neoplasia. *Lancet* **1971**, *2*, 163. [CrossRef]
18. Van Leeuwen, F.; Klip, H.; Mooij, T.M.; Van De Swaluw, A.; Lambalk, C.B.; Kortman, M.; Laven, J.; Jansen, C.; Helmerhorst, F.; Cohlen, B. Risk of borderline and invasive ovarian tumours after ovarian stimulation for in vitro fertilization in a large Dutch cohort. *Hum. Reprod.* **2011**, *26*, 3456–3465. [CrossRef]
19. Riman, T.; Dickman, P.W.; Nilsson, S.; Correia, N.; Nordlinder, H.; Magnusson, C.M.; Persson, I.R. Risk factors for epithelial borderline ovarian tumors: Results of a Swedish case–control study. *Gynecol. Oncol.* **2001**, *83*, 575–585. [CrossRef] [PubMed]
20. Mayr, D.; Hirschmann, A.; Löhrs, U.; Diebold, J. KRAS and BRAF mutations in ovarian tumors: A comprehensive study of invasive carcinomas, borderline tumors and extraovarian implants. *Gynecol. Oncol.* **2006**, *103*, 883–887. [CrossRef] [PubMed]
21. Ho, C.-L.; Kurman, R.J.; Dehari, R.; Wang, T.-L.; Shih, I.-M. Mutations of BRAF and KRAS precede the development of ovarian serous borderline tumors. *Cancer Res.* **2004**, *64*, 6915–6918. [CrossRef]
22. Anglesio, M.S.; Arnold, J.M.; George, J.; Tinker, A.V.; Tothill, R.; Waddell, N.; Simms, L.; Locandro, B.; Fereday, S.; Traficante, N. Mutation of ERBB2 provides a novel alternative mechanism for the ubiquitous activation of RAS-MAPK in ovarian serous low malignant potential tumors. *Mol. Cancer Res.* **2008**, *6*, 1678–1690. [CrossRef] [PubMed]
23. El-Balat, A.; Schmeil, I.; Gasimli, K.; Sänger, N.; Karn, T.; Ahr, A.; Becker, S.; Arsenic, R.; Holtrich, U.; Engels, K. Claudin-1 is linked to presence of implants and micropapillary pattern in serous borderline epithelial tumours of the ovary. *J. Clin. Pathol.* **2018**, *71*, 1060–1064. [CrossRef]
24. Malpica, A.; Wong, K.-K. The molecular pathology of ovarian serous borderline tumors. *Ann. Oncol.* **2016**, *27* (Suppl. S1), i16–i19. [CrossRef] [PubMed]

25. Ozretić, P.; Trnski, D.; Musani, V.; Maurac, I.; Kalafatić, D.; Orešković, S.; Levanat, S.; Sabol, M. Non-canonical Hedgehog signaling activation in ovarian borderline tumors and ovarian carcinomas. *Int. J. Oncol.* **2017**, *51*, 1869–1877. [CrossRef]
26. Hirst, J.; Crow, J.; Godwin, A. Ovarian cancer genetics: Subtypes and risk factors. In *Ovarian Cancer—From Pathogenesis to Treatment*; Devaja, O., Ed.; IntechOpen: London, UK, 2018.
27. Verhaak, R.G.; Tamayo, P.; Yang, J.-Y.; Hubbard, D.; Zhang, H.; Creighton, C.J.; Fereday, S.; Lawrence, M.; Carter, S.L.; Mermel, C.H. Prognostically relevant gene signatures of high-grade serous ovarian carcinoma. *J. Clin. Investig.* **2012**, *123*, 517–525. [CrossRef]
28. Ducie, J.; Dao, F.; Considine, M.; Olvera, N.; Shaw, P.A.; Kurman, R.J.; Shih, I.-M.; Soslow, R.A.; Cope, L.; Levine, D.A. Molecular analysis of high-grade serous ovarian carcinoma with and without associated serous tubal intra-epithelial carcinoma. *Nat. Commun.* **2017**, *8*, 1–9. [CrossRef] [PubMed]
29. Network, C.G.A.R. Integrated genomic analyses of ovarian carcinoma. *Nature* **2011**, *474*, 609. [CrossRef]
30. Cooke, S.L.; Ng, C.K.; Melnyk, N.; Garcia, M.J.; Hardcastle, T.; Temple, J.; Langdon, S.; Huntsman, D.; Brenton, J.D. Genomic analysis of genetic heterogeneity and evolution in high-grade serous ovarian carcinoma. *Oncogene* **2010**, *29*, 4905–4913. [CrossRef]
31. Javadi, S.; Ganeshan, D.M.; Qayyum, A.; Iyer, R.B.; Bhosale, P. Ovarian cancer, the revised FIGO staging system, and the role of imaging. *Am. J. Roentgenol.* **2016**, *206*, 1351–1360. [CrossRef]
32. Zeppernick, F.; Meinhold-Heerlein, I. The new FIGO staging system for ovarian, fallopian tube, and primary peritoneal cancer. *Arch. Gynecol. Obstet.* **2014**, *290*, 839–842. [CrossRef] [PubMed]
33. Yemelyanova, A.; Vang, R.; Kshirsagar, M.; Lu, D.; Marks, M.A.; Shih, I.M.; Kurman, R.J. Immunohistochemical staining patterns of p53 can serve as a surrogate marker for TP53 mutations in ovarian carcinoma: An immunohistochemical and nucleotide sequencing analysis. *Mod. Pathol.* **2011**, *24*, 1248–1253. [CrossRef]
34. Mota, A.; Triviño, J.C.; Rojo-Sebastian, A.; Martínez-Ramírez, Á.; Chiva, L.; González-Martín, A.; Garcia, J.F.; Garcia-Sanz, P.; Moreno-Bueno, G. Intra-tumor heterogeneity in TP53 null high grade serous ovarian carcinoma progression. *BMC Cancer* **2015**, *15*, 1–11. [CrossRef] [PubMed]
35. McAlpine, J.N.; Porter, H.; Köbel, M.; Nelson, B.H.; Prentice, L.M.; Kalloger, S.E.; Senz, J.; Milne, K.; Ding, J.; Shah, S.P. BRCA1 and BRCA2 mutations correlate with TP53 abnormalities and presence of immune cell infiltrates in ovarian high-grade serous carcinoma. *Mod. Pathol.* **2012**, *25*, 740–750. [CrossRef]
36. Brachova, P.; Thiel, K.W.; Leslie, K.K. The consequence of oncomorphic TP53 mutations in ovarian cancer. *Int. J. Mol. Sci.* **2013**, *14*, 19257–19275. [CrossRef]
37. Moschetta, M.; George, A.; Kaye, S.; Banerjee, S. BRCA somatic mutations and epigenetic BRCA modifications in serous ovarian cancer. *Ann. Oncol.* **2016**, *27*, 1449–1455. [CrossRef]
38. Pal, T.; Permuth-Wey, J.; Betts, J.A.; Krischer, J.P.; Fiorica, J.; Arango, H.; LaPolla, J.; Hoffman, M.; Martino, M.A.; Wakeley, K. BRCA1 and BRCA2 mutations account for a large proportion of ovarian carcinoma cases. *Cancer Interdiscip. Int. J. Am. Cancer Soc.* **2005**, *104*, 2807–2816.
39. Bai, H.; Cao, D.; Yang, J.; Li, M.; Zhang, Z.; Shen, K. Genetic and epigenetic heterogeneity of epithelial ovarian cancer and the clinical implications for molecular targeted therapy. *J. Cell. Mol. Med.* **2016**, *20*, 581–593. [CrossRef]
40. Tew, W.P.; Lacchetti, C.; Ellis, A.; Maxian, K.; Banerjee, S.; Bookman, M.; Jones, M.B.; Lee, J.-M.; Lheureux, S.; Liu, J.F. PARP inhibitors in the management of ovarian cancer: ASCO guideline. *Obstet. Gynecol. Surv.* **2020**, *75*, 739–741. [CrossRef]
41. Franzese, E.; Centonze, S.; Diana, A.; Carlino, F.; Guerrera, L.P.; Di Napoli, M.; De Vita, F.; Pignata, S.; Ciardiello, F.; Orditura, M. PARP inhibitors in ovarian cancer. *Cancer Treat. Rev.* **2019**, *73*, 1–9. [CrossRef] [PubMed]
42. Gadducci, A.; Guerrieri, M.E. PARP inhibitors in epithelial ovarian cancer: State of art and perspectives of clinical research. *Anticancer. Res.* **2016**, *36*, 2055–2064.
43. Gomez, M.K.; Illuzzi, G.; Colomer, C.; Churchman, M.; Hollis, R.L.; O'Connor, M.J.; Gourley, C.; Leo, E.; Melton, D.W. Identifying and Overcoming Mechanisms of PARP Inhibitor Resistance in Homologous Recombination Repair-Deficient and Repair-Proficient High Grade Serous Ovarian Cancer Cells. *Cancers* **2020**, *12*, 1503. [CrossRef]
44. Xie, H.; Wang, W.; Xia, B.; Jin, W.; Lou, G. Therapeutic applications of PARP inhibitors in ovarian cancer. *Biomed. Pharmacother.* **2020**, *127*, 110204. [CrossRef] [PubMed]
45. Takaya, H.; Nakai, H.; Takamatsu, S.; Mandai, M.; Matsumura, N. Homologous recombination deficiency status-based classification of high-grade serous ovarian carcinoma. *Sci. Rep.* **2020**, *10*, 1–8. [CrossRef] [PubMed]
46. Ahmed, N.; Kadife, E.; Raza, A.; Short, M.; Jubinsky, P.T.; Kannourakis, G. Ovarian cancer, cancer stem cells and current treatment strategies: A potential role of magmas in the current treatment methods. *Cells* **2020**, *9*, 719. [CrossRef] [PubMed]
47. Rose, M.; Burgess, J.T.; O'Byrne, K.; Richard, D.J.; Bolderson, E. PARP inhibitors: Clinical relevance, mechanisms of action and tumor resistance. *Front. Cell Dev. Biol.* **2020**, *8*, 8. [CrossRef] [PubMed]
48. Bonneau, C.; Rouzier, R.; Geyl, C.; Cortez, A.; Castela, M.; Lis, R.; Daraï, E.; Touboul, C. Predictive markers of chemoresistance in advanced stages epithelial ovarian carcinoma. *Gynecol. Oncol.* **2015**, *136*, 112–120. [CrossRef]
49. Roy, L.; Cowden Dahl, K.D. Can stemness and chemoresistance be therapeutically targeted via signaling pathways in ovarian cancer? *Cancers* **2018**, *10*, 241. [CrossRef]
50. Davidson, B.; Trope, C.G.; Reich, R. Epithelial–mesenchymal transition in ovarian carcinoma. *Front. Oncol.* **2012**, *2*, 33. [CrossRef]
51. Ashrafizadeh, M.; Zarrabi, A.; Hushmandi, K.; Kalantari, M.; Mohammadinejad, R.; Javaheri, T.; Sethi, G. Association of the epithelial–mesenchymal transition (EMT) with cisplatin resistance. *Int. J. Mol. Sci.* **2020**, *21*, 4002. [CrossRef]

52. Iwatsuki, M.; Mimori, K.; Yokobori, T.; Ishi, H.; Beppu, T.; Nakamori, S.; Baba, H.; Mori, M. Epithelial–mesenchymal transition in cancer development and its clinical significance. *Cancer Sci.* **2010**, *101*, 293–299. [CrossRef]
53. Haslehurst, A.M.; Koti, M.; Dharsee, M.; Nuin, P.; Evans, K.; Geraci, J.; Childs, T.; Chen, J.; Li, J.; Weberpals, J. EMT transcription factors snail and slug directly contribute to cisplatin resistance in ovarian cancer. *BMC Cancer* **2012**, *12*, 1–10. [CrossRef]
54. Ribatti, D.; Tamma, R.; Annese, T. Epithelial-mesenchymal transition in cancer: A historical overview. *Transl. Oncol.* **2020**, *13*, 100773. [CrossRef]
55. Voulgari, A.; Pintzas, A. Epithelial–mesenchymal transition in cancer metastasis: Mechanisms, markers and strategies to overcome drug resistance in the clinic. *Biochim. Biophys. Acta (BBA) Rev. Cancer* **2009**, *1796*, 75–90. [CrossRef]
56. Rohnalter, V.; Roth, K.; Finkernagel, F.; Adhikary, T.; Obert, J.; Dorzweiler, K.; Bensberg, M.; Müller-Brüsselbach, S.; Müller, R. A multi-stage process including transient polyploidization and EMT precedes the emergence of chemoresistant ovarian carcinoma cells with a dedifferentiated and pro-inflammatory secretory phenotype. *Oncotarget* **2015**, *6*, 40005. [CrossRef]
57. Loret, N.; Denys, H.; Tummers, P.; Berx, G. The role of epithelial-to-mesenchymal plasticity in ovarian cancer progression and therapy resistance. *Cancers* **2019**, *11*, 838. [CrossRef] [PubMed]
58. Chang, C.-M.; Chuang, C.-M.; Wang, M.-L.; Yang, Y.-P.; Chuang, J.-H.; Yang, M.-J.; Yen, M.-S.; Chiou, S.-H.; Chang, C.-C. Gene set− based integrative analysis revealing two distinct functional regulation patterns in four common subtypes of epithelial ovarian cancer. *Int. J. Mol. Sci.* **2016**, *17*, 1272. [CrossRef] [PubMed]
59. Chang, C.-M.; Chuang, C.-M.; Wang, M.-L.; Yang, M.-J.; Chang, C.-C.; Yen, M.-S.; Chiou, S.-H. Gene set-based functionome analysis of pathogenesis in epithelial ovarian serous carcinoma and the molecular features in different FIGO stages. *Int. J. Mol. Sci.* **2016**, *17*, 886. [CrossRef] [PubMed]
60. Chang, C.-M.; Wang, M.-L.; Lu, K.-H.; Yang, Y.-P.; Juang, C.-M.; Wang, P.-H.; Hsu, R.-J.; Yu, M.-H.; Chang, C.-C. Integrating the dysregulated inflammasome-based molecular functionome in the malignant transformation of endometriosis-associated ovarian carcinoma. *Oncotarget* **2018**, *9*, 3704. [CrossRef]
61. Chang, C.-M.; Yang, Y.-P.; Chuang, J.-H.; Chuang, C.-M.; Lin, T.-W.; Wang, P.-H.; Yu, M.-H.; Chang, C.-C. Discovering the deregulated molecular functions involved in malignant transformation of endometriosis to endometriosis-associated ovarian carcinoma using a data-driven, function-based analysis. *Int. J. Mol. Sci.* **2017**, *18*, 2345. [CrossRef]
62. Chang, C.-C.; Su, K.-M.; Lu, K.-H.; Lin, C.-K.; Wang, P.-H.; Li, H.-Y.; Wang, M.-L.; Lin, C.-K.; Yu, M.-H.; Chang, C.-M. Key immunological functions involved in the progression of epithelial ovarian serous carcinoma discovered by the gene ontology-based immunofunctionome analysis. *Int. J. Mol. Sci.* **2018**, *19*, 3311. [CrossRef] [PubMed]
63. Su, K.-M.; Lin, T.-W.; Liu, L.-C.; Yang, Y.-P.; Wang, M.-L.; Tsai, P.-H.; Wang, P.-H.; Yu, M.-H.; Chang, C.-M.; Chang, C.-C. The Potential Role of Complement System in the Progression of Ovarian Clear Cell Carcinoma Inferred from the Gene Ontology-Based Immunofunctionome Analysis. *Int. J. Mol. Sci.* **2020**, *21*, 2824. [CrossRef]
64. Chang, C.-M.; Li, Y.-F.; Lin, H.-C.; Lu, K.-H.; Lin, T.-W.; Liu, L.-C.; Su, K.-M.; Chang, C.-C. Dysregulated Immunological Functionome and Dysfunctional Metabolic Pathway Recognized for the Pathogenesis of Borderline Ovarian Tumors by Integrative Polygenic Analytics. *Int. J. Mol. Sci.* **2021**, *22*, 4105. [CrossRef]
65. Eddy, J.A.; Hood, L.; Price, N.D.; Geman, D. Identifying tightly regulated and variably expressed networks by Differential Rank Conservation (DIRAC). *PLoS Comput. Biol.* **2010**, *6*, e1000792. [CrossRef]
66. Benjamini, Y.; Hochberg, Y. Controlling the false discovery rate: A practical and powerful approach to multiple testing. *J. R. Stat. Soc. Ser. B (Methodol.)* **1995**, *57*, 289–300. [CrossRef]
67. Robin, X.; Turck, N.; Hainard, A.; Tiberti, N.; Lisacek, F.; Sanchez, J.-C.; Müller, M. pROC: An open-source package for R and S+ to analyze and compare ROC curves. *BMC Bioinform.* **2011**, *12*, 1–8. [CrossRef] [PubMed]
68. Van Diest, P.J.; van Dam, P.; Henzen-Logmans, S.C.; Berns, E.; Van der Burg, M.; Green, J.; Vergote, I. A scoring system for immunohistochemical staining: Consensus report of the task force for basic research of the EORTC-GCCG. European Organization for Research and Treatment of Cancer-Gynaecological Cancer Cooperative Group. *J. Clin. Pathol.* **1997**, *50*, 801. [CrossRef]
69. Charafe-Jauffret, E.; Tarpin, C.; Bardou, V.J.; Bertucci, F.; Ginestier, C.; Braud, A.C.; Puig, B.; Geneix, J.; Hassoun, J.; Birnbaum, D. Immunophenotypic analysis of inflammatory breast cancers: Identification of an 'inflammatory signature'. *J. Pathol.* **2004**, *202*, 265–273. [CrossRef]
70. Dessimoz, C.; Škunca, N. *The Gene Ontology Handbook*; Springer: Basingstoke, UK, 2017.
71. Liberzon, A.; Birger, C.; Thorvaldsdóttir, H.; Ghandi, M.; Mesirov, J.P.; Tamayo, P. The molecular signatures database hallmark gene set collection. *Cell Syst.* **2015**, *1*, 417–425. [CrossRef]
72. Zeisberg, M.; Neilson, E.G. Biomarkers for epithelial-mesenchymal transitions. *J. Clin. Investig.* **2009**, *119*, 1429–1437. [CrossRef]
73. Győrffy, B.; Lánczky, A.; Szállási, Z. Implementing an online tool for genome-wide validation of survival-associated biomarkers in ovarian-cancer using microarray data from 1287 patients. *Endocr. Relat. Cancer* **2012**, *19*, 197–208. [CrossRef]
74. Song, G.; Chen, L.; Zhang, B.; Song, Q.; Yu, Y.; Moore, C.; Wang, T.-L.; Shih, I.-M.; Zhang, H.; Chan, D.W. Proteome-wide tyrosine phosphorylation analysis reveals dysregulated signaling pathways in ovarian tumors*[S]. *Mol. Cell. Proteom.* **2019**, *18*, 448–460. [CrossRef] [PubMed]
75. Cheng, L.; Zheng, X.; Ling, R.; Gao, J.; Leung, K.-S.; Wong, M.-H.; Yang, S.; Liu, Y.; Dong, M.; Bai, H. Whole Transcriptome Analyses Identify Pairwise Gene Circuit Motif in Serous Ovarian Cancer. 2021. PREPRINT (Version 1). Available online: https://doi.org/10.21203/rs.3 (accessed on 20 July 2021).

76. Lassus, H.; Sihto, H.; Leminen, A.; Nordling, S.; Joensuu, H.; Nupponen, N.; Butzow, R. Genetic alterations and protein expression of KIT and PDGFRA in serous ovarian carcinoma. *Br. J. Cancer* **2004**, *91*, 2048–2055. [CrossRef]
77. Lee, Y.J.; Kim, D.; Shim, J.E.; Bae, S.J.; Jung, Y.J.; Kim, S.; Lee, H.; Kim, S.H.; Jo, S.B.; Lee, J.Y. Genomic profiling of the residual disease of advanced high-grade serous ovarian cancer after neoadjuvant chemotherapy. *Int. J. Cancer* **2020**, *146*, 1851–1861. [CrossRef] [PubMed]
78. Hanrahan, A.J.; Schultz, N.; Westfal, M.L.; Sakr, R.A.; Giri, D.D.; Scarperi, S.; Janikariman, M.; Olvera, N.; Stevens, E.V.; She, Q.-B. Genomic complexity and AKT dependence in serous ovarian cancer. *Cancer Discov.* **2012**, *2*, 56–67. [CrossRef]
79. Mabuchi, S.; Kuroda, H.; Takahashi, R.; Sasano, T. The PI3K/AKT/mTOR pathway as a therapeutic target in ovarian cancer. *Gynecol. Oncol.* **2015**, *137*, 173–179. [CrossRef] [PubMed]
80. Yu, T.; Wang, C.; Tong, R. ERBB2 gene expression silencing involved in ovarian cancer cell migration and invasion through mediating MAPK1/MAPK3 signaling pathway. *Eur. Rev. Med. Pharmacol. Sci.* **2020**, *24*, 5267–5280. [PubMed]
81. Schaner, M.E.; Ross, D.T.; Ciaravino, G.; Sørlie, T.; Troyanskaya, O.; Diehn, M.; Wang, Y.C.; Duran, G.E.; Sikic, T.L.; Caldeira, S. Gene expression patterns in ovarian carcinomas. *Mol. Biol. Cell* **2003**, *14*, 4376–4386. [CrossRef]
82. Tocci, P.; Cianfrocca, R.; Rosanò, L.; Sestito, R.; Di Castro, V.; Blandino, G.; Bagnato, A. Endothelin-1 receptor/β-arrestin1 is an actionable node that regulates YAP/TAZ signaling and chemoresistance in high-grade ovarian cancer. In Proceedings of the American Association for Cancer Research (AACR) Meeting, Washington, DC, USA, 1–5 April 2017.
83. Wu, M.; Sun, Y.; Wu, J.; Liu, G. Identification of Hub Genes in High-Grade Serous Ovarian Cancer Using Weighted Gene Co-Expression Network Analysis. *Med. Sci. Monit. Int. Med. J. Exp. Clin. Res.* **2020**, *26*, e922107. [CrossRef]
84. Nam, E.J.; Yoon, H.; Kim, S.W.; Kim, H.; Kim, Y.T.; Kim, J.H.; Kim, J.W.; Kim, S. MicroRNA expression profiles in serous ovarian carcinoma. *Clin. Cancer Res.* **2008**, *14*, 2690–2695. [CrossRef]
85. Hu, Y.; Pan, J.; Shah, P.; Ao, M.; Thomas, S.N.; Liu, Y.; Chen, L.; Schnaubelt, M.; Clark, D.J.; Rodriguez, H. Integrated proteomic and glycoproteomic characterization of human high-grade serous ovarian carcinoma. *Cell Rep.* **2020**, *33*, 108276. [CrossRef]
86. Ray, A.; Fornsaglio, J.; Dogan, S.; Hedau, S.; Naik, S.D.; De, A. Gynaecological cancers and leptin: A focus on the endometrium and ovary. *Facts Views Vis. ObGyn* **2018**, *10*, 5.
87. Zhang, S.; Lu, Z.; Mao, W.; Ahmed, A.A.; Yang, H.; Zhou, J.; Jennings, N.; Rodriguez-Aguayo, C.; Lopez-Berestein, G.; Miranda, R. CDK5 regulates paclitaxel sensitivity in ovarian cancer cells by modulating AKT activation, p21Cip1-and p27Kip1-mediated G1 cell cycle arrest and apoptosis. *PLoS ONE* **2015**, *10*, e0131833. [CrossRef] [PubMed]
88. Ouellet, V.; Provencher, D.M.; Maugard, C.M.; Le Page, C.; Ren, F.; Lussier, C.; Novak, J.; Ge, B.; Hudson, T.J.; Tonin, P.N. Discrimination between serous low malignant potential and invasive epithelial ovarian tumors using molecular profiling. *Oncogene* **2005**, *24*, 4672–4687. [CrossRef] [PubMed]
89. Xu, J.; Wu, R.-C.; O'malley, B.W. Normal and cancer-related functions of the p160 steroid receptor co-activator (SRC) family. *Nat. Rev. Cancer* **2009**, *9*, 615–630. [CrossRef] [PubMed]
90. Wiener, J.R.; Windham, T.C.; Estrella, V.C.; Parikh, N.U.; Thall, P.F.; Deavers, M.T.; Bast, R.C., Jr.; Mills, G.B.; Gallick, G.E. Activated SRC protein tyrosine kinase is overexpressed in late-stage human ovarian cancers. *Gynecol. Oncol.* **2003**, *88*, 73–79. [CrossRef] [PubMed]
91. Lui, G.Y.; Shaw, R.; Schaub, F.X.; Stork, I.N.; Gurley, K.E.; Bridgwater, C.; Diaz, R.L.; Rosati, R.; Swan, H.A.; Ince, T.A. BET, SRC, and BCL2 family inhibitors are synergistic drug combinations with PARP inhibitors in ovarian cancer. *EBioMedicine* **2020**, *60*, 102988. [CrossRef]
92. Beischlag, T.V.; Morales, J.L.; Hollingshead, B.D.; Perdew, G.H. The aryl hydrocarbon receptor complex and the control of gene expression. *Crit. Rev. ™ Eukaryot. Gene Expr.* **2008**, *18*, 207–250. [CrossRef] [PubMed]
93. Abel, J.; Haarmann-Stemmann, T. An introduction to the molecular basics of aryl hydrocarbon receptor biology. *Biol. Chem.* **2010**, *391*, 1235–1248. [CrossRef]
94. Larigot, L.; Juricek, L.; Dairou, J.; Coumoul, X. AhR signaling pathways and regulatory functions. *Biochim. Open* **2018**, *7*, 1–9. [CrossRef]
95. Wang, Z.; Snyder, M.; Kenison, J.E.; Yang, K.; Lara, B.; Lydell, E.; Bennani, K.; Novikov, O.; Federico, A.; Monti, S. How the AHR Became Important in Cancer: The Role of Chronically Active AHR in Cancer Aggression. *Int. J. Mol. Sci.* **2021**, *22*, 387. [CrossRef]
96. Paris, A.; Tardif, N.; Galibert, M.-D.; Corre, S. AhR and Cancer: From Gene Profiling to Targeted Therapy. *Int. J. Mol. Sci.* **2021**, *22*, 752. [CrossRef]
97. Kumar, M.B.; Perdew, G.H. Nuclear receptor coactivator SRC-1 interacts with the Q-rich subdomain of the AhR and modulates its transactivation potential. *Gene Expr. J. Liver Res.* **1999**, *8*, 273–286.
98. Beischlag, T.V.; Wang, S.; Rose, D.W.; Torchia, J.; Reisz-Porszasz, S.; Muhammad, K.; Nelson, W.E.; Probst, M.R.; Rosenfeld, M.G.; Hankinson, O. Recruitment of the NCoA/SRC-1/p160 family of transcriptional coactivators by the aryl hydrocarbon receptor/aryl hydrocarbon receptor nuclear translocator complex. *Mol. Cell. Biol.* **2002**, *22*, 4319. [CrossRef]
99. Tomkiewicz, C.; Herry, L.; Bui, L.; Metayer, C.; Bourdeloux, M.; Barouki, R.; Coumoul, X. The aryl hydrocarbon receptor regulates focal adhesion sites through a non-genomic FAK/Src pathway. *Oncogene* **2013**, *32*, 1811–1820. [CrossRef]
100. Choudhary, M.; Malek, G. The aryl hydrocarbon receptor: A mediator and potential therapeutic target for ocular and non-ocular neurodegenerative diseases. *Int. J. Mol. Sci.* **2020**, *21*, 6777. [CrossRef]
101. Feng, S.; Cao, Z.; Wang, X. Role of aryl hydrocarbon receptor in cancer. *Biochim. Biophys. Acta (BBA) Rev. Cancer* **2013**, *1836*, 197–210. [CrossRef] [PubMed]

102. Mulero-Navarro, S.; Fernandez-Salguero, P.M. New trends in aryl hydrocarbon receptor biology. *Front. Cell Dev. Biol.* **2016**, *4*, 45. [CrossRef]
103. Piotrowska, H.; Kucinska, M.; Murias, M. Expression of CYP1A1, CYP1B1 and MnSOD in a panel of human cancer cell lines. *Mol. Cell. Biochem.* **2013**, *383*, 95–102. [CrossRef] [PubMed]
104. Akhtar, S.; Hourani, S.; Therachiyil, L.; Al-Dhfyan, A.; Agouni, A.; Zeidan, A.; Uddin, S.; Korashy, H.M. Epigenetic Regulation of Cancer Stem Cells by the Aryl Hydrocarbon Receptor Pathway. *Semin. Cancer Biol.* **2020**. [CrossRef] [PubMed]
105. Safe, S.; Lee, S.-O.; Jin, U.-H. Role of the aryl hydrocarbon receptor in carcinogenesis and potential as a drug target. *Toxicol. Sci.* **2013**, *135*, 1–16. [CrossRef]
106. Khorram, O.; Garthwaite, M.; Golos, T. Uterine and ovarian aryl hydrocarbon receptor (AHR) and aryl hydrocarbon receptor nuclear translocator (ARNT) mRNA expression in benign and malignant gynaecological conditions. *Mol. Hum. Reprod.* **2002**, *8*, 75–80. [CrossRef] [PubMed]
107. Tsuchiya, M.; Katoh, T.; Motoyama, H.; Sasaki, H.; Tsugane, S.; Ikenoue, T. Analysis of the AhR, ARNT, and AhRR gene polymorphisms: Genetic contribution to endometriosis susceptibility and severity. *Fertil. Steril.* **2005**, *84*, 454–458. [CrossRef] [PubMed]
108. Beedanagari, S.R.; Taylor, R.T.; Bui, P.; Wang, F.; Nickerson, D.W.; Hankinson, O. Role of epigenetic mechanisms in differential regulation of the dioxin-inducible human CYP1A1 and CYP1B1 genes. *Mol. Pharmacol.* **2010**, *78*, 608–616. [CrossRef] [PubMed]
109. Salani, R.; Backes, F.J.; Fung, M.F.K.; Holschneider, C.H.; Parker, L.P.; Bristow, R.E.; Goff, B.A. Posttreatment surveillance and diagnosis of recurrence in women with gynecologic malignancies: Society of Gynecologic Oncologists recommendations. *Am. J. Obstet. Gynecol.* **2011**, *204*, 466–478. [CrossRef] [PubMed]
110. Pokhriyal, R.; Hariprasad, R.; Kumar, L.; Hariprasad, G. Chemotherapy resistance in advanced ovarian cancer patients. *Biomark. Cancer* **2019**, *11*, 1179299X19860815. [CrossRef]
111. Jing, Y.; Han, Z.; Zhang, S.; Liu, Y.; Wei, L. Epithelial-Mesenchymal Transition in tumor microenvironment. *Cell Biosci.* **2011**, *1*, 1–7. [CrossRef]
112. Gao, D.; Vahdat, L.T.; Wong, S.; Chang, J.C.; Mittal, V. Microenvironmental regulation of epithelial–mesenchymal transitions in cancer. *Cancer Res.* **2012**, *72*, 4883–4889. [CrossRef]
113. Jung, H.-Y.; Fattet, L.; Yang, J. Molecular pathways: Linking tumor microenvironment to epithelial–mesenchymal transition in metastasis. *Clin. Cancer Res.* **2015**, *21*, 962–968. [CrossRef]
114. Mladinich, M.; Ruan, D.; Chan, C.-H. Tackling cancer stem cells via inhibition of EMT transcription factors. *Stem Cells Int.* **2016**, *2016*, 1–10. [CrossRef]
115. Kurrey, N.; Amit, K.; Bapat, S. Snail and Slug are major determinants of ovarian cancer invasiveness at the transcription level. *Gynecol. Oncol.* **2005**, *97*, 155–165. [CrossRef]
116. Ganesan, R.; Mallets, E.; Gomez-Cambronero, J. The transcription factors Slug (SNAI2) and Snail (SNAI1) regulate phospholipase D (PLD) promoter in opposite ways towards cancer cell invasion. *Mol. Oncol.* **2016**, *10*, 663–676. [CrossRef] [PubMed]
117. Kim, Y.-S.; Hwang, K.-A.; Hyun, S.-H.; Nam, K.-H.; Lee, C.-K.; Choi, K.-C. Bisphenol A and nonylphenol have the potential to stimulate the migration of ovarian cancer cells by inducing epithelial–mesenchymal transition via an estrogen receptor dependent pathway. *Chem. Res. Toxicol.* **2015**, *28*, 662–671. [CrossRef]
118. Oral, D.; Erkekoglu, P.; Kocer-Gumusel, B.; Chao, M.-W. Epithelial-mesenchymal transition: A special focus on phthalates and bisphenol a. *J. Environ. Pathol. Toxicol. Oncol.* **2016**, *35*, 43–58. [CrossRef]
119. Xu, Z.; Ding, W.; Deng, X. PM2. 5, fine particulate matter: A novel player in the epithelial-mesenchymal transition? *Front. Physiol.* **2019**, *10*, 1404. [CrossRef] [PubMed]
120. Lee, G.-A.; Hwang, K.-A.; Choi, K.-C. Roles of dietary phytoestrogens on the regulation of epithelial-mesenchymal transition in diverse cancer metastasis. *Toxins* **2016**, *8*, 162. [CrossRef] [PubMed]
121. Moretti, S.; Nucci, N.; Menicali, E.; Morelli, S.; Bini, V.; Colella, R.; Mandarano, M.; Sidoni, A.; Puxeddu, E. The aryl hydrocarbon receptor is expressed in thyroid carcinoma and appears to mediate epithelial-mesenchymal-transition. *Cancers* **2020**, *12*, 145. [CrossRef]

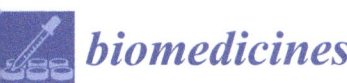

Article

Preliminary Study on the Expression of Testin, p16 and Ki-67 in the Cervical Intraepithelial Neoplasia

Aneta Popiel [1,*], Aleksandra Piotrowska [1], Patrycja Sputa-Grzegrzolka [2], Beata Smolarz [3], Hanna Romanowicz [3], Piotr Dziegiel [1,4], Marzenna Podhorska-Okolow [5] and Christopher Kobierzycki [1]

[1] Division of Histology and Embryology, Department of Human Morphology and Embryology, Wroclaw Medical University, 50-368 Wroclaw, Poland; aleksandra.piotrowska@umed.wroc.pl (A.P.); piotr.dziegiel@umed.wroc.pl (P.D.); christopher.kobierzycki@umed.wroc.pl (C.K.)
[2] Division of Anatomy, Department of Human Morphology and Embryology, Wroclaw Medical University, 50-368 Wroclaw, Poland; patrycja.sputa-grzegrzolka@umed.wroc.pl
[3] Department of Pathology, Polish Mother's Memorial Hospital Research Institute, 93-338 Lodz, Poland; smolbea@wp.pl (B.S.); hanna-romanowicz@wp.pl (H.R.)
[4] Department of Physiotherapy, University School of Physical Education, 51-612 Wroclaw, Poland
[5] Division of Ultrastructural Research, Wroclaw Medical University, 50-368 Wroclaw, Poland; marzenna.podhorska-okolow@umed.wroc.pl
* Correspondence: popielaneta1@gmail.com

Abstract: Cervical cancer is one of the most common malignant cancers in women worldwide. The 5-year survival rate is 65%; nevertheless, it depends on race, age, and clinical stage. In the oncogenesis of cervical cancer, persistent HPV infection plays a pivotal role. It disrupts the expression of key proteins as Ki-67, p16, involved in regulating the cell cycle. This study aimed to identify the potential role of testin in the diagnosis of cervical precancerous lesions (CIN). The study was performed on selected archival paraffin-embedded specimens of CIN1 (31), CIN2 (75), and CIN3 (123). Moderate positive correlation was observed between testin and Ki-67 as well as testin and p16 expression in all dysplastic lesions ($r = 0.4209$, $r = 0.5681$; $p < 0.0001$ for both). Statistical analysis showed stronger expression of the testin in dysplastic lesions vs. control group ($p < 0.0001$); moreover, expression was significantly higher in HSIL than LSIL group ($p < 0.0024$). In addition, a significantly stronger expression of testin was observed in CIN3 vs. CIN1 and CIN3 vs. CIN2. In our study, expression of Ki-67, p16, and testin increased gradually as the lesion progressed from LSIL to HSIL. The three markers complemented each other effectively, which may improve test sensitivity and specificity when used jointly.

Keywords: testin; p16 protein; cervical cancer; cervical neoplasia; immunohistochemistry

1. Introduction

Cervical cancer is one of the most common malignant cancers in women worldwide. Each year, over 580,000 new cases of cervical cancer are diagnosed [1]. The American Cancer Society estimates that 4290 women will die due to cervical cancer in 2021 in the United States. In 2018, the number of deaths worldwide was 311,000, 90% of which occurred in low- and middle-income countries. The 5-year survival rate is 65%; nevertheless, it depends on race, age, and clinical stage. In developing countries in Africa, Asia, and South America, cervical cancer causes over 50% of early deaths in women of childbearing age. The WHO (World Health Organization) invests great effort into decreasing mortality and morbidity by means of promoting both primary and secondary preventive care for cervical cancer. In May 2018, WHO announced its project to eliminate cervical cancer as a public health issue between 2020 and 2030, reducing the age-correlated incidence rate to 4/100,000. WHO developed a triple intervention plan, which includes scaling up vaccination against HPV, twice-lifetime cervical screenings up to 70%, and treatment of preinvasive lesions and invasive cancer to 90% [2]. Informing patients that HPV is an important cause of cervical cancer has led to significant advances in the primary and secondary prevention of cervical cancer. Ten years ago, the WHO introduced vaccines against two of the most cancerogenic types, HPV16 and HPV18. They are highly effective at preventing HPV infections when administered before sexual activity. Nowadays there are available vaccines against seven carcinogenic HPV types and two non-cancer types that cause warts [3]. Cervical cancer is most often diagnosed in women aged 35–44, whereas it rarely occurs before 20 years of age. Over 15% of all cases occur in women above 65 years of age; however, it is rare in women who undergo regular screening. The main risk factor of cervical cancer is persistent HPV infection. It promotes impaired growth and differentiation of cells, leading to dysplasia (cervical intraepithelial neoplasia, CIN) [4]. We distinguished three grades of cervical dysplasia: CIN1 (LSIL; low-grade squamous intraepithelial lesion), CIN2, and CIN3 (classified together as HSIL; high-grade squamous intraepithelial lesion). The risk of developing invasive cervical cancer from HSIL is approximately 20% (10–40% according to literature) [5–7]. In the oncogenesis of cervical cancer, persistent HPV infection plays a pivotal role as it is necessary for CIN changes to occur. In assessing the risk of progression of lesions and the proper selection of treatment, techniques of viral DNA identification are used, which may be helpful in the triage of patients with cytological diagnosis of atypical squamous cells of undetermined significance (ASCUS). HPV DNA tests are highly sensitive, but the specificity of HPV tests is low due to most HPV infections being naturally cleared [8]; this creates the need to search for more specific diagnostic methods. More specific markers of cervical cancer have been identified from HPV-induced oncogenesis studies. The oncogenic HPV viruses disrupt the expression of key proteins as Ki-67, p16 involved in regulating the cell cycle. Our study aimed to identify the potential role of testin protein in the diagnosis of cervical precancerous lesions. Research points to its possible role in cervical cancer, whereas in CIN it has not been analyzed yet [9,10]. In this article, we focus on the correlation between testin and known markers used in the diagnosis of cervical intraepithelial changes.

2. Materials and Methods

2.1. Material

The study was performed on selected archival paraffin-embedded specimens of CIN1 (31), CIN2 (75), and CIN3 (123). Patients aged from 25 to 86 years old were female (Table 1). The control group consisted of 125 cases of normal cervical tissue possessed from patients who underwent total hysterectomy due to uterine leiomyomas. Patients were operated on between 2014 and 2017 in the Polish Mother's Memorial Hospital in Lodz.

Table 1. Clinicopathological features of study group patients.

Feature	N	%
Age		
<35	119	51.97
35–45	75	32.75
>45	35	15.28
Cytology result		
CIN 1	31	13.5
CIN 2	75	32.8
CIN 3	123	53.7
Histology result		
LSIL	31	13.5
HSIL	198	86.5

2.2. TMA Construction

Hematoxylin and eosin-stained (HE) 6-μm thick paraffin sections were prepared to verify the histopathological diagnosis and assess the suitability of the sample for further analysis. In short, slides were scanned utilizing histologic scanner Pannoramic MIDI

(3DHistech Ltd., Sysmex Suisse AG, Horgen, Switzerland). Afterward, scans were examined by two independent pathologists who chose and electronically labeled areas of the CIN in the changed epithelium of the cervix. For TMA construction, from the corresponding paraffin donor blocks, triplicate tissue core punches (2 mm) for every case were obtained (TMA Grand Master; 3DHistech, Budapest, Hungary). The normal epithelial tissue of the cervix was marked as a control group.

2.3. Immunohistochemistry (IHC)

Immunohistochemical reactions were performed on 4 μm paraffin sections obtained from TMA blocks in an automated staining platform, Autostainer Link48 (Dako, Glostrup, Denmark). Deparaffinization, rehydration, and antigen retrieval was performed using EnVision FLEX Target Retrieval Solution (97 °C, 20 min; pH 6 for Ki-67 and pH 9 for p16 and testin) in PT-Link. The activity of endogenous peroxidase was blocked by 5 min exposure to a peroxidase-blocking reagent (Dako). Monoclonal mouse anti-p16 antibody (1:100+linker, 550834, BP Pharmingen, San Diego, CA, USA), anti-Ki-67 (ready to use, IR626, Dako), and polyclonal rabbit anti-testin (1:400, NBP1-87987, Novus Biologicals, Centennial, CO, USA) were used as the primary antibody (20 min incubation) followed by incubation with a secondary antibody conjugated with horseradish peroxidase (EnVision™ FLEX/HRP—20 min incubation). 3,3′-diaminobenzidine (DAB) was utilized as the peroxidase substrate, and the sections were incubated for 10 min. Finally, all sections were counterstained with EnVision FLEX Hematoxylin (Dako) for 5 min. After dehydration in graded ethanol concentrations (70%, 96%, absolute) and xylene, all slides were closed with coverslips in SUB-X Mounting Medium in a coverslipper.

The slides were scanned using a histologic scanner, Pannoramic MIDI (3DHistech). Reactions were evaluated (Ki-67) with the use of Quant Center software (3DHistech) under researcher supervision. For every case, three TMA cores were quantified by the algorithm SCORE (range = 0–8), and the final result was an average count. Expression of testin was assessed using a Pannoramic Viewer Digital image analysis as well as a routinely used immunoreactive scale (IRS) by Remmele and Stegner, presented in Table 2. The expression of p16 antigen was evaluated by two parameters, a percentage of p16-positive cells, and reaction intensity. The percentage of positive cells was evaluated in the highest expression area ("hot spot") and graded as follows (grade 0) when no cells stained, positive cells >0–5% (grade 1), positive cells >5–25% (grade 2), positive cells >25% (grade 3). The intensity of the reaction was scored as negative (0), weak (1), moderate (2), and strong (3). The reaction was considered as positive when nuclear, or nuclear and cytoplasmic, strong, and diffuse p16 staining beginning from the basal cell layer of the epithelium was observed. Whereas non-specific patterns, focal, wispy, small clusters of cells and a complete lack of staining qualified as negative p16 expression. Testin cytoplasmatic expression was scored as follows:

Table 2. Immunoreactive scale scoring system.

Score	Positively Stained Cells (PP)	Intensity of Staining (SI)	IRS Points (PP × SI)	IRS Classification
0	no staining	no color reaction	0–1	Negative
1	<10%	mild reaction	2–3	Positive, mild expression
2	10–50%	moderate reaction	4–8	Positive, moderate expression
3	51–80%	strong reaction	9–12	Positive, strong expression
4	>80%			

2.4. Statistical Analysis

The results were statistically analyzed using GraphPad Prism 5.0 software using Spearman correlation, Kruskal–Wallis, Dunn's multiple comparison, and Mann–Whitney tests. In all analyzed cases, the associations were considered statistically significant for $p < 0.05$.

3. Results

Expression of Ki-67 was observed in 100%, p16 in 84.6%, and testin in 98.25% of cervical dysplasia cases (Figure 1).

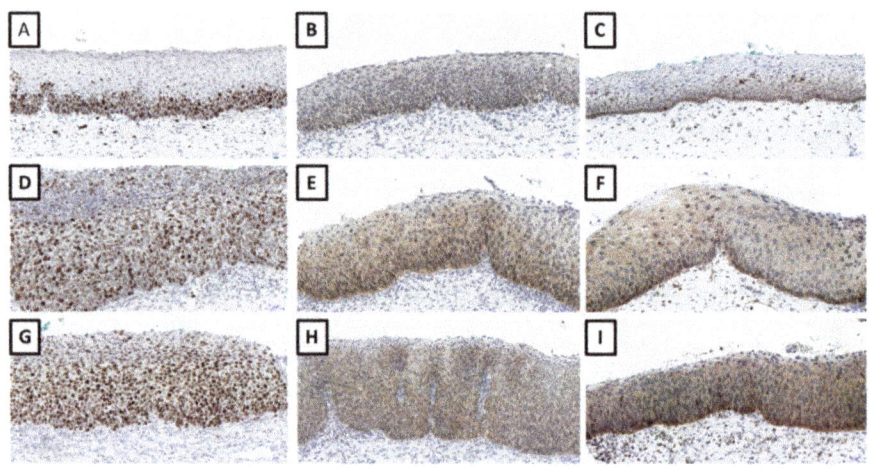

Figure 1. Immunohistochemical expression of Ki-67 ((**A**), CIN1; (**D**), CIN2; (**G**), CIN3); p16 protein ((**B**), CIN1; (**E**), CIN2; (**H**), CIN3), and testin ((**C**), CIN1; (**F**), CIN2; (**I**), CIN3). Magnification ×200.

A moderate positive correlation was observed between testin and Ki-67 as well testin and p16 expression in all dysplastic lesions (r = 0.4209, r = 0.5681; $p < 0.0001$ for both; Spearman correlation test). The relationships subdivided according to CINs are presented in Table 3.

Table 3. Spearman correlation test results.

	CIN1		CIN2		CIN3	
	Ki-67	p16	Ki-67	p16	Ki-67	p16
testin	r = 0.3678 p < 0.0418	NS	r = 0.3441 p < 0.0025	r = 0.6348 p < 0.0001	r = 0.3406 p < 0.0001	r = 0.4364 p < 0.0001
Ki-67		r = 0.5342 p < 0.0028		r = 0.6032 p < 0.0001		r = 0.3802 p < 0.0001

Statistical analysis showed stronger expression for testin in dysplastic lesions vs. control group ($p < 0.0001$; Mann–Whitney test; Figure 2A). Moreover, the expression was significantly higher in HSIL than the LSIL group ($p < 0.0024$; Mann–Whitney test; Figure 2B). Expression of p16 and Ki-67 was stronger in all dysplastic lesions vs. control group ($p < 0.0001$; Mann–Whitney test; Figure 2 C,D), and the expression of these two markers was higher in HSIL than in LSIL ($p < 0.0001$; Mann–Whitney test). The expression of p16 does not show statistically significant differences between normal cervical tissue and CIN1 ($p > 0.05$; Dunn's multiple comparison test). The expression of Ki-67 in normal cervical tissue was significantly lower than in CIN1 ($p < 0.05$; Dunn's multiple comparison test). In addition, significantly stronger expression of testin was observed in CIN3 vs. CIN1 and CIN3 vs. CIN2 cases ($p < 0.05$ respectively; Dunn's multiple comparison test). There were no statistically significant differences in testin expression between CIN1 and CIN2 as well as in p16 expression between CIN2 and CIN3 ($p > 0.05$; Dunn's Multiple Comparison test). Additionally, moderate positive correlation was observed between the expression of testin and Ki67, testin and p16 also between Ki-67 and p16 in all dysplastic lesions ($p < 0.0001$, $r = 0.3917$; $p < 0.0001$, $r = 0.5681$; $p < 0.0001$, $r = 0.5655$ Spearmann correlation test; Figure 3A–C). No differences in the relationship between age groups and type of CIN were observed. The highest percentage of HSIL lesions occurred in the <35 age group (Table 4). In addition, there was no statistically significant relationship between age groups and Ki-67 (Figure 4) or p16 median (Figure 5), but the relationship between age group and testin was close to being statistically significant (Chi-square test; $p = 0.0667$; Table 5).

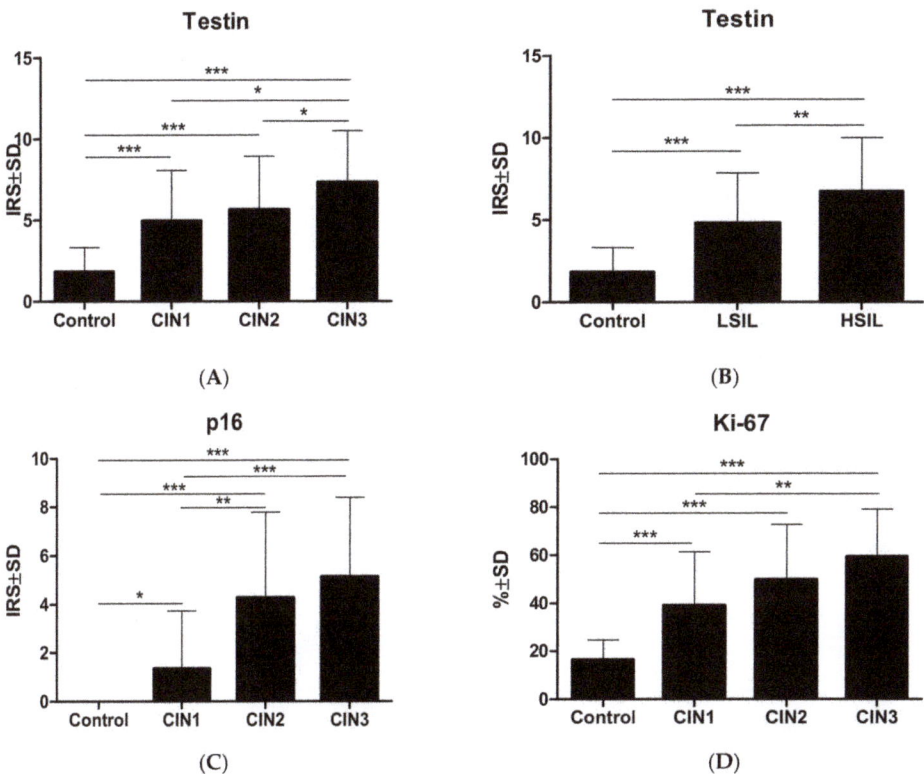

Figure 2. Immunohistochemical reaction in cervical intraepithelial neoplasia: (**A**) testin expression in CIN lesions; (**B**) testin expression in LSIL and HSIL lesions; (**C**) p16 expression in CIN lesions; (**D**) Ki-67 expression in CIN lesions. * $p < 0.05$, ** $p < 0.01$ and *** $p < 0.001$.

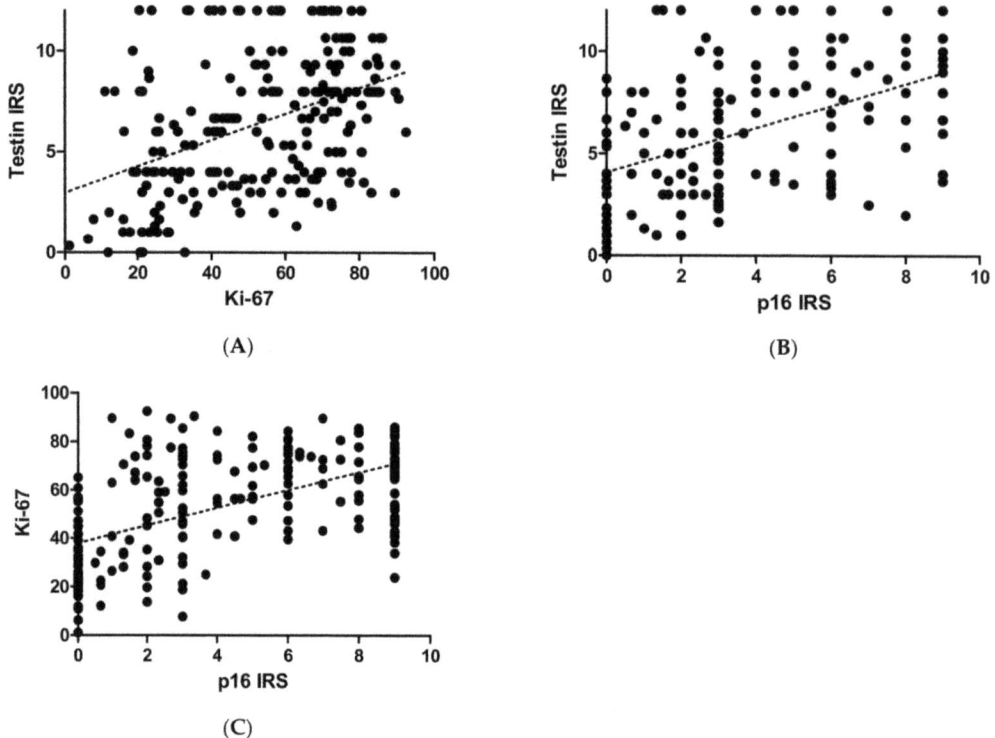

Figure 3. Immunohistochemical reaction in cervical intraepithelial neoplasia: (**A**) testin and Ki-67 correlation in CIN lesions; (**B**) testin and p16 correlation in CIN lesions; (**C**) Ki-67 and p16 correlation in CIN lesions.

Table 4. LSIL and HSIL in specific age groups.

	LSIL	HSIL
<35	13	106
35–45	13	62
>45	5	30

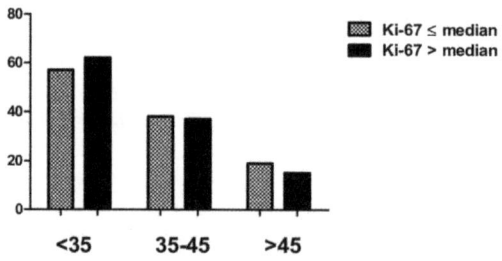

Figure 4. Median of the Ki-67 expression in age groups of CIN lesions.

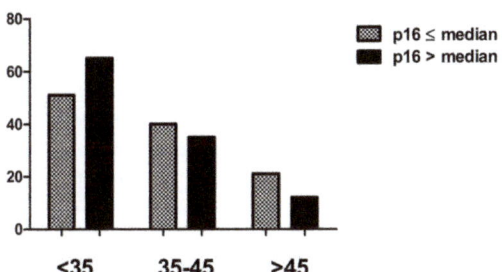

Figure 5. Median of the p16 expression in age groups of CIN lesions.

Table 5. Median of the testin expression in age groups of CIN lesions.

	Testin < Median	Testin > Median
<35	58	61
35–45	49	26
>45	18	17

4. Discussion

The term dysplasia refers to the replacement of normal squamous stratified epithelium by abnormal cells with pathological morphology spreading on successive layers of the epithelium. In the early 1980s, this term was changed into cervical intraepithelial neoplasia by the International Society of Gynecological Pathologists [11]. The terminology change was dictated by a detailed understanding of cervical cancerogenesis. All changes in the epithelium leading to the formation of CIN1, CIN2, CIN3, and cervical cancer are a series of related events, not isolated actions as previously believed. For clinicians, the most important aspect of diagnostics for CIN is to differentiate LSIL from HSIL. For this reason, many currently ongoing studies search for new markers that may streamline the diagnostic process. In this study, we focused on the correlation between testin and Ki-67 as a marker of proliferation and p16, indicating the impact of the HPV infection on the cervical epithelium. The latest report indicates that the TES gene is a tumor suppressor gene that can contribute to cancerogenesis, but the mechanism of the loss of TES gene expression is still unknown. HPV infection leads to the overexpression of E6 and E7 oncoproteins which disrupt the normal function of the tumor suppressor gene [12]. There is a lack of studies that analyze the expression of testin in LSIL and HSIL. The expression of this producer in CIN may prove an important factor in the development of cervical lesions.

P16, also known as p16INK4a, is encoded by the cyclin-dependent kinase inhibitor 2A (CDKN2A) gene located on chromosome 9p21.3. It is a cell cycle protein that regulates cell proliferation in the G1-S phase due to the reciprocal relationship with another tumor suppressor protein-Rb. In persistent HPV infection, oncogenic proteins E6 and E7 bind to host regulatory proteins. In HPV, E6 oncoproteins lead to the dysfunction of the p53 suppressor gene through direct protein–protein interaction, inducing p53 protein degradation [13]. On the other hand, E7 oncoproteins form a complex with retinoblastoma (Rb) protein that blocks the phosphorylation of Rb protein, thereby increasing free E2F; this results in both abnormal cell cycle progression and overexpression of p16 protein. Overexpression of p16 is commonly found in cells infected by HPV. Currently, IHC expression of p16 together with the expression of Ki-67 is routinely used to improve diagnosis of cervical lesions [14–16]. In the present study, the correlation between the grade of cervical lesions and the expression of p16 was strong ($p < 0.0001$). A similar correlation was observed according to the expression of Ki-67. It directly confirms the observation of other authors' research and indicates the validity of using commercial kits (CINtec PLUS Kit) to diagnose LSIL and HSIL [17–20]. Our study confirms the results of other research and indicates that p16 expression positively correlates with the degree of cervical lesions [21]. This study also shows no statistically significant difference between the expression of p16 in normal cervical tissue and CIN1, suggesting that p16 does not fully reflect the degree of cervical lesions. The absence of p16 expression can be used to eliminate associated high-grade squamous intraepithelial lesions in biopsy material. There is one limitation of p16 analysis as a CIN marker. P16 expression can sometimes be focal or diffuse in benign endocervical intercalated columnar cells, tubal metaplasia of the endometrium, and cervical endometriosis [22]. Despite that, the expression of p16 in these cells does not have the premalignant potential [23].

Ki-67 is a cellular marker of proliferation, detected in the non-G0 phase of the cell cycle [24]. In normal squamous cervical epithelium, Ki-67 is present only in basal and parabasal layers. In dysplasia and carcinoma, their expression extends above the basal one-third of squamous epithelium [25]. Many studies have shown that the elevated expression of Ki-67 is closely related to cell mitosis and cell proliferation [26–29]. Some scientists highlight this marker's role in distinguishing different degrees of cervical lesion [21,28,29]. The results of this study showed that the expression of Ki-67 was higher in the CIN1, CIN2, and CIN3 groups than in the control group ($p < 0.05$). The expression level of Ki-67 was significantly higher in HSIL than LSIL ($p < 0.05$), indicating that the expression level increased with the development of the HSIL lesions. Moreover, there is a significant difference in Ki-67 expression between normal cervical tissue and CIN1. Some studies show that Ki-67 is expressed in proliferative non-cancerous tissue, and in this study, patients with LSIL also have a positive expression of Ki-67 [30]. High expression of Ki-67 is associated with the severity of cervical lesions but not with HPV infection [31]. There is evidence that Ki-67 has a prognostic value superior to the standard histopathological grading to prognosticate CIN progression. Several studies have shown that diffuse expression of Ki-67 is present in almost all cases of HSIL or cervical cancer [32–34].

Testin is a protein with molecular mass 47kDa. The human TES gene is localized on the fragile site FRA7G at 7q31.2 [35]. Testin protein comprises three LIM (Linl-1, Isl-1, Mec-3) domains, and each consists of two zinc fingers linked by two amino acid spacers [36]. It was observed that the N- and C-terminal parts could interact with each other and create open and close conformations in cells. When expressed separately in cells, these two halves show partially different subcellular localizations with a dominant role of LIM domains targeting focal adhesion. Testin is localized along the actin stress fibers at the cell–cell junction and focal adhesion. Testin can interact with cytoskeletal proteins such as zyxin, talin, and VASP [9,37]. Together, they play a significant role in cell motility and adhesion. In chicken and human fibroblast, testin notably activates cell spreading, but there is a loss of testin increased cell motility. These suggest that testin appears crucial in regulating cellular migration, invasion, and process of epithelial-mesenchymal transition. Additionally, testin is involved in the cell cycle. The expression of testin protein positively correlates with a percentage of cells in the G1 phase; however, overexpression can induce apoptosis and decreased colony-forming ability. The expression of testin has been described in many types of human malignancies, but there is fewer data about the expression of testin in cervical intraepithelial neoplasia. The mechanism and pathways of testin's influence on cancerogenesis are still unknown. Some of the authors point out hypermethylation of the gene as the main factor. [35,36,38–43]. In this study, the expression of testin was significantly stronger in all dysplastic lesions compared to the control group. Testin expressed stronger in HSIL than LSIL; this indicates testin as a good diagnostic marker for distinguishing cervical lesions (CIN1 vs. CIN2 and CIN3). Zhong et al. support that testin has open and close conformations in cells by detecting the anti-TES serum in the nucleolus and anti-TESC as well anti-TESN sera in the cytoplasm. Cellular location is important for protein function because many phosphates, kinases, and transcription factors regulate their activity by controlling subcellular distribution [44]. Testin shuttling among cellular compartments may have divergent functions with different interacting partner proteins. The multiple conformational states and different locations in cellular compartments impact various expressions of testin protein; this may be the factor that suggests low testin expression in HSIL lesions. Future studies should be performed to find functions correlating with different cellular locations [45]. We plan on expanding our research with further studies to include cancer tissue. We plan on researching correlations between testin and lymphovascular space invasion, nodes metastasis, angiogenesis, and epithelial-mesenchymal transition markers in the upcoming months.

5. Conclusions

In our study, the expressions of Ki-67, p16, and testin gradually increased as the lesion progressed from LSIL to HSIL. The three markers complemented each other effectively, which may improve test sensitivity and specificity when used jointly.

Author Contributions: Conceptualization, A.P. (Aneta Popiel) and C.K.; methodology, A.P. (Aleksandra Piotrowska); software, P.S.-G.; validation, A.P. (Aneta Popiel), P.D., and M.P.-O.; formal analysis, A.P. (Aneta Popiel); investigation, A.P. (Aleksandra Piotrowska); resources, H.R. and B.S.; data curation, A.P. (Aneta Popiel); writing—original draft preparation, A.P. (Aneta Popiel); writing—review and editing, C.K.; visualization, P.S.-G.; supervision, P.D.; project administration, M.P.-O.; funding acquisition, A.P. (Aneta Popiel). All authors have read and agreed to the published version of the manuscript.

Funding: This research was funded by the National Science Centre, Poland grant number, 2018/29/N/NZ5/01911. The APC was funded by the National Science Centre.

Institutional Review Board Statement: The study was conducted according to the guidelines of the Declaration of Helsinki and approved by the Ethics Committee of the Medical University in Wroclaw (6 May 2019; protocol code 411/2019).

Informed Consent Statement: Patient consent was waived due to use of anonymized archival material, which in no way influenced the diagnostic and therapeutic process.

Data Availability Statement: The data presented in this study are available upon request from the corresponding author. The data are not publicly available due to privacy issue.

Conflicts of Interest: The authors declare no conflict of interest.

References

1. Cubie, H.A.; Campbell, C. Cervical cancer screening—The challenges of complete pathways of care in low-income countries: Focus on Malawi. *Women's Health* **2020**, *16*, 1745506520914804. [CrossRef]
2. Canfell, K.; Kim, J.J.; Brisson, M.; Keane, A.; Simms, K.T.; Caruana, M.; Burger, E.A.; Martin, D.; Nguyen, D.T.N.; Bénard, É.; et al. Mortality impact of achieving WHO cervical cancer elimination targets: A comparative modelling analysis in 78 low-income and lower-middle-income countries. *Lancet* **2020**, *395*, 591–603. [CrossRef]
3. Wentzensen, N.; Schiffman, M.; Palmer, T.; Arbyn, M. Triage of HPV positive women in cervical cancer screening. *J. Clin. Virol. Off. Publ. Pan Am. Soc. Clin. Virol.* **2016**, *76*, 49–55. [CrossRef] [PubMed]
4. Moreno-Acosta, P.; Romero-Rojas, A.; Vial, N.; Huertas, A.; Acosta, J.; Mayorga, D.; Schyrly, C.; Molano, M.; Gamboa, O.; Cotes, M.; et al. Persistent High-Risk HPV Infection and Molecular Changes Related to the Development of Cervical Cancer. *Case Rep. Obstet. Gynecol.* **2020**, *2020*, 6806857. [CrossRef]
5. Tao, L.; Han, L.; Li, X.; Gao, Q.; Pan, L.; Wu, L.; Luo, Y.; Wang, W.; Zheng, Z.; Guo, X. Prevalence and risk factors for cervical neoplasia: A cervical cancer screening program in Beijing. *BMC Public Health* **2014**, *14*, 1185. [CrossRef]
6. Kim, H.Y.; Kim, S.M.; Seo, J.-H.; Park, E.-H.; Kim, N.; Lee, D.-H. Age-specific prevalence of serrated lesions and their subtypes by screening colonoscopy: A retrospective study. *BMC Gastroenterol.* **2014**, *14*, 82. [CrossRef] [PubMed]
7. Raab, S.S.; Bishop, N.S.; Zaleski, M.S. Long-term outcome and relative risk in women with atypical squamous cells of undetermined significance. *Am. J. Clin. Pathol.* **1999**, *112*, 57–62. [CrossRef] [PubMed]
8. Naucler, P.; Ryd, W.; Törnberg, S.; Strand, A.; Wadell, G.; Elfgren, K.; Rådberg, T.; Strander, B.; Forslund, O.; Hansson, B.G.; et al. Efficacy of HPV DNA testing with cytology triage and/or repeat HPV DNA testing in primary cervical cancer screening. *J. Natl. Cancer Inst.* **2009**, *101*, 88–99. [CrossRef] [PubMed]
9. Gu, Z.; Ding, G.; Liang, K.; Zhang, H.; Guo, G.; Zhang, L.; Cui, J. TESTIN suppresses tumor growth and invasion via manipulating cell cycle progression in endometrial carcinoma. *Med. Sci. Monit.* **2014**, *20*, 980–987. [CrossRef] [PubMed]
10. Dong, R.; Pu, H.; Wang, Y.; Yu, J.; Lian, K.; Mao, C. TESTIN was commonly hypermethylated and involved in the epithelial-mesenchymal transition of endometrial cancer. *Apmis* **2015**, *123*, 394–400. [CrossRef]
11. Buckley, C.; Butler, E.; Fox, H. Cervical intraepithelial neoplasia. *J. Clin. Pathol.* **1982**, *35*, 1–13. [CrossRef] [PubMed]

12. Balasubramaniam, S.D.; Balakrishnan, V.; Oon, C.E.; Kaur, G. Key molecular events in cervical cancer development. *Medicina* **2019**, *55*, 384. [CrossRef]
13. Lu, D.W.; El-Mofty, S.K.; Wang, H.L. Expression of p16, Rb, and p53 proteins in squamous cell carcinomas of the anorectal region harboring human papillomavirus DNA. *Mod. Pathol.* **2003**, *16*, 692–699. [CrossRef] [PubMed]
14. Hebbar, A.; Murthy, V.S. Role of p16/INK4a and Ki-67 as specific biomarkers for cervical intraepithelial neoplasia: An institutional study. *J. Lab. Phys.* **2017**, *9*, 104–110. [CrossRef] [PubMed]
15. Kanthiya, K.; Khunnarong, J.; Tangjitgamol, S.; Puripat, N.; Tanvanich, S. Expression of the p16 and Ki67 in cervical squamous intraepithelial lesions and cancer. *Asian Pac. J. Cancer Prev.* **2016**, *17*, 3201–3206.
16. de Melo, F.L.P.; Lancellotti, C.L.P.; da Silva, M.A.L.G. Expression of the Immunohistochemical Markers p16 and Ki-67 and Their Usefulness in the Diagnosis of Cervical Intraepithelial Neoplasms. *Rev. Bras. Ginecol. Obstet.* **2016**, *38*, 82–87. [CrossRef]
17. Takacs, F.Z.; Radosa, J.C.; Bochen, F.; Juhasz-Böss, I.; Solomayer, E.F.; Bohle, R.M.; Breitbach, G.P.; Schick, B.; Linxweiler, M. Sec62/Ki67 and p16/Ki67 dual-staining immunocytochemistry in vulvar cytology for the identification of vulvar intraepithelial neoplasia and vulvar cancer: A pilot study. *Arch. Gynecol. Obstet.* **2019**, *299*, 825–833. [CrossRef]
18. Desai, F.; Singh, L.S.; Majachunglu, G.; Kamei, H. Diagnostic accuracy of conventional Cell Blocks along with p16INK4 and Ki67 biomarkers as triage tests in resource-poor organized cervical cancer screening programs. *Asian Pac. J. Cancer Prev.* **2019**, *20*, 917. [CrossRef]
19. Miyamoto, S.; Hasegawa, J.; Morioka, M.; Hirota, Y.; Kushima, M.; Sekizawa, A. The association between p16 and Ki-67 immunohistostaining and the progression of cervical intraepithelial neoplasia grade 2. *Int. J. Gynecol. Obstet.* **2016**, *134*, 45–48. [CrossRef]
20. Sangwaiya, A.; Gill, M.; Bairwa, S.; Chaudhry, M.; Sen, R.; Prakash Kataria, S. Utility of P16/INK4a and KI-67 in preneoplastic and neoplastic lesions of cervix. *Iran. J. Pathol.* **2018**, *13*, 308–316. [PubMed]
21. Nam, E.J.; Kim, J.W.; Hong, J.W.; Jang, H.S.; Lee, S.Y.; Jang, S.Y.; Lee, D.W.; Kim, S.W.; Kim, J.H.; Kim, Y.T.; et al. Expression of the p16INK4a and Ki-67 in relation to the grade of cervical intraepithelial neoplasia and high-risk human papillomavirus infection. *J. Gynecol. Oncol.* **2008**, *19*, 162–168. [CrossRef]
22. Tringler, B.; Gup, C.J.; Singh, M.; Groshong, S.; Shroyer, A.L.; Heinz, D.E.; Shroyer, K.R. Evaluation of p16INK4a and pRb expression in cervical squamous and glandular neoplasia. *Hum. Pathol.* **2004**, *35*, 689–696. [CrossRef]
23. Silva, D.C.; Gonçalves, A.K.; Cobucci, R.N.; Mendonça, R.C.; Lima, P.H.; Júnior, G.C. Immunohistochemical expression of p16, Ki-67 and p53 in cervical lesions—A systematic review. *Pathol. Res. Pract.* **2017**, *213*, 723–729. [CrossRef]
24. Min, Z.; Pu, X.; Gu, Z. Correlative analysis of the expression of IL-10 and Ki-67 in human cervical cancer and cervical intraepithelial neoplasias and human papillomavirus infection. *Oncol. Lett.* **2018**, *16*, 7189–7194. [CrossRef]
25. Ancuţa, E.; Ancuţa, C.; Cozma, L.G.; Iordache, C.; Anghelache-Lupaşcu, I.; Anton, E.; Carasevici, E.; Chirieac, R. Tumor biomarkers in cervical cancer: Focus on Ki-67 proliferation factor and E-cadherin expression. *Rom. J. Morphol. Embryol.* **2008**, *50*, 413–418.
26. Li, L.T.; Jiang, G.; Chen, Q.; Zheng, J.N. Predic Ki67 is a promising molecular target in the diagnosis of cancer (Review). *Mol. Med. Rep.* **2015**, *11*, 1566–1572. [CrossRef]
27. Juríková, M.; Danihel, L'.; Polák, Š.; Varga, I. Ki67, PCNA, and MCM proteins: Markers of proliferation in the diagnosis of breast cancer. *Acta Histochem.* **2016**, *118*, 544–552. [CrossRef]
28. Denkert, C.; Budczies, J.; von Minckwitz, G.; Wienert, S.; Loibl, S.; Klauschen, F. Strategies for developing Ki67 as a useful biomarker in breast cancer. *Breast* **2015**, *24*, 67–72. [CrossRef] [PubMed]
29. Ma, X.; Wu, Y.; Zhang, T.; Song, H.; Jv, H.; Guo, W.; Ren, G. Ki67 proliferation index as a histopathological predictive and prognostic parameter of oral mucosal melanoma in patients without distant metastases. *J. Cancer* **2017**, *18*, 3828. [CrossRef]
30. Shi, Q.; Xu, L.; Yang, R.; Meng, Y.; Qiu, L. Ki-67 and P16 proteins in cervical cancer and precancerous lesions of young women and the diagnostic value for cervical cancer and precancerous lesions. *Oncol. Lett.* **2019**, *18*, 1351–1355. [CrossRef] [PubMed]
31. Davidson, B.; Goldberg, I.; Lerner-Geva, L.; Gotlieb, W.H.; Ben-Baruch, G.; Novikov, I.; Kopolovic, J. Expression of topoisomerase II and Ki-67 in cervical carcinoma-clinicopathological study using immunohistochemistry. *Apmis* **2000**, *108*, 209–215. [CrossRef] [PubMed]
32. Qian, Q.P.; Zhang, X.; Ding, B.; Jiang, S.W.; Li, Z.M.; Ren, M.L.; Shen, Y. Performance of P16/Ki67 dual staining in triaging hr-HPV-positive population during cervical Cancer screening in the younger women. *Clin. Chim. Acta* **2018**, *483*, 281–285. [CrossRef] [PubMed]
33. Li, Y.; Liu, J.; Gong, L.; Sun, X.; Long, W. Combining HPV DNA load with p16/Ki-67 staining to detect cervical precancerous lesions and predict the progression of CIN1-2 lesions. *Virol. J.* **2019**, *16*, 1–9. [CrossRef] [PubMed]
34. Piri, R.; Ghaffari, A.; Azami-Aghdash, S.; Ali-Akbar, Y.P.; Saleh, P.; Naghavi-Behzad, M. Ki-67/MIB-1 as a prognostic marker in cervical cancer—a systematic review with meta-analysis. *Asian Pac. J. Cancer Prev.* **2015**, *16*, 6997–7002.
35. Sarti, M.; Sevignani, C.; Calin, G.A.; Aqeilan, R.; Shimizu, M.; Pentimalli, F.; Picchio, M.C.; Godwin, A.; Rosenberg, A.; Drusco, A.; et al. Adenoviral Transduction of testin Gene into Breast and Uterine Cancer Cell Lines Promotes Apoptosis and Tumor Reduction In vivo. *Clin. Cancer Res.* **2005**, *11*, 806–813. [PubMed]
36. Tobias, E.S.; Hurlstone, A.F.L.; Mackenzie, E.; MacFarlane, R.; Black, D.M. The TES gene at 7q31. 1 is methylated in tumours and encodes a novel growth-suppressing LIM domain protein. *Oncogene* **2001**, *20*, 2844–2853. [CrossRef]
37. Popiel, A.; Kobierzycki, C.; Dzięgiel, P. The Role of Testin in Human Cancers. *Pathol. Oncol. Res.* **2019**, *25*, 1279–1284. [CrossRef]

38. Li, H.; Huang, K.; Gao, L.; Wang, L.; Niu, Y.; Liu, H.; Wang, Z.; Wang, L.; Wang, G.; Wang, J. TES inhibits colorectal cancer progression through activation of p38. *Oncotagret* **2016**, *7*, 45819. [CrossRef]
39. Ma, H.; Weng, D.; Chen, Y.; Huang, W.; Pan, K.; Wang, H.; Sun, J.; Wang, Q.; Zhou, Z.; Wang, H.; et al. Extensive analysis of D7S486 in primary gastric cancer supports TESTIN as a candidate tumor suppressor gene. *Mol. Cancer* **2010**, *9*, 190. [CrossRef]
40. Chêne, L.; Giroud, C.; Desgrandchamps, F.; Boccon-Gibod, L.; Cussenot, O.; Berthon, P.; Latil, A. Extensive analysis of the 7q31 region in human prostate tumors supports TES as the best candidate tumor suppressor gene. *Int. J. Cancer* **2004**, *111*, 798–804. [CrossRef]
41. Sarti, M.; Pinton, S.; Limoni, C.; Carbone, G.M.; Pagani, O.; Cavalli, F.; Catapano, C.V. Differential expression of testin and survivin in breast cancer subtypes. *Oncol. Rep.* **2013**, *30*, 824–832. [CrossRef]
42. Wang, M.; Wang, Q.; Peng, W.; Hu, J. Testin is a tumor suppressor in non-small cell lung cancer. *Oncol. Rep.* **2017**, *37*, 1027–1035. [CrossRef] [PubMed]
43. Qiu, H.; Zhu, J.; Yuan, C.; Yan, S.; Yang, Q.; Kong, B. Frequent hypermethylation and loss of heterozygosity of the testis derived transcript gene in ovarian cancer. *Cancer Sci.* **2010**, *101*, 1255–1260. [CrossRef]
44. Szymańska-Chabowska, A.; Juzwiszyn, J.; Jankowska-Polańska, B.; Tański, W.; Chabowski, M. Chitinase 3-Like 1, Nestin, and Testin Proteins as Novel Biomarkers of Potential Clinical Use in Colorectal Cancer: A Review. *Health Med.* **2020**, *1279*, 1–8.
45. Zhong, Y.; Zhu, J.; Wang, Y.; Zhou, J.; Ren, K.; Ding, X.; Zhang, J. LIM domain protein TES changes its conformational states in different cellular compartments. *Mol. Cell. Biochem.* **2009**, *320*, 85–92. [CrossRef] [PubMed]

NK Cell-Mediated Eradication of Ovarian Cancer Cells with a Novel Chimeric Antigen Receptor Directed against CD44

Rüdiger Klapdor [1,2,3,4,*,†], Shuo Wang [1,2,†], Michael A. Morgan [2,3,4], Katharina Zimmermann [2,3,4], Jens Hachenberg [1,2,4], Hildegard Büning [2,3,4], Thilo Dörk [1,4], Peter Hillemanns [1,4] and Axel Schambach [2,3,4,5,*]

1. Department of Gynecology and Obstetrics, Hannover Medical School, 30625 Hannover, Germany; wangshuo1022@gmail.com (S.W.); hachenberg.jens@mh-hannover.de (J.H.); doerk.thilo@mh-hannover.de (T.D.); Hillemanns.Peter@mh-hannover.de (P.H.)
2. Institute for Experimental Hematology, Hannover Medical School, 30625 Hannover, Germany; morgan.michael@mh-hannover.de (M.A.M.); zimmermann.katharina@mh-hannover.de (K.Z.); buening.hildegard@mh-hannover.de (H.B.)
3. REBIRTH Center for Translational Regenerative Medicine, Hannover Medical School, 30625 Hannover, Germany
4. Comprehensive Cancer Center Niedersachsen, CCC Hannover, Hannover Medical School, 30625 Hannover, Germany
5. Division of Hematology/Oncology, Boston Children's Hospital, Harvard Medical School, Boston, MA 02115, USA
* Correspondence: Klapdor.ruediger@mh-hannover.de (R.K.); schambach.axel@mh-hannover.de (A.S.)
† Both authors contributed equally and share responsibility for first authorship.

Abstract: Ovarian cancer is the most common cause of gynecological cancer-related death in the developed world. Disease recurrence and chemoresistance are major causes of poor survival rates in ovarian cancer patients. Ovarian cancer stem cells (CSCs) were shown to represent a source of tumor recurrence owing to the high resistance to chemotherapy and enhanced tumorigenicity. Chimeric antigen receptor (CAR)-based adoptive immunotherapy represents a promising strategy to reduce the risk for recurrent disease. In this study, we developed a codon-optimized third-generation CAR to specifically target CD44, a marker widely expressed on ovarian cancer cells and associated with CSC-like properties and intraperitoneal tumor spread. We equipped NK-92 cells with the anti-CD44 CAR (CD44NK) and an anti-CD19 control CAR (CD19NK) using lentiviral SIN vectors. Compared to CD19NK and untransduced NK-92 cells, CD44NK showed potent and specific cytotoxic activity against CD44-positive ovarian cancer cell lines (SKOV3 and OVCAR3) and primary ovarian cancer cells harvested from ascites. In contrast, CD44NK had less cytotoxic activity against CD44-negative A2780 cells. Specific activation of engineered NK cells was also demonstrated by interferon-γ (IFNγ) secretion assays. Furthermore, CD44NK cells still demonstrated cytotoxic activity under cisplatin treatment. Most importantly, the simultaneous treatment with CD44NK and cisplatin showed higher anti-tumor activity than sequential treatment.

Keywords: chimeric antigen receptor; ovarian cancer; CD44; adoptive immunotherapy; NK cells

1. Introduction

Ovarian cancer remains the most lethal among gynecological cancers [1]. Unfortunately, because localized ovarian cancer is generally asymptomatic and screening tests have not been successfully implemented, 75% of patients present with advanced tumor stages (FIGO stages III–IV) at the time of diagnosis [2]. Therefore, there is an urgent need for the development of novel and effective therapeutic strategies. It is well-known that the immune system plays an important role in monitoring tumor development and progression [3]. Compelling clinical evidence shows that the presence of tumor-infiltrating lymphocytes (TILs) is associated with a favorable prognosis in ovarian cancer [4–7]. These studies suggest that the immune system plays a substantial role in controlling ovarian cancer progression and that immunotherapy might present an effective therapeutic option.

Chimeric antigen receptor (CAR)-modified T and natural killer (NK) cells have gained recent attention in ovarian cancer treatment [8,9]. CARs are synthetic receptors that consist of a single-chain variable fragment (scFv) for antigen recognition, a transmembrane domain and a cytoplasmic domain to activate the NK cells. Second and third-generation CARs were developed, which additionally contain one or two co-stimulatory domains, such as those derived from CD28 and/or 4-1BB, to improve survival and proliferation of the effector cells [10,11].

Recurrence followed by chemoresistance is one of the main contributing factors to the poor prognosis in ovarian cancer patients. Many researchers have demonstrated the existence of ovarian cancer stem cells (CSCs) with increased tumorigenicity, differentiating capacity and chemoresistance [12,13]. Therefore, targeted therapy against CSCs has emerged as a promising strategy in combination with conventional chemotherapy in ovarian cancer. CD44 expression has been shown to be associated with CSC-like properties in a variety of tumors [14,15], including ovarian cancer [16]. In addition, CD44 is known to be the major receptor for hyaluronan (HA), which is implicated in cell–cell and cell–matrix interactions and is associated with the promotion of cancer metastasis [17,18]. The binding of HA to CD44 was shown to mediate ovarian cancer cell adhesion to peritoneal mesothelial cells [19,20]. Collectively, CD44 could be a promising target molecule for immunotherapy in ovarian cancer.

In this study, we developed a novel CD44-specific third-generation CAR and analyzed its anti-tumor activity in ovarian cancer cell lines and primary patient-derived ovarian cancer cells. To maximize the benefits of anti-CD44 CAR expressing NK cells, the cytotoxicity was also evaluated in combination with chemotherapy.

2. Material and Methods

2.1. Cell Lines

Human embryonic kidney 293T cells (HEK-293T, ATCC CRL-3216) were used for lentiviral vector production and grown in Dulbecco's modified Eagle's medium (Biochrom, Berlin, Germany) supplemented with 10% heat inactivated FBS, 100 U/mL penicillin, 100 mg/mL streptomycin, and 10 mmol/L HEPES. NK-92 cells were cultured in RPMI-1640 medium (Sigma-Aldrich, Steinheim, Germany) supplemented with stable L-Glutamine, 10% FBS, 100 U/mL penicillin, 100 mg/mL streptomycin, and 200 IU/mL IL-2 (Proleukin S; Novartis Pharma GmbH, Nürnberg, Germany). Ovarian cancer cell lines A2780, SKOV3, and OVCAR3 were stably equipped with EGFP by lentiviral transduction and cultured in RPMI-1640 medium supplemented with stable L-Glutamine, 10% FBS, 100 U/mL penicillin, and 100 mg/mL streptomycin. After obtaining informed consent, primary ovarian cancer cells (P1, P2 and P3) were harvested from sequential ascites samples of an ovarian cancer patient and cultured in the same condition as ovarian cancer cell lines in low-attachment flasks (Corning, Wiesbaden, Germany).

Cloning of Vectors and Lentiviral Vector Production

The sequence of CD44 scFv was selected from a fully human anti-CD44 monoclonal antibody (mAb) called PF-03475952 [21]. All sequences underwent optimization of codon usage and GC content to increase the efficiency of transcriptional processing and protein expression. The recognition sequences of restriction enzymes (AgeI, NotI, SalI, and BsrgI) were removed, and then the DNA synthesis was performed by GeneArt (Thermo Fisher, Regensburg, Germany). Our anti-CD44 CAR was generated from an already published third-generation anti-CD19 CAR [22] by replacing the scFv fragment. This anti-CD19 CAR contains CD28, 4-1BB and CD3ζ domains and served as a control in further experiments. After producing a third-generation lentiviral SIN vector, an internal ribosomal entry site (IRES)-driven dTomato expression cassette was inserted between SalI sites to allow co-expression and facilitate detection of transduced cells.

To produce lentiviral vectors, HEK-293T cells were transfected using a calcium phosphate method. HEK-293T cells (5×10^6) were seeded in 10 cm dishes and cultured overnight. The following plasmids for each dish were mixed and diluted in water with the desired volume: 12 µg of the vector plasmid, 12 µg of pcDNA3.GP.4 × CTE (gag/pol), 5 µg of pRSV-Rev and 2 µg of RD114/TR envelope plasmids. The purified lentiviral packaging plasmids were purchased from Plasmid Factory (Bielefeld, Germany). Viral supernatants were harvested 36 h after transfection, filtered through MillexGP 0.22 µm filters (Millipore, Schwalbach, Germany), concentrated via ultracentrifugation, and stored at −80 °C until use.

2.2. Transduction of NK Cells

NK-92 cells were equipped with CAR constructs by Retronectin-assisted transduction. Briefly, 48-well plates were coated with Retronectin (Takara, Shiga, Otsu, Japan) (210 µL of 24 µg/mL in PBS per well) overnight at 4 °C or 2 h at room temperature. Retronectin was then removed. The wells were blocked with sterile-filtered PBS containing 2% BSA for 30 min at room temperature. After washing with HBSS/HEPES (Biochrom, Berlin, Germany), viral supernatants were then added into the Retronectin-precoated plates and centrifuged for 30 min at $400 \times g$ and 4 °C. Afterwards, 5×10^4 NK-92 cells were added and incubated for 24 h. Then, the cells were transferred to uncoated plates.

2.3. IFNγ Release Assays

IFNγ release assays were performed in triplicate by co-culture of NK cells and target cells at an E/T ratio of 5:1 in 96-well plates in a final volume of 200 µL of NK cell media containing 200 IU/mL IL-2. After 24 h, cell fraction-free co-culture supernatants were assayed for presence of IFNγ using DuoSet Ancillary Reagent Kit (R&D Systems, Minneapolis, MN, USA), according to the manufacturer's instructions. The average zero standard optical density (O.D.) was measured by the microplate spectrophotometer at a wavelength of 450 nm, and correction was set to 540 nm.

2.4. Cytotoxicity Assays

2.4.1. Live Cell Imaging Using Fluorescent Microscopy

GFP expressing ovarian cancer cells were seeded in 48-well plates and cultured overnight. The effector NK cells were then added at an effector-target (E/T) ratio of 5:1. Time-lapse imaging was immediately started with temperature and gas control. Phase-contrast and fluorescent images of each position were taken every 15 min. The positions were selected and saved by the software before addition of NK cells; the acquisition focal plane was quickly set afterwards.

2.4.2. Analysis of Cytotoxicity by Fluoroskan Ascent™ FL

Ovarian cancer cells were seeded in flat-bottom 96-well plates (Sarstedt, Nürmbrecht, Germany) at appropriate densities (A2780, 2×10^4 cells/well; SKOV3 and OVCAR3, 1.5×10^4 cells/well) and cultured overnight. NK-92 and CAR-NK-92 cells were added at an E/T ratio of 5:1 on the following day. At several time points, culture medium containing NK cells and cell debris was completely removed by inverting the plates and blotting them against clean paper towels. After adding 200 µL 5% (w/v) SDS into each well, the fluorescence intensities of GFP in the cell homogenate, which corresponds to the cell numbers, was measured at excitation 485 nm/emission 520 nm using Fluoroskan Ascent™ FL (Thermo Fisher Scientific, Waltham, MA, USA).

2.4.3. Analysis of Cytotoxicity by xCELLigence

To estimate the anti-tumor activity of NK cells against unmarked primary ovarian cancer cells, the xCELLigence RTCA SP instrument (ACEA Biosciences, San Diego, CA, USA) was used according to the instructions of the supplier. To achieve equilibrium of E-Plate 96 surface (ACEA Biosciences), 100 µL of cell culture media were added to each of the 96 wells before seeding the target cells. The plates were then left in the cell culture hood for 30 min at room temperature. Afterwards, the background impedance of cell culture media was measured for calculation of the cell index value. Next, the E-Plate 96 was removed from the incubator and the desired cells were added in 50 μL medium. The cell suspension was properly prepared for the appropriate cell concentrations previously determined by a titration experiment (A2780: 2×10^4; OVCAR3: 1.5×10^4; SKOV3 and primary ovarian cancer cells: 1×10^4). The plate was left in the culture hood for 30 min to allow the cells to settle to the bottom of the well. Then, the E-Plate 96 was reinserted, and the impedance of each well was measured every 15 min. The next day, when the cells reached the logarithmic growth phase, E-Plate 96 was removed from the incubator and effector NK cells were added in 50 μL medium at the desired E/T ratio. Then, the impedance was measured every 1 min for 8 h and every 15 min thereafter. The experiments were manually stopped 48 to 72 h after the addition of effector cells.

2.5. Chemotoxicity Assays

A2780 or primary ovarian cancer cells P3 were seeded in 48-well plates in the appropriate cell number. NK cells at an E/T ratio of 2:1 and cisplatin at the previously determined IC_{50} concentration (Sigma Aldrich, St. Louis, MO, USA) were added in 200 μL medium. Total incubation time was 96 h. In the sequential treatment groups, co-incubation with NK cells was performed for 24 h and cisplatin treatment for 72 h. Cells were washed twice before changing conditions to ensure no NK cells or cisplatin remained. Controls were analyzed at each step to reduce systematic bias. After treatment, all wells were washed twice and analyzed with the CellTiter 96® AQueous One Solution Cell Proliferation Assay (Promega, Fitchburg, WI, USA) following the manufacturer's protocol.

2.6. Statistical Analysis

Data from the experiments are expressed as means ± standard deviations. Two-way ANOVA combined with Tukey's multiple comparisons test was used to analyze Fluoroskan results. One-way ANOVA combined with Tukey's multiple comparisons test was used for comparison of differences among indicated groups. A $p <0.05$ was considered significant.

3. Results

3.1. Generation of a New Codon-Optimized Anti-CD44 CAR

The CAR sequence was cloned into a third-generation lentiviral SIN vector (pRRL.PPT) [23]. After production of lentiviral vector, retronectin-mediated transduction was performed on human NK-92 cells. The design of the CAR is shown in Figure 1A.

A2780, SKOV3 and OVCAR3 cell lines were used as target cells. Surface CD44 expression levels of these human ovarian cancer cell lines were evaluated by flow cytometry. SKOV3 and OVCAR3 were shown to have high CD44 expression (98.8% and 85.3%, respectively), whereas A2780 lacked CD44 expression (Figure 1B).

3.2. CD44NK Cells Show Specific Cytotoxicity against Ovarian Cancer Cell Lines

To directly visualize the CAR-NK-92 cell-killing process, ovarian cancer cell lines expressing EGFP were co-cultured with CAR-NK-92 cells at an E/T ratio of 5:1. As soon as NK cells were added, a series of images were taken every 15 min by fluorescence microscopy. Figure 2A shows the morphological changes of the cell death induced by CAR-NK cells.

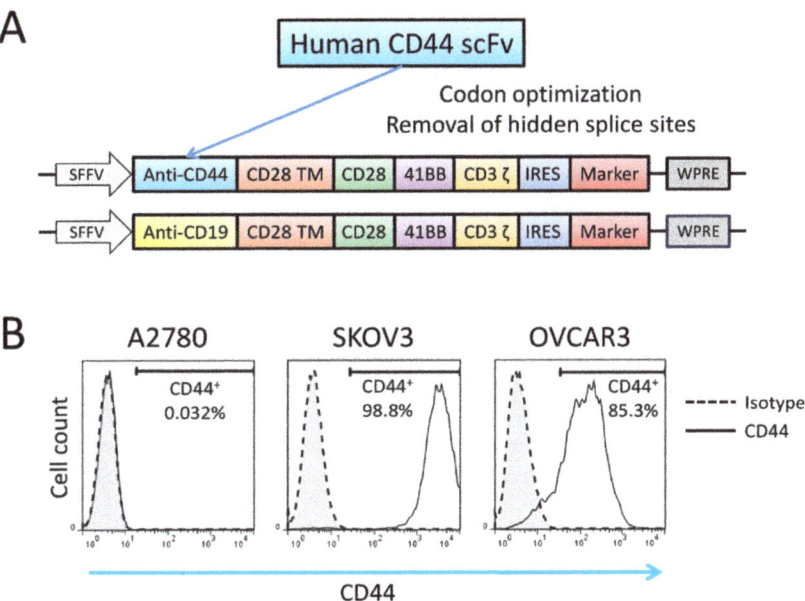

Figure 1. The structure of the new codon-optimized anti-CD44-CAR and antigen expression on target cells. (**A**) Schematic illustration of the modular architecture of newly developed third-generation CARs. (**B**) Flow cytometric analyses of the antigen expression of CD44 on ovarian cancer cell lines.

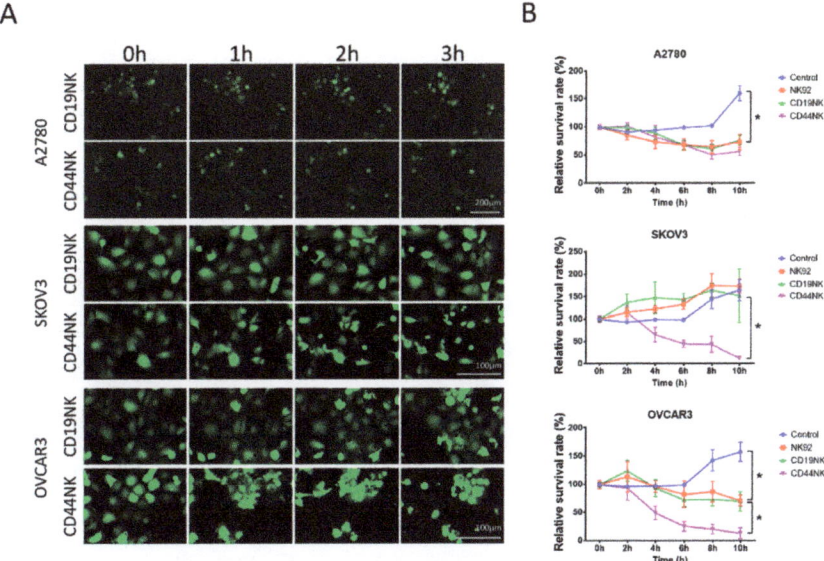

Figure 2. (**A**) Visualization of killing by CAR-NK-92 cells by fluorescence microscopy. A2780, SKOV3, and OVCAR3 cells were co-cultured with effector NK cells at an E/T ratio of 5:1. CD19NK cells were used as an antigen-specificity control. During the early process of death, the cells became smaller in size with condensed cytoplasm and tightly packed organelles. After cell shrinkage, massive membrane blebbing occurred, followed by separation of cell fragments into apoptotic bodies and

subsequently loss of the GFP signal. (**B**) Fluoroskan results showing the killing effect of the CAR-NK-92 cells in ovarian cancer cell lines. GFP-expressing A2780, SKOV3, and OVCAR3 cells were seeded in flat-bottom 96-well plates at previously determined densities (A2780, 2×10^4 cells/well; SKOV3 and OVCAR3 1.5×10^4 cells/well). On the next day, NK-92 and CAR-NK-92 cells were added at the effector/target (E/T) ratio of 5:1. After removing culture medium containing NK cells and cell debris, residual attached cells were lysed with SDS, and fluorescence intensity was measured at excitation 485 nm/emission 520 nm using Fluoroskan Ascent™ FL. * indicates a significant difference calculated by two-way ANOVA, $p < 0.05$. Values represent the mean from two separate experiments each containing three samples.

To quantify the cytotoxicity of CAR-NK-92 cells, a fluorescence-based cell survival assay was used. CAR-NK-92 cells and NK-92 cells were co-incubated with GFP expressing ovarian cancer cells (E/T ratio of 5:1). The GFP intensities were measured with the Fluoroskan reader every 2 h. Compared to A2780 and OVCAR3 cells cultured alone, viability of these cancer cells was significantly reduced by co-culture with untransduced NK-92 cells ($p < 0.0001$) (Figure 2B). However, the nonspecific cytotoxicity of NK-92 and control CD19NK cells did not affect the survival rate of SKOV3 cells as compared to SKOV3 cells cultured alone ($p = 0.939$). On the contrary, the survival rate in SKOV3 cells was significantly decreased by CD44NK cells ($p < 0.0001$). Significant cytotoxicity of CD44NK cells was also observed in OVCAR3 cells. No enhanced cytotoxicity of CD44NK cells was observed in CD44-negative A2780 cells. No differences in survival of all three cell lines were observed between those co-incubated with CD19NK cells or NK-92 cells. To further test the capacity of CD44NK cells to specifically eliminate target cells, a CD44-expressing lentiviral vector (co-expressing eGFP) was introduced into the CD44-negative A2780 cells. As shown in Figure S1, enforced expression of CD44 resulted in more efficient elimination of the CD44-modified A2780 cells by CD44NK cells. This was also shown by fluorescence microscopy of these co-cultures (Figure S2).

3.3. CD44NK Cells Specifically Kill Primary Patient-Derived Ovarian Cancer Cells

To analyze the killing activity of CAR-NK-92 cells against primary cancer cells, three patient-derived ovarian cancer cell samples (P1-3) were used. These cells were harvested from ascites of one patient at three different time points during chemotherapy. P1 was obtained before paclitaxel treatment, P2 and P3 were collected 20 and 30 days after initiation of paclitaxel treatment, respectively. The cells were characterized by high EPCAM and mesothelin expression (see Figure S3). The ascites cells also showed high CD44 expression, which did not decrease during or after chemotherapy (Figure 3A). We used the xCELLigence analyzer to measure the cytotoxicity of engineered NK cells, as the primary ovarian cancer cells were not labeled with fluorescence markers. Co-incubation of primary cells with CD44NK cells resulted in pronounced and dose-dependent lysis of cancer cells over time (Figure 3B–D). A complete lysis of target cells was already observed in P1 and P3 at an E/T ratio of 5:1, target cells reached baseline CI values after 4 h in P1 and 9 h in P3. A higher E/T ratio (10:1) led to an accelerated lysis of P3 within 4 h. Adding CD44NK cells at the E/T ratio of 1:1 caused a significant CI value reduction within 9 h in P3 (Figure 3C). To verify killing after co-incubation, microscopic images of P3 cells before and 2 h after co-incubation with control NK-92 or CAR-engineered NK cells at the E/T ratio with 5:1 are shown in Figure 3E.

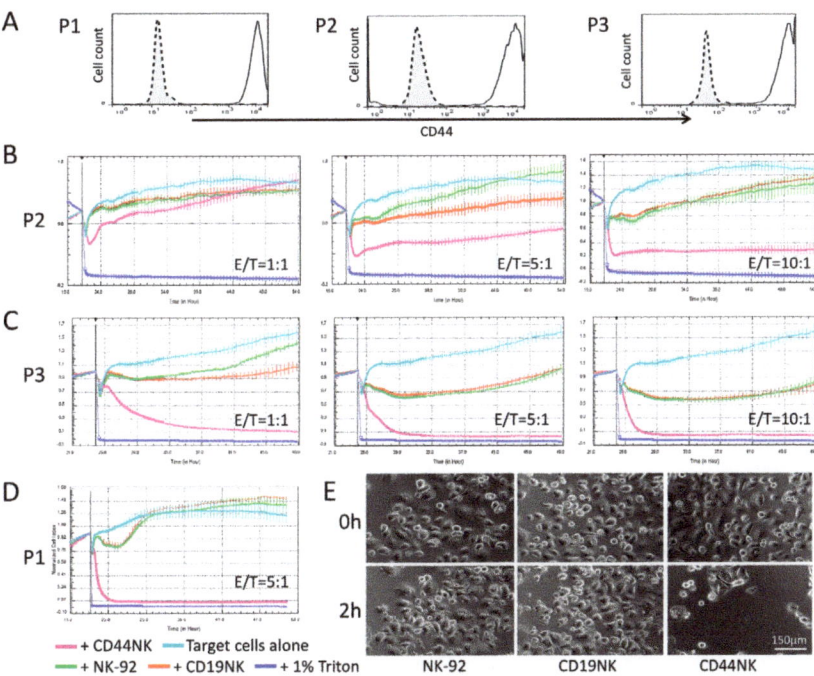

Figure 3. CD44NK cells specifically kill primary patient-derived ovarian cancer cells. (**A**) Flow cytometric analyses of expression levels of CD44 on three different primary ovarian cancer cell samples collected from one patient before chemotherapy (P1) or during chemotherapy (P2 and P3). Cytotoxic effects of engineered NK-92 cells on primary ovarian cancer cells P2 (**B**), P3 (**C**), and P1 (**D**) as measured by xCELLigence. E/T indicates the specific effector/target cell ratios. (**E**) Sequential microscopic images of the co-culture of CD19NK or CD44NK cells with primary ovarian cancer cells with an E/T ratio of 5:1.

3.4. Determination of CAR-NK-92 Activity by IFNγ Quantification

To quantify IFNγ secretion, NK-92 and CAR-NK-92 cells were either cultured alone or co-cultured with target cells at an E/T ratio of 5:1. After 24 h, cell-free supernatants were harvested and measured for IFNγ secretion using an ELISA. As shown in Figure 4, NK-92 and CAR-NK-92 cells spontaneously produced negligible or low levels of IFNγ when incubated alone. CD44NK cells were strongly activated by CD44 high expressing SKOV3, OVCAR3 and primary cells, and produced significantly increased IFNγ ($p < 0.0001$). Compared to CD19NK, co-incubation with CD44NK cells resulted in a 174- and 111-fold increase in IFNγ secretion level in P1 and P3, respectively. A five-fold increase in IFNγ secretion level was also shown in co-culture of A2780 cells with CD44NK cells compared to A2780 cells co-cultured with CD19NK cells. This may be due to the very low expression of CD44 on A2780 cells.

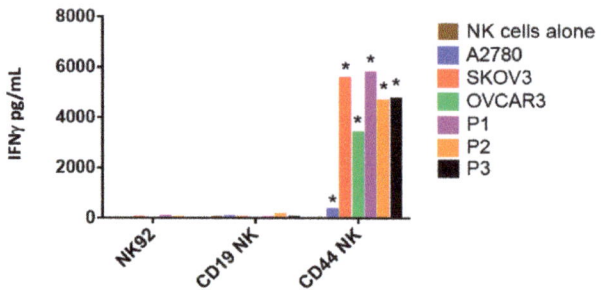

Figure 4. Quantification of IFNγ produced by NK-92 and CAR-NK-92 cells. IFNγ concentration in the cell-free supernatant after co-culture for 24 h with an E/T ratio of 5:1 was measured by ELISA. Values represent the mean ± standard deviation from two separate experiments, each containing three samples. * $p < 0.05$ compared to CD19NK.

3.5. Additive Anti-Tumor Activity of CD44NK Cells in Combination with Cisplatin Treatment

Platinum-based chemotherapy remains the core of primary treatment of advanced-stage ovarian cancer. In an attempt to maximize the benefits of the current therapy, the anti-tumor effect of combinatorial treatment of cisplatin and CAR-NK-92 cells was evaluated. CD44-negative A2780 and CD44-positive P3 cells were used as target cells. Co-incubation was performed for 4 days with NK cells at an E/T ratio of 2:1 and with the previously determined cisplatin IC_{50} dose. For the sequential treatment, co-incubation with NK cells and cisplatin was performed over 24 and 72 h, respectively. Relative survival rates were calculated by dividing the results obtained from each group by the results of cisplatin monotherapy (Figure 5A,B). CAR-NK-92 and untransduced NK-92 cells were still cytotoxic under cisplatin treatment. (Figure 5B). Compared to CD19NK and untransduced NK-92 cells, CD44NK cells significantly enhanced anti-tumor effects when applied as monotherapy ($p < 0.05$) and with simultaneous treatment using cisplatin ($p < 0.005$) (Figure 5B). Notably, this effect was not observed in CD44 negative A2780 cells under all designated conditions ($p > 0.31$) (Figure 5A).

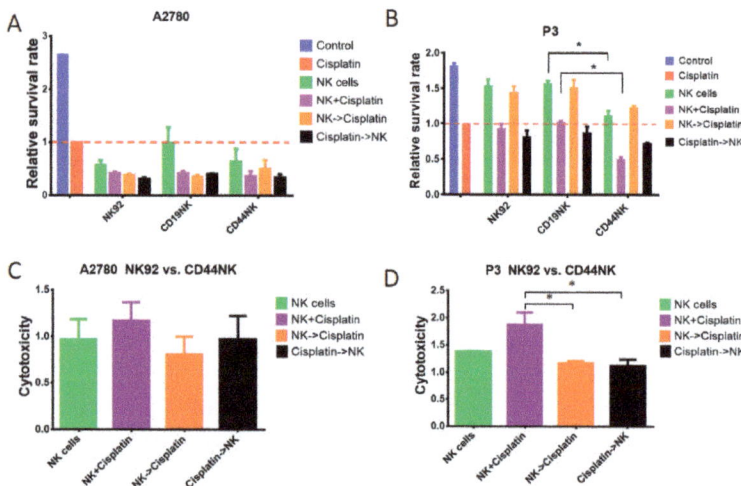

Figure 5. Additive anti-tumor activity of CD44NK cells in combination with cisplatin treatment. A2780 (**A**) and P3 (**B**) cells were treated for 4 days (cisplatin treatment for 72 h, NK-92 or CAR-NK-92 treatment 24 h) with the previously determined IC_{50} dose of cisplatin and an E/T ratio of 2:1. Relative

survival rate was calculated by dividing the results obtained from each group by the results of cisplatin monotherapy. Tumor cell loss of A2780 (**C**) and P3 (**D**) was calculated by dividing the results of CD44NK cells by the results of untransduced NK-92 cells for the designated conditions. * indicates a significant difference calculated by one-way ANOVA, $p < 0.05$. Values represent the mean from two separate experiments each containing three samples.

To further evaluate the benefit of incorporating CD44NK cells in the treatment of ovarian cancer, we calculated the relative cytotoxicity of CD44NK cells in relation to the unspecific NK-92 cells to rule out possible unspecific killing effects (Figure 5C,D). As expected, no significant differences were observed in CD44 negative A2780 cells (Figure 5C). CD44NK cells showed significantly higher anti-tumor activity in the simultaneous treatment with cisplatin than in sequential treatment ($p < 0.05$) (Figure 5D). The simultaneous treatment with CD44NK cells and cisplatin also resulted in the lowest survival rate in the P3 primary ovarian cancer sample ($p < 0.05$) (Figure 5B).

4. Discussion

In this work, we describe a novel anti-CD44 third-generation CAR directed against ovarian cancer. The increased efficiency of anti-ovarian cancer activity by CD44NK cells led to specific killing activity against ovarian cancer cell lines and patient-derived ovarian cancer cells in various assays. Concurrent therapy with cisplatin increased the killing effect compared to the respective monotherapy or a sequential therapy. Thus, the combination of immunotherapy with cisplatin could be a promising treatment strategy for advanced or relapsed ovarian cancer.

CD44 and its variants represent promising targets for ovarian cancer immunotherapy. The expression of CD44 was shown to be more pronounced in the recurrent and metastatic ovarian cancer tissues, when compared with its primary counterparts. Most ovarian cancer cells are initially chemosensitive. However, there is a population of highly chemoresistant cells with stem cell properties that survives initial therapy [24]. The exact surface markers characterizing ovarian CSCs remain controversial, but CD133, CD44, and CD24 are widely described as ovarian CSC markers in current studies [25]. Importantly, a correlation between the poor outcome of ovarian cancer patients and the expression of these CSC markers has been observed [26,27]. Contrary to other CSC markers, i.e., CD133, CD44 is widely expressed in ovarian cancer cells and was highly expressed in the samples analyzed in this study. Interestingly, several studies found CD44 expression to be associated with CSC-like properties of ovarian cancer cells. For example, ALDH1-bright cells from ovarian cancer cell lines show increased CD44 expression [28] and inhibition of CD44 was shown to inhibit growth of sphere-forming ovarian cancer cells [29]. However, the role of CD44 as a stem cell marker is still controversial and needs to be investigated in further studies.

Independently from its role as a CSC marker, a significant correlation was demonstrated between CD44 expression and disease-free survival and overall survival [27]. It was reported that peritoneal cells produce several extracellular matrix molecules that interact with CD44 [30,31]. CD44 was shown to mediate ovarian cancer cell adhesion to peritoneal mesothelial cells by binding cell surface HA, and thus promotes intraperitoneal ovarian cancer spread [19,20,32]. Downregulation of CD44 expression dramatically decreased the migratory potentials and invasiveness of ovarian cancer cells in vitro and suppressed tumor growth and peritoneal dissemination of human ovarian cancer xenograft in nude mice [27,33]. Interestingly, a recent study demonstrated that ovarian cancer-derived exosomes could transfer CD44 to human peritoneal mesothelial cells (HPMCs) and induce morphologic change in HPMCs to a mesenchymal, spindle phenotype. These exosomes increased CD44 expression in HPMCs, which facilitated cancer invasion by inducing the HPMCs to secrete matrix metalloproteinase-9 (MMP9) [34]. Furthermore, CD44 expression was shown to be significantly higher in the paclitaxel-resistant ovarian cell lines than in the drug-sensitive parental cell lines. Overexpression of CD44 was found in relapsed/recurrent tumors in a xenograft mouse model treated with paclitaxel [27]. CD44 targeted therapy was shown to effectively inhibit ovarian cancer dissemination, abrogate ascites, and prolong survival time [35,36]. All of these pieces of evidence suggest that developing new strategies to target CD44 in ovarian cancer may prevent disease recurrence, metastasis, and chemoresistance.

CAR-based immunotherapy has shown outstanding results in hematological malignancies [37]. Ovarian cancer is an immunogenic tumor with several tumor-specific antigens, which makes it an excellent target for CAR therapy. Sun et al. developed a humanized HER2 CAR containing chA21 scFv and T-cell intracellular signaling chains made up of CD28 and CD3ζ. They demonstrated that anti-HER2 CAR T cells were able to recognize and kill ovarian cancer cells ex vivo [38]. CAR-modified MUC-CD-targeted T cells infused through either intravenous or intraperitoneal injection showed either delayed progression or fully eradicated disease in SCID-Beige mice bearing orthotopic human MUC-CD-positive ovarian carcinoma tumors [9]. However, an early phase I study using anti-FRα CAR T cells in ovarian cancer patients reported that tumor burden was not significantly reduced in any patient. CAR T cells were present in the circulation in large numbers for the first 2 days after transfer, but rapidly declined to barely detectable levels one month later in most patients [39]. Although robust anti-tumor activity of anti-FRα CAR T cells was shown in vitro, they were unable to show tumor regression in clinical settings in patients due to their inability to persist in the tumor microenviroment. To overcome this limitation, Song and colleagues developed a new anti-FRα CAR in combination with a 4-1BB co-stimulatory motif and demonstrated that 4-1BB improved CAR T cell persistence in vivo [10]. Carpenito et al. equipped T cells with a third-generation mesothelin-specific CAR consisting of CD28 and 4-1BB as co-stimulators, and transferred them intratumorally and intravenously into mice engrafted with pre-established tumors. After infusion of those CAR T cells, tumor burden was reduced, and complete eradication of the tumors was observed in some cases [40]. However, a CAR with mouse origin scFvs has limited anti-tumor effect due to transgene immunogenicity. Therefore, a second-generation fully human anti-mesothelin CAR (P4 CAR) was developed. Primary human T cells expressing P4 CAR efficiently killed mesothelin-expressing tumors in vitro and in vivo [8]. A phase I trial for infusion of anti-mesothelin CAR T cells in patients with recurrent serous ovarian cancer was shown to be feasible and safe [41].

In contrast to other studies that used T cells in CAR therapy for ovarian cancer [8,9,38–42], we chose NK-92 as effector cells in this study. NK-92 cells were established from a patient with non-Hodgkin's lymphoma and their safety and anti-tumor capability were shown in clinical trials [43,44]. NK-92 cells were shown to be generally safe with moderate and transient toxicities in advanced cancer patients, and large-scale expansion of these cells is feasible [44]. Importantly, NK-92 cells express a relatively large number of activating receptors and lack most of the killer inhibitory receptors (KIRs) that are normally expressed on NK cells. Furthermore, NK-92 express high levels of molecules involved in the perforin-granzyme cytolytic pathway and additional cytotoxic effector molecules, indicating the potential of alternative anti-tumor mechanisms [45]. This confers NK-92 cells with superior cytotoxicity against a broad spectrum of tumor targets. Kloess and colleagues compared the function of CD123-CAR-expressing NK-92 cells and primary human donor NK (dNK) cells. They demonstrated that CAR-NK-92 cells had significantly stronger cytotoxic activity against leukemia cells as compared to CAR-dNK cells. The cytokine secretion profiles of CAR-NK-92 and CAR-dNK cells were shown to be very different [46]. However, it is important to note that CAR-NK-92 cells also exhibited significantly higher potential for adverse side effects against non-target cells [46]. Notably, NK-92 cells can be easily expanded in cultures with short doubling times to generate potent clinical-grade NK-92 effectors [47] and require only minimal manipulation without the need for cell-selection procedures. Thus, NK-92 cells offer an attractive platform for future study of novel NK-cell-based therapy.

In this study, we chose CD44 as a promising target and developed a novel third-generation anti-CD44 CAR incorporating a fully human anti-CD44 scFv linked to CD28 and 4-1BB as co-stimulators and a CD3ζ signaling domain. NK-92 cells equipped with the anti-CD44 CAR exhibited potent cytotoxic activity against CD44-positive ovarian cancer cell lines and primary ovarian cancer cells. Among these target cancer cells, A2780, OVCAR3, P2 and P3 cells also appeared to be sensitive to nonspecific cytotoxicity of CD19NK and NK-92 cells. However, CAR-restricted killing induced by CD44NK occurred more rapidly and more potently in CD44-positive OVCAR3, P2 and P3 cells. In parallel, the measurement of NK cell activation by IFNγ secretion assays confirmed these observations. Meanwhile, this significantly increased CAR-restricted cytotoxicity of CD44NK was hardly observed in CD44-low-expressing A2780 cells. Interestingly, we detected a slightly increased IFNγ level in co-culture of A2780 cells with CD44NK cells compared to that with CD19NK cells. This may be due to the very low expression of CD44 on A2780 cells, and the death of those cells was not detected by fluorescent microscopy or Fluoroskan measurements. Notably, P1 cells exhibited high resistance to nonspecific cytotoxicity of CD19NK and NK-92 cells even with a higher E/T ratio of 10:1 (data not shown), but these primary cancer cells strongly activated CD44NK cells and were largely eliminated by CD44NK cells with a lower E/T ratio of 5:1. In this study, we tested the killing effect of CD44NK cells against three primary samples isolated from one patient at different time points. Therefore, we cannot predict cytotoxic effects against all ovarian cancer cells in general. Since CD44NK cells showed activity against all tested cell lines and primary cells that express CD44, we assume that the CD44NK cells will also be effective against other ovarian cancer cells that express CD44. However, we also know that the cytotoxic activity of CAR-T or CAR-NK cells depends on susceptibility of the individual cells as shown in Figure 3. Thus, each patient has to be screened for CD44 expression before CAR therapy can be considered.

A previous study indicated that carboplatin induced CD44 expressing ovarian cancer cells to produce HA, which can contribute to chemoresistance by regulating ATP binding cassette transporter expression [48]. This highlights the importance of combinatorial treatment of chemotherapy and CD44-targeted therapy in ovarian cancer. To investigate the feasibility of combinatorial treatment of cytoreductive chemotherapy and specific elimination of CD44-positive highly chemoresistant tumor cells by CD44NK cells, we tested the anti-tumor activity of cisplatin and CAR-NK-92 cells in monotherapy, simultaneous, and sequential treatment. To mimic clinical settings and reduce the nonspecific cytotoxicity of NK cells, we used a low E/T ratio of 2:1. Compared to cisplatin monotherapy, simultaneous treatment with CD44NK cells and cisplatin resulted in a significant additive anti-tumor effect on P3 cells (27.1% more cell reduction). In contrast, simultaneous treatment with control NK cells and cisplatin did not show any additive effect in P3 primary ovarian cancer cells.

However, CAR-based therapy for solid tumors is faced with many challenges. In hematological malignancies, circulating CAR-engineered effector cells in the bloodstream have already reached the majority of their target cancer cells. In solid tumors, there are multiple barriers that hinder therapeutically sufficient tumor infiltration by CAR effector cells (reviewed in [49]). Regional CAR effector cell administration is one method to facilitate NK cell interaction with the tumor and potentially reduce off-tumor toxicity. A study of intraperitoneal (i.p.) injection of pan-ErbB/IL-4 CAR T cells targeting patient-derived malignant pleural mesotheliomas xenografts in SCID mice showed tumor regression or cure in all mice [50]. Katz and colleagues showed that i.p. delivery of CAR T cells resulted in superior protection against peritoneal tumors, when compared with systemically infused CAR T cells. I.p. infusion also provided prolonged protection against i.p. tumor relapse and demonstrated an increased effector memory phenotype over time [51]. Further in vivo studies are required to evaluate the efficacy and safety of CD44NK treatment.

CD44 is also widely distributed in normal tissues, e.g., central nervous system, lung, and hematopoietic cells [52]. The potential toxicity of CD44NK cells on normal tissues should be investigated in further studies. Strategies to prevent possible side effects, e.g., by using bispecific CARs, are already being evaluated in our lab.

In summary, we developed a novel third-generation CAR against CD44. The CAR-restricted killing effect of CD44NK cells was demonstrated in vitro. Additionally, we investigated combinatorial treatment strategies of CD44NK cells and cisplatin therapy and showed that CD44NK cells retained cytotoxicity during cisplatin incubation. The most potent anti-tumor effect was achieved by simultaneous treatment with CD44NK cells and cisplatin. This study will be the basis for further in vivo studies and future clinical developments.

Supplementary Materials: The following are available online at https://www.mdpi.com/article/10.3390/biomedicines9101339/s1, Figure S1. CD44NK effectively kill A2780 cells that were modified to express CD44, Figure S2. CD44-specific killing capacity of CD44NK cells. CD44NK cells were co-cultured with A2780 eGFP cells, A2780 CD44iGFP cells or OVCAR3 eGFP cells at an effector to target (E:T) ratio of 5:1, Figure S3. Flow cytometric analyses of EPCAM and Mesothelin expression levels on the three different primary ovarian cancer cell samples.

Author Contributions: Conceptualization, R.K., A.S., S.W.; Methodology, R.K., A.S., S.W., M.A.M., K.Z.; Software, R.K., S.W.; Validation, R.K., A.S., T.D., P.H., M.A.M.; Formal Analysis, R.K., A.S., M.A.M., P.H., H.B., S.W., K.Z.; Investigation, R.K., S.W., K.Z.; Resources,, A.S., R.K., T.D., P.H., H.B., M.A.M.; Data Curation, R.K., S.W., K.Z.; Writing—Original Draft Preparation, S.W., R.K.; Writing—Review and Editing, A.S., M.A.M., P.H., H.B., S.W., J.H., K.Z.; Visualization, R.K., S.W.; Supervision, A.S., P.H., T.D., M.A.M., H.B.; Project Administration, A.S., R.K.; Funding Acquisition, A.S., R.K., P.H. All authors have read and agreed to the published version of the manuscript.

Funding: This study was supported by HILF (Hochschulinterne Leistungsförderung, Hannover Medical School) and the Young Academy (Hannover Medical School; both granted to Dr. Rüdiger Klapdor) as well as DFG (SFB738, Cluster of Excellence REBIRTH and KFO 286) and Lower Saxony Ministry of Science and Culture (MWK).

Institutional Review Board Statement: The study was conducted according to the guidelines of the Declaration of Helsinki. Only anonymized samples were used.

Informed Consent Statement: See Material and Methods section. Informed consent was obtained from patients.

Data Availability Statement: Data is contained within the article and supplementary material.

Acknowledgments: We thank the Claudia-von-Schilling-Foundation for funding the xCELLigence RTCA SP instrument. We gratefully acknowledge the technical assistance of Britta Wieland and helpful advice of Kristine Bousset. We thank Ulrich Hacker for providing primary ovarian cancer cells.

Conflicts of Interest: The authors declare no conflict of interest.

References

1. Bray, F.; Ferlay, J.; Soerjomataram, I.; Siegel, R.L.; Torre, L.A.; Jemal, A. Global cancer statistics 2018: GLOBOCAN estimates of incidence and mortality worldwide for 36 cancers in 185 countries. *CA Cancer J. Clin.* **2018**, *68*, 394–424. [CrossRef]
2. Heintz, A.; Odicino, F.; Maisonneuve, P.; A Quinn, M.; Benedet, J.L.; Creasman, W.T.; Ngan, H.Y.S.; Pecorelli, S.; Beller, U. Carcinoma of the Ovary. *Int. J. Gynecol. Obstet.* **2006**, *95*, S161–S192. [CrossRef]
3. Galon, J.; Angell, H.K.; Bedognetti, D.; Marincola, F.M. The Continuum of Cancer Immunosurveillance: Prognostic, Predictive, and Mechanistic Signatures. *Immunity* **2013**, *39*, 11–26. [CrossRef] [PubMed]
4. Zhang, L.; Conejo-Garcia, J.R.; Katsaros, D.; Gimotty, P.A.; Massobrio, M.; Regnani, G.; Makrigiannakis, A.; Gray, H.; Schlienger, K.; Liebman, M.N.; et al. Intratumoral T Cells, Recurrence, and Survival in Epithelial Ovarian Cancer. *N. Engl. J. Med.* **2003**, *348*, 203–213. [CrossRef] [PubMed]
5. Sato, E.; Olson, S.H.; Ahn, J.; Bundy, B.; Nishikawa, H.; Qian, F.; Jungbluth, A.A.; Frosina, D.; Gnjatic, S.; Ambrosone, C.; et al. Intraepithelial CD8+ tumor-infiltrating lymphocytes and a high CD8+/regulatory T cell ratio are associated with favorable prognosis in ovarian cancer. *Proc. Natl. Acad. Sci. USA* **2005**, *102*, 18538–18543. [CrossRef] [PubMed]
6. Hwang, W.-T.; Adams, S.F.; Tahirovic, E.; Hagemann, I.; Coukos, G. Prognostic significance of tumor-infiltrating T cells in ovarian cancer: A meta-analysis. *Gynecol. Oncol.* **2012**, *124*, 192–198. [CrossRef] [PubMed]
7. Li, J.; Wang, J.; Chen, R.; Bai, Y.; Lu, X. The prognostic value of tumor-infiltrating T lymphocytes in ovarian cancer. *Oncotarget* **2017**, *8*, 15621–15631. [CrossRef]
8. Lanitis, E.; Poussin, M.; Hagemann, I.; Coukos, G.; Sandaltzopoulos, R.; Scholler, N.; Powell, D.J. Redirected Antitumor Activity of Primary Human Lymphocytes Transduced with a Fully Human Anti-mesothelin Chimeric Receptor. *Mol. Ther.* **2012**, *20*, 633–643. [CrossRef]

9. Chekmasova, A.A.; Rao, T.D.; Nikhamin, Y.; Park, K.; Levine, D.A.; Spriggs, D.R.; Brentjens, R.J. Successful Eradication of Established Peritoneal Ovarian Tumors in SCID-Beige Mice following Adoptive Transfer of T Cells Genetically Targeted to the MUC16 Antigen. *Clin. Cancer Res.* **2010**, *16*, 3594–3606. [CrossRef]
10. Song, D.-G.; Ye, Q.; Carpenito, C.; Poussin, M.; Wang, L.-P.; Ji, C.; Figini, M.; June, C.H.; Coukos, G.; Powell, D.J., Jr. In Vivo Persistence, Tumor Localization, and Antitumor Activity of CAR-Engineered T Cells Is Enhanced by Costimulatory Signaling through CD137 (4-1BB). *Cancer Res.* **2011**, *71*, 4617–4627. [CrossRef]
11. Klapdor, R.; Wang, S.; Hacker, U.; Büning, H.; Morgan, M.; Dörk, T.; Hillemanns, P.; Schambach, A. Improved Killing of Ovarian Cancer Stem Cells by Combining a Novel Chimeric Antigen Receptor–Based Immunotherapy and Chemotherapy. *Hum. Gene Ther.* **2017**, *28*, 886–896. [CrossRef]
12. Foster, R.; Buckanovich, R.J.; Rueda, B.R. Ovarian cancer stem cells: Working towards the root of stemness. *Cancer Lett.* **2013**, *338*, 147–157. [CrossRef]
13. Latifi, A.; Abubaker, K.; Castrechini, N.; Ward, A.; Liongue, C.; Dobill, F.; Kumar, J.; Thompson, E.W.; Quinn, M.; Findlay, J.K.; et al. Cisplatin treatment of primary and metastatic epithelial ovarian carcinomas generates residual cells with mesenchymal stem cell-like profile. *J. Cell. Biochem.* **2011**, *112*, 2850–2864. [CrossRef]
14. Takaishi, S.; Okumura, T.; Tu, S.; Wang, S.S.; Shibata, W.; Vigneshwaran, R.; Gordon, S.A.; Shimada, Y.; Wang, T.C. Identification of Gastric Cancer Stem Cells Using the Cell Surface Marker CD44. *STEM CELLS* **2009**, *27*, 1006–1020. [CrossRef]
15. Prince, M.E.; Sivanandan, R.; Kaczorowski, A.; Wolf, G.T.; Kaplan, M.J.; Dalerba, P.; Weissman, I.L.; Clarke, M.F.; Ailles, L.E. Identification of a subpopulation of cells with cancer stem cell properties in head and neck squamous cell carcinoma. *Proc. Natl. Acad. Sci. USA* **2007**, *104*, 973–978. [CrossRef]
16. Zhang, S.; Balch, C.; Chan, M.; Lai, H.-C.; Matei, D.; Schilder, J.M.; Yan, P.S.; Huang, T.H.-M.; Nephew, K.P. Identification and Characterization of Ovarian Cancer-Initiating Cells from Primary Human Tumors. *Cancer Res.* **2008**, *68*, 4311–4320. [CrossRef]
17. Orian-Rousseau, V. CD44, a therapeutic target for metastasising tumours. *Eur. J. Cancer* **2010**, *46*, 1271–1277. [CrossRef] [PubMed]
18. Zöller, M. CD44: Can a cancer-initiating cell profit from an abundantly expressed molecule? *Nat. Rev. Cancer* **2011**, *11*, 254–267. [CrossRef] [PubMed]
19. Lessan, K.; Aguiar, D.J.; Oegema, T.; Siebenson, L.; Skubitz, A.P. CD44 and β1 Integrin Mediate Ovarian Carcinoma Cell Adhesion to Peritoneal Mesothelial Cells. *Am. J. Pathol.* **1999**, *154*, 1525–1537. [CrossRef]
20. A Cannistra, S.; Kansas, G.S.; Niloff, J.; Defranzo, B.; Kim, Y.; Ottensmeier, C. Binding of ovarian cancer cells to peritoneal mesothelium in vitro is partly mediated by CD44H. *Cancer Res.* **1993**, *53*, 3830–3838. [PubMed]
21. Runnels, H.A.; Weber, G.L.; Min, J.; Kudlacz, E.M.; Zobel, J.F.; Donovan, C.B.; Thiede, M.A.; Zhang, J.; Alpert, R.B.; Salafia, M.A.; et al. PF-03475952: A potent and neutralizing fully human anti-CD44 antibody for therapeutic applications in inflammatory diseases. *Adv. Ther.* **2010**, *27*, 168–180. [CrossRef] [PubMed]
22. Suerth, J.D.; Morgan, M.A.; Kloess, S.; Heckl, D.; Neudörfl, C.; Falk, C.S.; Koehl, U.; Schambach, A. Efficient generation of gene-modified human natural killer cells via alpharetroviral vectors. *J. Mol. Med.* **2016**, *94*, 83–93. [CrossRef]
23. Dull, T.; Zufferey, R.; Kelly, M.; Mandel, R.J.; Nguyen, M.; Trono, D.; Naldini, L. A Third-Generation Lentivirus Vector with a Conditional Packaging System. *J. Virol.* **1998**, *72*, 8463–8471. [CrossRef]
24. Albini, A.; Bruno, A.; Gallo, C.; Pajardi, G.E.; Noonan, U.M.; Dallaglio, K. Cancer stem cells and the tumor microenvironment: Interplay in tumor heterogeneity. *Connect. Tissue Res.* **2015**, *56*, 414–425. [CrossRef]
25. Garson, K.; Vanderhyden, B.C. Epithelial ovarian cancer stem cells: Underlying complexity of a simple paradigm. *Reproduction* **2015**, *149*, R59–R70. [CrossRef]
26. Steffensen, K.D.; Alvero, A.B.; Yang, Y.; Waldstrøm, M.; Hui, P.; Holmberg, J.C.; Silasi, D.-A.; Jakobsen, A.; Rutherford, T.; Mor, G. Prevalence of Epithelial Ovarian Cancer Stem Cells Correlates with Recurrence in Early-Stage Ovarian Cancer. *J. Oncol.* **2011**, *2011*, 1–12. [CrossRef] [PubMed]
27. Gao, Y.; Foster, R.; Yang, X.; Feng, Y.; Shen, J.K.; Mankin, H.J.; Hornicek, F.J.; Amiji, M.M.; Duan, Z. Up-regulation of CD44 in the development of metastasis, recurrence and drug resistance of ovarian cancer. *Oncotarget* **2015**, *6*, 9313–9326. [CrossRef]
28. Wang, Y.-C.; Yo, Y.-T.; Lee, H.-Y.; Liao, Y.-P.; Chao, T.-K.; Su, P.-H.; Lai, H.-C. ALDH1-Bright Epithelial Ovarian Cancer Cells Are Associated with CD44 Expression, Drug Resistance, and Poor Clinical Outcome. *Am. J. Pathol.* **2012**, *180*, 1159–1169. [CrossRef]
29. Du, Y.-R.; Chen, Y.; Gao, Y.; Niu, X.-L.; Li, Y.-J.; Deng, W.-M. Effects and Mechanisms of Anti-CD44 Monoclonal Antibody A3D8 on Proliferation and Apoptosis of Sphere-Forming Cells with Stemness From Human Ovarian Cancer. *Int. J. Gynecol. Cancer* **2013**, *23*, 1367–1375. [CrossRef]
30. Dimitroff, C.J.; Lee, J.Y.; Fuhlbrigge, R.C.; Sackstein, R. A distinct glycoform of CD44 is an L-selectin ligand on human hematopoietic cells. *Proc. Natl. Acad. Sci. USA* **2000**, *97*, 13841–13846. [CrossRef] [PubMed]
31. Dimitroff, C.J.; Lee, J.Y.; Rafii, S.; Fuhlbrigge, R.C.; Sackstein, R. Cd44 Is a Major E-Selectin Ligand on Human Hematopoietic Progenitor Cells. *J. Cell Biol.* **2001**, *153*, 1277–1286. [CrossRef] [PubMed]
32. Carpenter, P.M.; Dao, A.V. The role of hyaluronan in mesothelium-induced motility of ovarian carcinoma cells. *Anticancer Res.* **2003**, *23*, 3985–3990.
33. Cheng, W.; Liu, T.; Wan, X.; Gao, Y.; Wang, H. MicroRNA-199a targets CD44 to suppress the tumorigenicity and multidrug resistance of ovarian cancer-initiating cells. *FEBS J.* **2012**, *279*, 2047–2059. [CrossRef] [PubMed]

34. Nakamura, K.; Sawada, K.; Kinose, Y.; Yoshimura, A.; Toda, A.; Nakatsuka, E.; Hashimoto, K.; Mabuchi, S.; Morishige, K.-I.; Kurachi, H.; et al. Exosomes Promote Ovarian Cancer Cell Invasion through Transfer of CD44 to Peritoneal Mesothelial Cells. *Mol. Cancer Res.* **2016**, *15*, 78–92. [CrossRef]
35. De Stefano, I.; Battaglia, A.; Zannoni, G.F.; Prisco, M.G.; Fattorossi, A.; Travaglia, D.; Baroni, S.; Renier, D.; Scambia, G.; Ferlini, C.; et al. Hyaluronic acid–paclitaxel: Effects of intraperitoneal administration against CD44(+) human ovarian cancer xenografts. *Cancer Chemother. Pharmacol.* **2011**, *68*, 107–116. [CrossRef]
36. Lee, S.J.; Ghosh, S.C.; Han, H.D.; Stone, R.L.; Bottsford-Miller, J.; Shen, D.Y.; Auzenne, E.J.; Lopez-Araujo, A.; Lu, C.; Nishimura, M.; et al. Metronomic Activity of CD44-Targeted Hyaluronic Acid-Paclitaxel in Ovarian Carcinoma. *Clin. Cancer Res.* **2012**, *18*, 4114–4121. [CrossRef] [PubMed]
37. Park, J.H.; Geyer, M.B.; Brentjens, R.J. CD19-targeted CAR T-cell therapeutics for hematologic malignancies: Interpreting clinical outcomes to date. *Blood* **2016**, *127*, 3312–3320. [CrossRef] [PubMed]
38. Sun, M.; Shi, H.; Liu, C.; Liu, J.; Liu, X.; Sun, Y. Construction and evaluation of a novel humanized HER2-specific chimeric receptor. *Breast Cancer Res.* **2014**, *16*, R61. [CrossRef]
39. Kershaw, M.H.; Westwood, J.A.; Parker, L.L.; Wang, G.; Eshhar, Z.; Mavroukakis, S.A.; White, D.E.; Wunderlich, J.R.; Canevari, S.; Rogers-Freezer, L.; et al. A Phase I Study on Adoptive Immunotherapy Using Gene-Modified T Cells for Ovarian Cancer. *Clin. Cancer Res.* **2006**, *12*, 6106–6115. [CrossRef]
40. Carpenito, C.; Milone, M.C.; Hassan, R.; Simonet, J.C.; Lakhal, M.; Suhoski, M.M.; Varela-Rohena, A.; Haines, K.M.; Heitjan, D.F.; Albelda, S.M.; et al. Control of large, established tumor xenografts with genetically retargeted human T cells containing CD28 and CD137 domains. *Proc. Natl. Acad. Sci. USA* **2009**, *106*, 3360–3365. [CrossRef]
41. Tanyi, J.L.; Haas, A.R.; Beatty, G.L.; Stashwick, C.J.; O'Hara, M.; Morgan, M.A.; Porter, D.L.; Melenhorst, J.J.; Plesa, G.; Lacey, S.F.; et al. Anti-mesothelin chimeric antigen receptor T cells in patients with epithelial ovarian cancer. *J. Clin. Oncol.* **2016**, *34*, 5511. [CrossRef]
42. Koneru, M.; Purdon, T.; Spriggs, D.; Koneru, S.; Brentjens, R.J. IL-12 secreting tumor-targeted chimeric antigen receptor T cells eradicate ovarian tumorsin vivo. *OncoImmunology* **2015**, *4*, e994446. [CrossRef]
43. Tonn, T.; Becker, S.; Esser, R.; Schwabe, D.; Seifried, E. Cellular Immunotherapy of Malignancies Using the Clonal Natural Killer Cell Line NK-92. *J. Hematother.* **2001**, *10*, 535–544. [CrossRef]
44. Arai, S.; Meagher, R.; Swearingen, M.; Myint, H.; Rich, E.; Martinson, J.; Klingemann, H. Infusion of the allogeneic cell line NK-92 in patients with advanced renal cell cancer or melanoma: A phase I trial. *Cytotherapy* **2008**, *10*, 625–632. [CrossRef] [PubMed]
45. Maki, G.; Klingemann, H.-G.; Martinson, J.A.; Tam, Y.K. Factors Regulating the Cytotoxic Activity of the Human Natural Killer Cell Line, NK-92. *J. Hematother.* **2001**, *10*, 369–383. [CrossRef] [PubMed]
46. Kloess, S.; Oberschmidt, O.; Dahlke, J.; Vu, X.-K.; Neudoerfl, C.; Kloos, A.; Gardlowski, T.; Matthies, N.; Heuser, M.; Meyer, J.; et al. Preclinical Assessment of Suitable Natural Killer Cell Sources for Chimeric Antigen Receptor Natural Killer–Based "Off-the-Shelf" Acute Myeloid Leukemia Immunotherapies. *Hum. Gene Ther.* **2019**, *30*, 381–401. [CrossRef]
47. Tam, Y.; Martinson, J.; Doligosa, K.; Klingernann, H.-G. Ex vivo expansion of the highly cytotoxic human natural killer cell line NK-92 under current good manufacturing practice conditions for clinical adoptive cellular immunotherapy. *Cytotherapy* **2003**, *5*, 259–272. [CrossRef] [PubMed]
48. Ricciardelli, C.; Ween, M.P.; A Lokman, N.; A Tan, I.; E Pyragius, C.; Oehler, M.K. Chemotherapy-induced hyaluronan production: A novel chemoresistance mechanism in ovarian cancer. *BMC Cancer* **2013**, *13*, 476. [CrossRef]
49. Vignali, D.; Kallikourdis, M. Improving homing in T cell therapy. *Cytokine Growth Factor Rev.* **2017**, *36*, 107–116. [CrossRef]
50. Klampatsa, A.; Achkova, D.Y.; Davies, D.M.; Parente-Pereira, A.C.; Woodman, N.; Rosekilly, J.; Osborne, G.; Thayaparan, T.; Bille, A.; Sheaf, M.; et al. Intracavitary 'T4 immunotherapy' of malignant mesothelioma using pan-ErbB re-targeted CAR T-cells. *Cancer Lett.* **2017**, *393*, 52–59. [CrossRef]
51. Katz, S.; Point, G.R.; Cunetta, M.; Thorn, M.; Guha, P.; Espat, N.J.; Boutros, C.; Hanna, N.; Junghans, R.P. Regional CAR-T cell infusions for peritoneal carcinomatosis are superior to systemic delivery. *Cancer Gene Ther.* **2016**, *23*, 142–148. [CrossRef] [PubMed]
52. Fox, S.; Fawcett, J.; Jackson, D.G.; Collins, I.; Gatter, K.C.; Harris, A.; Gearing, A.; Simmons, D.L. Normal human tissues, in addition to some tumors, express multiple different CD44 isoforms. *Cancer Res.* **1994**, *54*, 4539–4546.

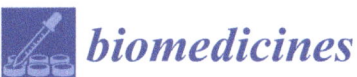

Article

A DNA Damage Response Gene Panel for Different Histologic Types of Epithelial Ovarian Carcinomas and Their Outcomes

Ying-Cheng Chiang [1,2], Po-Han Lin [3,4], Tzu-Pin Lu [5], Kuan-Ting Kuo [6], Yi-Jou Tai [2,7], Heng-Cheng Hsu [7,8], Chia-Ying Wu [2,7], Chia-Yi Lee [7,8], Hung Shen [7,8], Chi-An Chen [1,2,*,†] and Wen-Fang Cheng [1,2,7,9,*,†]

1 Department of Obstetrics and Gynecology, College of Medicine, National Taiwan University, Taipei 100226, Taiwan; ycchiang@ntuh.gov.tw
2 Department of Obstetrics and Gynecology, National Taiwan University Hospital, Taipei 100226, Taiwan; stilabry@gmail.com (Y.-J.T.); ascheetah@msn.com (C.-Y.W.)
3 Department of Medical Genetics, National Taiwan University Hospital, Taipei 100226, Taiwan; pohanlin01@gmail.com
4 Graduate Institute of Medical Genomics and Proteomics, College of Medicine, National Taiwan University, Taipei 100025, Taiwan
5 Institute of Epidemiology and Preventive Medicine, Department of Public Health, National Taiwan University, Taipei 100025, Taiwan; tbenlu@gmail.com
6 Department of Pathology, College of Medicine, National Taiwan University, Taipei 100225, Taiwan; pathologykimo@gmail.com
7 Graduate Institute of Clinical Medicine, College of Medicine, National Taiwan University, Taipei 100225, Taiwan; b101092037@gmail.com (H.-C.H.); plzfixthecar@gmail.com (C.-Y.L.); shkt0802@gmail.com (H.S.)
8 Department of Obstetrics and Gynecology, National Taiwan University Hospital, Hsin-Chu Branch, Hsin-Chu 30059, Taiwan
9 Graduate Institute of Oncology, College of Medicine, National Taiwan University, Taipei 100025, Taiwan
* Correspondence: chianchen@ntu.edu.tw (C.-A.C.); wenfangcheng@yahoo.com (W.-F.C.); Tel.: +886-2-2312-3456 (ext. 71964) (W.-F.C.)
† Equal contribution.

Abstract: DNA damage response (DDR) is important for maintaining genomic integrity of the cell. Aberrant DDR pathways lead to accumulation of DNA damage, genomic instability and malignant transformations. Gene mutations have been proven to be associated with epithelial ovarian cancer, and the majority of the literature has focused on *BRCA*. In this study, we investigated the somatic mutation of DNA damage response genes in epithelial ovarian cancer patients using a multiple-gene panel with next-generation sequencing. In all, 69 serous, 39 endometrioid and 64 clear cell carcinoma patients were enrolled. Serous carcinoma patients (69.6%) had higher percentages of DDR gene mutations compared with patients with endometrioid (33.3%) and clear cell carcinoma (26.6%) ($p < 0.001$, chi-squared test). The percentages of DDR gene mutations in patients with recurrence (53.9 vs. 32.9% $p = 0.006$, chi-squared test) or cancer-related death (59.2 vs. 34.4% $p = 0.001$, chi-squared test) were higher than those without recurrence or living patients. In endometrioid carcinoma, patients with ≥2 DDR gene mutations had shorter PFS ($p = 0.0035$, log-rank test) and OS ($p = 0.015$, log-rank test) than those with one mutation or none. In clear cell carcinoma, patients with ≥2 DDR gene mutations had significantly shorter PFS ($p = 0.0056$, log-rank test) and OS ($p = 0.0046$, log-rank test) than those with 1 DDR mutation or none. In the EOC patients, somatic DDR gene mutations were associated with advanced-stage tumor recurrence and tumor-related death. Type I EOC patients with DDR mutations had an unfavorable prognosis, especially for clear cell carcinoma.

Keywords: epithelial ovarian cancer; DNA damage response; somatic mutation; clear cell carcinoma

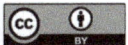

1. Introduction

Epithelial ovarian carcinoma (EOC) is a major cause of death in women worldwide, and patients are usually diagnosed at an advanced stage with a 5-year survival of less than 50% [1–4]. Clinical prognostic factors include cancer stage, histological subtypes, tumor grade, residual tumor size after debulking surgery and response to chemotherapy. Despite an initial good response to primary treatments of debulking surgery and adjuvant platinum-based chemotherapy, the majority of patients experience a cancer relapse that is resistant to salvage treatments and eventually die of the disease [4,5].

Precision medicine is the current direction for cancer management depending on the specific genetic or molecular features of cancer. There are several subtypes of EOC—high-grade serous, clear cell, endometrioid, mucinous and low-grade serous—that could be viewed as distinct diseases for their differences in clinical course and pathological features [6,7]. To date, the most promising target therapies for EOC are anti-angiogenesis agents and poly ADP-ribose polymerase inhibitors (PARPi). Bevacizumab in combination with chemotherapy has demonstrated improved progression-free survival, and an overall survival benefit in high-risk patients [8–10]. Maintenance therapy with PARPi has revised the management of EOC in newly diagnosed and recurrent diseases. The identification of *BRCA* mutations or homologous recombination deficiency (HRD) status is critical for selecting potential patients, but both positive and negative patients as defined by current HRD assays benefited from PARPi [11–15].

DNA damage response (DDR) is important for maintaining a cell's genomic integrity, and the DDR pathway is composed of various molecules that detect DNA damage, activate cell-cycle checkpoints, trigger apoptosis, and coordinate DNA repair [16–18]. Several exogenous or endogenous sources (e.g., oxidative damage, radiation, ultraviolet light, cytotoxic materials, replication errors) may result in DNA damage that may eventually lead to genomic instability and cell death [19]. DDR consists of several pathways, including base excision (BER), mismatch (MMR) and nucleotide excision repair (NER); translesion synthesis (TLS) for single-strand break repair; homologous recombination (HR) and nonhomologous DNA end joining (NHEJ) for double-strand break repair; and cell cycle regulation (CCR) (27, 28). Homologous recombination is an error-proof repair pathway to restore the original sequence at the double-strand DNA break. *BRCA* 1/2 genes participating in HR and maintaining PARPi therapy for *BRCA*-mutated EOC is a good example of synthetic lethality [20]. Several other DDR genes have been identified as potential targets for novel cancer therapy under clinical investigation [16,17]. Understanding the complex DDR pathways is helpful for exploring the feasibility of novel DDR inhibitors in clinical practice. In the study, we investigated the somatic mutations of DDR genes in 172 EOC patients using a targeted DDR gene panel using a next-generation sequencing method. The correlation of the somatic DDR gene mutations, clinical parameters and outcomes was analysed.

2. Materials and Methods

2.1. Patients and Specimens

The study protocol was approved by the National Taiwan University Hospital Research Ethics Committee (201509042RINA, approved on 24 November 2015 and 201608025RINA, approved on 07 October 2016). Informed consent from all participants was obtained and the methods were performed in accordance with the guidelines and regulations. From December 2015 to October 2018, 172 women diagnosed with epithelial ovarian cancer who had received debulking surgery and adjuvant chemotherapy were enrolled. The cancerous tissue specimens collected during debulking surgery were immediately frozen in liquid nitrogen and stored at −70 °C. A portion of the tissue specimens were sent for pathological examinations to confirm the diagnosis and ensure tumorous tissue sufficient for the following experiments. Clinical data were obtained from medical records, including age, cancer stage, the findings during debulking surgery, treatment course and recurrence. Optimal debulking surgery was defined as a maximal residual tumor size <1 cm following surgery. The tumor grade based on International Union Against Cancer criteria, and cancer stage was based on International Federation of Gynecology and Obstetrics (FIGO) criteria [21]. All patients received platinum-based adjuvant chemotherapy and regular follow-ups after primary treatments. Recurrence was defined as abnormal results from imaging studies (including computerized tomography or magnetic resonance imaging), elevated CA-125 (more than twice the upper normal limit) for two consecutive tests in 2-week intervals, or a biopsy-proven disease. Progression-free survival (PFS) was defined as the time from the date of primary treatment completion to the date of confirmed recurrence, disease progression or last follow-up. Overall survival (OS) was defined as the period from surgery to the date of death related to EOC or the date of last follow-up.

2.2. The Panel of DNA Damage Repair Genes

We selected 60 genes involved in DNA damage response (DDR) for the gene panel (Table 1), including genes of homologous recombination (HR), nonhomologous DNA end joining (NHEJ), base excision repair (BER), mismatch repair (MMR), nucleotide excision repair (NER), translesion synthesis (TLS) and cell cycle regulation (CCR) [16,17].

Table 1. List of the DNA damage response (DDR) gene panel.

Gene	DDR Pathway	Gene	DDR Pathway
ATM	CCR	ku70/XRCC6	NHEJ
BARD1	HR	ku80/XRCC5	NHEJ
BRCA1	HR	MDM4	CCR
BRCA2/FANCD1	HR	MLH1	MMR
BRIP1/FANCJ	HR	MLH3	MMR
CHEK2	CCR	MRE11	HR
DDB1	NER	MSH2	MMR
DDB2	NER	MSH3	MMR
ERCC1	NER	MSH6	MMR
ERCC2/XPD	NER	MUTYH	BER
ERCC3/XPB	NER	NBN	HR
ERCC4	NER	NBS1	HR
ERCC5/BIVM	NER	OGG1	BER
ERCC6/CSB	NER	PMS1	MMR
ERCC8/CSA	NER	PMS2	MMR
FANCA	HR	POLD1	TLS
FANCB	HR	POLE	TLS
FANCC	HR	POLB	TLS
FANCD1/BRCA2	HR	POLH	TLS
FANCD2	HR	POLK	TLS
FANCE	HR	RAD50	HR
FANCF	HR	RAD51	HR
FANCG/XRCC	HR	RAD51C/FANCO	HR
FANCI	HR	RAD51D	HR
FANCJ/BRIP1	HR	TP53	CCR
FANCL/PHF9	HR	XPA	NER
FANCM	HR	XPC	NER
FANCN/PALB2	HR	XRCC2	NHEJ
FANCO/RAD51C	HR	XRCC3	NHEJ
FANCP/SLX4	HR	XRCC4	NHEJ

Note: BER: base excision repair; CCR: cell cycle regulation; DDR: DNA damage repair; HR: homologous recombination; MMR: mismatch repair; NER: nucleotide excision repair; NHEJ: nonhomologous DNA end joining; TLS: translesion synthesis.

2.3. Genomic DNA Extraction

Genomic DNA was isolated using a QIAGEN Genomic DNA extraction kit according to the manufacturer's instructions (Qiagen Inc., Valencia, CA, US). The purity and concentration of the genomic DNA were checked by agarose gel electrophoresis and the $OD_{260/280}$ ratio.

2.4. Library Preparation, Next-Generation Sequencing, and Sequence Mapping

The genomic DNA was fragmented with Covaris fragmentation protocol (Covaris, Inc., Woburn, MA, US). The size of the fragmented genomic DNA was checked by Agilent Bioanalyzer 2100 (Agilent Technologies, Inc., Santa Clara, CA, US) and NanoDrop spectrophotometer (Thermo Fisher Scientific, Inc., Wilmington, DE, US). The target gene library was generated with NimblGen capture kits (Roche NimblGen, Inc. Hacienda Dr Pleasanton, CA, US). The samples were sequenced by Illumina MiSeq with paired-end reads of 300 nucleotides.

The analysis algorithm was conducted according to our previous protocol [22]. Briefly, the raw sequencing data were aligned with the reference human genome (Feb. 2009, GRCh37/hg19) with Burrows–Wheeler Aligner software (version 0.5.9) [23]. SAM tools (version 0.1.18) was used for data conversion, sorting, and indexing [24]. For single nucleotide polymorphisms (SNPs) and small insertion/deletions (indels), Genome Analysis Toolkit (GATK; version 2.7) was used for variant calling with Base/indel-calibrator and HaplotypeCaller. Pindel or Breakdancer software were used for structural variants larger than 100 bp which cannot be identified by GATK, such as large deletions, insertions and duplications [25]. After variant calling, ANNOVAR was used for annotation of the genetic variants [26,27]. The dbSNP, Exome sequencing Project 6500 (ESP6500) and the 1000 Genomes variant dataset were used to filter common variants of sequencing results.

2.5. Variant Classification

The sequence variants were classified according to the IARC variant classification [28]. The pathogenic mutations were defined as large-scale deletion, frame-shift mutation, nonsense mutation, genetic variants associated with uncorrected splicing and mutations affecting protein function demonstrated by functional analyses. The pathogenic and likely pathogenic mutations were used as deleterious mutations in our study. An allele frequency greater than 0.01 in the general population in the 1000 Genomes variant dataset or ESP6500 database were considered benign or likely benign genetic variants. Silent and intronic variants that did not affect splicing were also considered benign or likely benign. Other variants, mainly missense mutations without known functional data, were considered as variants of uncertain significance (VUSs). To reduce their number, bioinformatics analyses, including PolyPhen2 and SIFT, were used to evaluate potential pathogenicity [29–31]. The VUSs were suspected of being deleterious mutations if they met two criteria: (1) a population frequency of less than 0.01 in the 1000 Genomes and ESP6500 databases and (2) a bioinformatics analysis result with a SIFT score less than 0.05 and a polyphen2 score greater than 0.95.

2.6. Statistical Analysis

All statistical analyses were performed using the Statistical Package for Social Sciences software package (IBM SPSS Statistics for Windows, Version 22.0. IBM Corp. Armonk, NY, US) and R (version 3.1.2, The R Foundation for Statistical Computing, Institute for Statistics and Mathematics, Wirtschaftsuniversität Wien, Welthandelsplatz Vienna, Austria). One-way ANOVA was used to compare continuous variables and a chi-squared test was used for categorical variables. Survival curves were generated using the Kaplan–Meier method, and differences were calculated using the log-rank test. A multivariate Cox's regression model was used to evaluate the prognostic factors for progression-free survival (PFS) and overall survival (OS). Statistical significance was set as a p value of less than 0.05.

3. Results

3.1. Clinical Characteristics of the Patients

There were 172 EOC patients enrolled: 69 serous, 39 endometrioid and 64 clear cell carcinomas (Table 2). There were 68 high-grade serous carcinomas (type II tumor) and 104 type I tumors. The median age was 52, and the median pre-treatment CA125 value was 400 U/mL; 59.9% were diagnosed at an advanced cancer stage, and 65.1% had undergone optimal debulking surgery; 59.3% had disease recurrence, and 44.2% died of EOC. All patients received adjuvant platinum and paclitaxel chemotherapy.

Table 2. Characteristics of the epithelial ovarian cancer patients.

Patient Numbers	172
Median Age (years old)	52 (29–85)
Median CA 125 (U/mL)	400 (12–7265)
Histology	
Serous carcinoma	69 (40.1%)
Endometrioid carcinoma	39 (22.7%)
Clear cell carcinoma	64 (37.2%)
FIGO stage	
Early	69 (40.1%)
Advanced	103 (59.9%)
Grade	
Low	29 (16.9%)
High	143 (83.1%)
Debulking surgery	
Optimal	112 (65.1%)
Suboptimal	60 (34.9%)
Recurrence	
Yes	102 (59.3%)
No	70 (40.7%)
Death	
Yes	76 (44.2%)
No	96 (55.8%)

3.2. Deleterious DDR Gene Mutations

As shown in Table 3, 114 deleterious somatic mutations were identified from 26 genes of our 60-gene DDR panel in 78 EOC patients: 27 nonsense mutations in 23 patients, 28 frameshift mutations in 20, 28 missense mutations in 26 patients and 31 mutations involving uncorrected splicing in 29 patients. There were single-gene mutations in 57 patients, and multiple-gene mutations in 21: 2 mutations in 14 patients, 3 mutations in 2, 4 mutations in 3, 5 mutations in 1 and 6 mutations in 1 patient (Figure 1). We also identified 109 missense mutations classified as variants of uncertain significance (VUSs) with the potential of being deleterious mutations after searching the database (http://www.ncbi.nlm.nih.gov/snp, accessed on 28 September 2021) and bioinformatic analyses (Table S1 and Figure S1).

The pattern of prevalent mutated DDR genes was different among the histological subtypes (Figure 1). The proportion of wild type DDR genes was 54.7% in all EOC patients; 30.4% in serous carcinoma, 66.7% in endometrioid carcinoma and 73.4% in clear cell carcinoma. The top three prevalent mutated DDR genes were *TP53* (27.9%), *MUTYH* (6.4%) and *BRCA2* (5.8%) for all patients. Serous carcinoma—*TP53* (56.5%), *BRCA2* (5.8%) and *RAD51C* (5.8%); endometrioid carcinoma—*TP53* (15.4%), *ATM* (12.8%) and *MSH2* (7.7%); clear cell carcinoma—*MUTYH* (9.4%), *TP53* (4.7%), *BRCA2* (3.1%) and *ERCC8* (3.1%). The top three prevalent mutated subgroups of DDR genes were CCR (30.8%), HR (10.5%) and BER (7.0%) for all patients. Serous carcinoma—CCR (58.05%), HR (15.9%) and BER (5.8%); endometrioid carcinoma—CCR (23.1%), MMR (15.4%) and HR (7.7%); clear cell carcinoma—BER (9.4%), CCR (6.3%) and HR (6.3%). For detailed information, please refer to Table S2 and Figure S2.

Table 3. The deleterious DDR gene mutations in the patients.

Gene	Mutation	Transcript	gDNA/cDNA	Amino Acid	Reported/Novel
ATM	frameshift deletion	NM_000051	c.1402_1403del	p.K468fs	rs587781347
ATM	frameshift deletion	NM_000051	c.8426delA	p.Q2809fs	rs587782558
ATM	frameshift insertion	NM_000051	c.4736dupA	p.Q1579fs	rs864622164
ATM	missense mutation	NM_000051	c.C6200A	p.A2067D	rs397514577
ATM	nonsense mutation	NM_000051	c.C5188T	p.R1730X	rs764389018
ATM	nonsense mutation	NM_000051	c.C850T	p.Q284X	rs757782702
BARD1	frameshift insertion	NM_000465	c.70_71insGT	p.P24fs	NA
BRCA1	nonsense mutation	NM_007294	c.3531dupT	p.S1178_K1179delinsX	NA
BRCA1	nonsense mutation	NM_007294	c.G2635T	p.E879X	rs80357251
BRCA2	frameshift deletion	NM_000059	c.1585delT	p.F529fs	NA
BRCA2	frameshift insertion	NM_000059	c.7407dupT	p.T2469fs	rs397507916
BRCA2	nonsense mutation	NM_000059	c.4965delC	p.Y1655X	rs80359475
BRCA2	nonsense mutation	NM_000059	c.A5623T	p.K1875X	NA
BRCA2	nonsense mutation	NM_000059	c.C2590T	p.Q864X	rs1060502414
BRCA2	nonsense mutation	NM_000059	c.C6952T	p.R2318X	rs80358920
BRCA2	nonsense mutation	NM_000059	c.G3922T	p.E1308X	rs80358638
BRIP1	frameshift insertion	NM_032043	c.394dupA	p.T132fs	rs587781416
CHEK2	splicing	NM_007194	g. 29130716 C>G		NA
ERCC8	frameshift deletion	NM_000082	c.191_195del	p.S64fs	NA
ERCC8	splicing	NM_000082	c.1123-2->T		NA
ERCC8	splicing	NM_000082	c.1123-2->T		NA
ERCC8	splicing	NM_000082	c.1123-2->T		NA
ERCC8	splicing	NM_000082	c.1123-2->T		rs777444521
FANCC	nonsense mutation	NM_000136	c.G1225T	p.E409X	NA
FANCG	splicing	NM_004629	c.511-2->C		NA
FANCI	splicing	NM_001113378	c.3187-2A>G		NA
FANCM	frameshift deletion	NM_020937	c.3998delA	p.Q1333fs	rs746983128
MLH1	frameshift deletion	NM_000249	c.1771delG	p.D591fs	NA
MLH1	splicing	NM_000249	c.2104-2A>G		rs267607889
MLH1	splicing	NM_000249	c.790+2T>C		rs267607790
MLH3	missense mutation	NM_001040108	c.G2221T	p.V741F	rs28756990
MLH3	missense mutation	NM_001040108	c.G2221T	p.V741F	rs28756990
MLH3	missense mutation	NM_001040108	c.G2221T	p.V741F	rs28756990
MLH3	missense mutation	NM_001040108	c.G2221T	p.V741F	rs28756990
MRE11	frameshift insertion	NM_005590	c.1222dupA	p.T408fs	rs774440500
MSH2	nonsense mutation	NM_000251	c.C226T	p.Q76X	rs63750042
MSH2	nonsense mutation	NM_000251	c.G1738T	p.E580X	rs63751411
MSH2	splicing	NM_000251	c.943-1G>C		rs12476364
MSH3	frameshift deletion	NM_002439	c.1141delA	p.K381fs	rs587776701
MSH6	frameshift insertion	NM_001281492	c.2916dupT	p.T972fs	NA
MSH6	nonsense mutation	NM_001281492	c.G726A	p.W242X	NA
MSH6	splicing	NM_001281492	g. 48033792_48033795 del TAAC		NA
MUTYH	missense mutation	NM_001128425	c.G1187A	p.G396D	rs36053993
MUTYH	nonsense mutation	NM_001128425	c.G467A	p.W156X	rs762307622
MUTYH	splicing	NM_001128425	c.576+1G>C		NA
MUTYH	splicing	NM_001128425	c.934-2A>G		rs77542170
MUTYH	splicing	NM_001128425	c.934-2A>G		rs77542170
MUTYH	splicing	NM_001128425	c.934-2A>G		rs77542170
MUTYH	splicing	NM_001128425	c.934-2A>G		rs77542170
MUTYH	splicing	NM_001128425	c.934-2A>G		rs77542170
MUTYH	splicing	NM_001128425	c.934-2A>G		rs77542170
MUTYH	splicing	NM_001128425	c.934-2A>G		rs77542170
MUTYH	splicing	NM_001128425	c.934-2A>G		rs77542170
OGG1	nonsense mutation	NM_016819	c.A974G	p.X325W	NA
POLD1	splicing	NM_002691	c.2954-1G>-		NA
RAD50	frameshift deletion	NM_005732	c.2157delA	p.L719fs	NA
RAD50	frameshift deletion	NM_005732	c.536delT	p.I179fs	NA

Table 3. Cont.

Gene	Mutation	Transcript	gDNA/cDNA	Amino Acid	Reported/Novel
RAD50	frameshift insertion	NM_005732	exon13:c.2157dupA	p.L719fs	rs397507178
RAD51C	frameshift insertion	NM_058216	c.390dupA	p.G130fs	rs730881940
RAD51C	nonsense mutation	NM_058216	c.T833G	p.L278X	NA
RAD51C	splicing	NM_058216	c.905-2A>C		NA
RAD51C	splicing	NM_058216	c.905-2A>C		NA
RAD51D	splicing	NM_002878	c.480+1G>A		NA
TP53	frameshift deletion	NM_000546	c.102delC	p.P34fs	NA
TP53	frameshift deletion	NM_000546	c.121delG	p.D41fs	NA
TP53	frameshift deletion	NM_000546	c.216delC	p.P72fs	NA
TP53	frameshift deletion	NM_000546	c.257_272del	p.A86fs	NA
TP53	frameshift deletion	NM_000546	c.501delG	p.Q167fs	NA
TP53	frameshift deletion	NM_000546	c.539_549del	p.E180fs	NA
TP53	frameshift insertion	NM_000546	c.102dupC	p.L35fs	NA
TP53	frameshift insertion	NM_000546	c.455dupC	p.P152fs	NA
TP53	frameshift insertion	NM_000546	c.498dupA	p.Q167fs	NA
TP53	frameshift insertion	NM_000546	c.889dupG	p.H297fs	NA
TP53	missense mutation	NM_000546	c.A488G	p.Y163C	rs148924904
TP53	missense mutation	NM_000546	c.A578G	p.H193R	rs786201838
TP53	missense mutation	NM_000546	c.A659C	p.Y220S	rs121912666
TP53	missense mutation	NM_000546	c.A659G	p.Y220C	rs121912666
TP53	missense mutation	NM_000546	c.A659G	p.Y220C	rs121912666
TP53	missense mutation	NM_000546	c.A736G	p.M246V	rs483352695
TP53	missense mutation	NM_000546	c.A838G	p.R280G	rs753660142
TP53	missense mutation	NM_000546	c.C380T	p.S127F	rs730881999
TP53	missense mutation	NM_000546	c.C451T	p.P151S	rs28934874
TP53	missense mutation	NM_000546	c.C844T	p.R282W	rs28934574
TP53	missense mutation	NM_000546	c.C844T	p.R282W	rs28934574
TP53	missense mutation	NM_000546	c.G412C	p.A138P	rs28934875
TP53	missense mutation	NM_000546	c.G524A	p.R175H	rs28934578
TP53	missense mutation	NM_000546	c.G524A	p.R175H	rs28934578
TP53	missense mutation	NM_000546	c.G638T	p.R213L	rs587778720
TP53	missense mutation	NM_000546	c.G730A	p.G244S	rs1057519989
TP53	missense mutation	NM_000546	c.G743A	p.R248Q	rs11540652
TP53	missense mutation	NM_000546	c.G743A	p.R248Q	rs11540652
TP53	missense mutation	NM_000546	c.G818A	p.R273H	rs28934576
TP53	missense mutation	NM_000546	c.G818A	p.R273H	rs28934576
TP53	missense mutation	NM_000546	c.G836A	p.G279E	rs1064793881
TP53	missense mutation	NM_000546	c.G856A	p.E286K	rs786201059
TP53	nonsense mutation	NM_000546	c.588_589insTGA	p.V197delinsX	NA
TP53	nonsense mutation	NM_000546	c.912dupT	p.K305_R306delinsX	NA
TP53	nonsense mutation	NM_000546	c.C430T	p.Q144X	NA
TP53	nonsense mutation	NM_000546	c.C499T	p.Q167X	NA
TP53	nonsense mutation	NM_000546	c.C574T	p.Q192X	NA
TP53	nonsense mutation	NM_000546	c.C586T	p.R196X	rs397516435
TP53	nonsense mutation	NM_000546	c.C637T	p.R213X	rs397516436
TP53	nonsense mutation	NM_000546	c.G272A	p.W91X	NA
TP53	nonsense mutation	NM_000546	c.G438A	p.W146X	NA
TP53	nonsense mutation	NM_000546	c.G859T	p.E287X	NA
TP53	nonsense mutation	NM_000546	c.G880T	p.E294X	rs1057520607
TP53	splicing	NM_000546	c.376-1G>T		NA
TP53	splicing	NM_000546	c.672+1G>A		rs863224499
TP53	splicing	NM_000546	c.993+2T>G		NA
TP53	splicing	NM_000546	c.993+2T>G		NA
TP53	splicing	NM_000546	c.993+1G>T		rs11575997
TP53	splicing	NM_000546	g.7577493_7577497 del CCTGA		NA
XRCC4	frameshift deletion	NM_003401	c.810delA	p.R270fs	NA
XRCC6	splicing	NM_001469	c.589+1G>T		NA

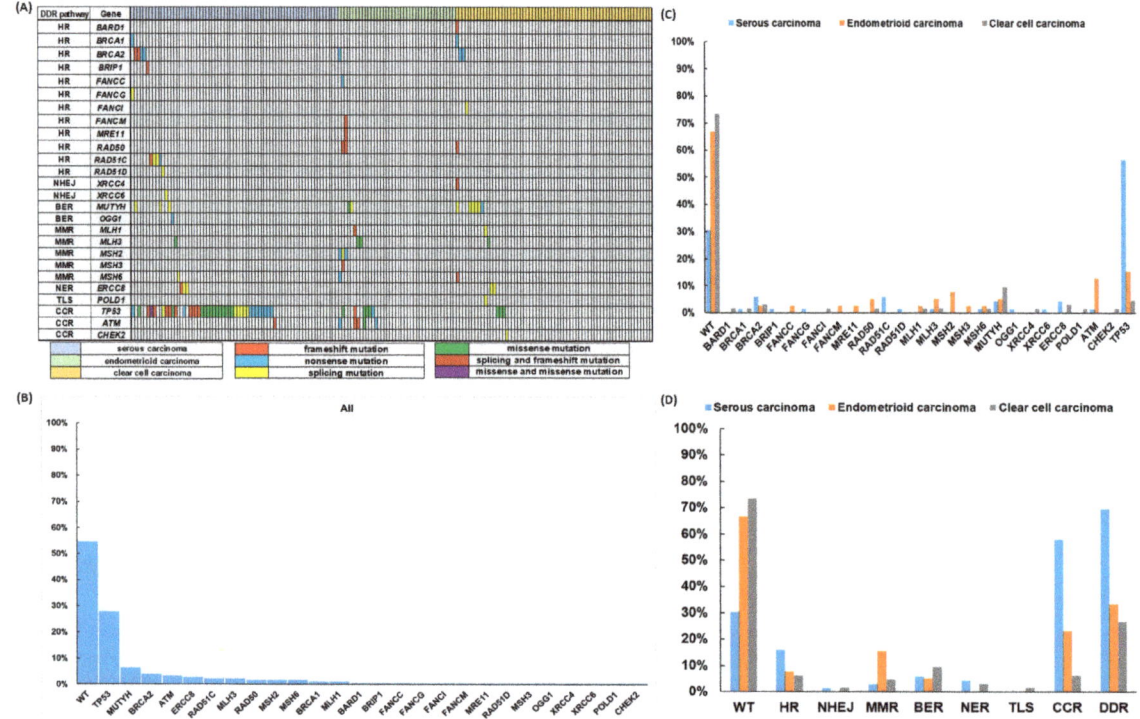

Figure 1. Deleterious DNA damage response (DDR) gene mutations in 172 epithelial ovarian carcinoma (EOC) patients (**A**) The pattern of DDR mutations of different histologic subtypes. (**B**) The percentages of DDR mutations in all 172 EOC patients. (**C**) The percentages of DDR mutations in different histologic subtypes. (**D**) The percentages of DDR mutations classified by different pathways in different histologic subtypes.

3.3. Correlation of DDR Gene Mutations with Clinical Outcomes of the EOC Patients

We evaluated the correlations between the mutation of DDR genes, the clinicopathologic parameters and outcome of the EOC patients. As shown in Table 4, type II tumors had a higher percentage of HR gene mutations than type I tumors (16.18 vs. 6.73%, $p = 0.048$, chi-squared test). Endometrioid carcinoma (15.38%) had a higher percentage of MMR mutations than those of serous carcinoma (2.90%) and clear cell carcinoma (4.69%) ($p = 0.03$, chi-squared test). Low-grade tumors had a higher percentage of MMR mutations compared with high-grade tumors (17.24 vs. 4.20%, $p = 0.009$, chi-squared test). Type II tumors had a higher percentage of DSBR mutations than type I tumors (17.65 vs. 6.73%, $p = 0.026$, chi-squared test). Serous carcinoma (57.97%) had a higher percentage of CCR mutations than those of endometrioid carcinoma (23.08%) and clear cell carcinoma (6.25%) ($p < 0.001$, chi-squared test). Type II tumors had higher percentage of CCR mutations than those of type I tumors (58.82 vs. 12.50%, $p < 0.001$, chi-squared test). The advanced-stage patients had a higher percentage of CCR mutations than the early-stage patients (42.72 vs. 13.04%, $p < 0.001$, chi-squared test). The recurrent patients had a higher percentage of CCR mutations than those without recurrence (39.22% vs. 18.57%, $p = 0.004$, chi-squared test). Patients who died of EOC had higher percentages of CCR mutations than living patients (40.79 vs. 22.92%, $p = 0.012$, chi-squared test). Serous carcinoma (69.57%) had higher percentage of DDR mutations than those of endometrioid carcinoma (33.33%) and clear cell carcinoma (26.56%) ($p < 0.001$, chi-squared test). Type II tumors had a higher percentage of DDR mutations than type I tumors (70.59 vs. 28.85%, $p < 0.001$, chi-squared test). The advanced stage patients had higher percentage of DDR mutations than the early-stage patients (57.28 vs. 27.54%, $p < 0.001$, chi-squared test). Recurring patients had a higher percentage of DDR mutations than those without recurrence (53.92 vs. 32.86%, $p = 0.006$, chi-squared test). Patients who died of EOC had a higher percentage of DDR mutations than living patients (59.21 vs. 34.38%, $p = 0.001$, chi-squared test).

EOC patients without DDR gene mutation had longer progression-free survival (PFS) ($p = 0.0072$, log-rank test, Figure 2A) and overall survival (OS) ($p = 0.022$, log-rank test, Figure 2B) than those with 1 DDR or ≥ 2 DDR mutations. In serous carcinoma, patients with or without DDR mutations had similar PFS ($p = 0.56$, log-rank test, Figure 2C). Patients with ≥ 2 DDR mutations had a trend of better OS than those with 1 mutation or none, but it was not statistically significant ($p = 0.47$, log-rank test, Figure 2D). In endometrioid carcinoma, patients with ≥ 2 DDR gene mutations had shorter PFS ($p = 0.0035$, log-rank test, Figure 2E) and OS ($p = 0.015$, log-rank test, Figure 2F) than those with 1 mutation or none. In clear cell carcinoma, patients with ≥ 2 DDR gene mutations had significantly shorter PFS ($p = 0.0056$, log-rank test, Figure 2G) and OS ($p = 0.0046$, log-rank test, Figure 2H) than those with 1 DDR mutation or none.

Tumor recurrence with CCR gene mutation (HR: 1.68 (1.12–2.50), $p = 0.011$), 1 DDR gene mutation (HR: 1.71 (1.12–2.60), $p = 0.013$), endometrioid carcinoma (HR: 0.17 (0.08–0.37), $p < 0.001$), type II tumor (HR: 2.69 (1.81–4.00), $p < 0.001$), advanced-stage carcinoma (HR: 5.29 (3.16–8.85), $p < 0.001$), high-grade tumor (HR: 5.57 (2.26–13.70), $p < 0.001$) and optimal debulking surgery (HR: 0.28 (0.18–0.41), $p < 0.001$) were significant in the univariate Cox regression model (Table 5). Advanced-stage carcinoma (HR: 3.08 (1.63–5.80), $p = 0.001$) and optimal debulking surgery (HR: 0.51 (0.32–0.80), $p = 0.004$) were important prognostic factors in the multivariate analysis. Cancer-related death with TLS gene mutation (HR: 33.76 (3.95–289.00), $p = 0.001$), 1 DDR gene mutation (HR: 1.96 (1.20–3.20), $p = 0.007$), endometrioid carcinoma (HR: 0.12 (0.04–0.38), $p < 0.001$), type II tumor (HR: 1.88 (1.19–2.96), $p = 0.007$), advanced-stage carcinoma (HR: 6.84 (3.28–14.25), $p < 0.001$), high-grade tumor (HR: 17.97 (2.50–129.29), $p = 0.004$) and optimal debulking surgery (HR: 0.26 (0.16–0.41), $p < 0.001$) were significant in the univariate Cox regression model. Type II tumor (HR: 0.35 (0.20–0.60), $p < 0.001$), TLS gene mutation (HR: 9.57 (1.08–84.83), $p = 0.042$), advanced-stage carcinoma (HR: 4.82 (2.09–11.09), $p < 0.001$) and optimal debulking surgery (HR: 0.38 (0.22–0.64), $p < 0.001$) were important prognostic factors in the multivariate analysis.

Table 4. The correlation of DDR gene mutations with clinical parameters in the epithelial ovarian cancer patients.

Genes		Histology			Type		FIGO Stage		Tumor Grade		Recurrence		Death	
		OSA	OEA	OCCA	I	II	Early	Advanced	Low	High	No	Yes	No	Yes
Total	172	69	39	64	104	68	69	103	29	143	70	102	96	76
HR														
Wild type	154 89.53%	58 84.06%	36 92.31%	60 93.75%	97 93.27%	57 83.82%	64 92.75%	90 87.38%	26 89.66%	128 89.51%	64 91.43%	90 88.24%	89 92.71%	65 85.53%
Mutation	18 10.47%	11 15.94%	3 7.69%	4 6.25%	7 6.73%	11 16.18%	5 7.25%	13 12.62%	3 10.34%	15 10.49%	6 8.57%	12 11.76%	7 7.29%	11 14.47%
p value *			0.154			0.048		0.259		0.981		0.502		0.126
NHEJ														
Wild type	170 98.84%	68 98.55%	39 100.00%	63 98.44%	103 99.04%	67 98.53%	69 100.00%	101 98.06%	29 100.00%	141 98.60%	70 100.00%	100 98.04%	96 100.00%	74 97.37%
Mutation	2 1.16%	1 1.45%	0 0.00%	1 1.56%	1 0.96%	1 1.47%	0 0.00%	2 1.94%	0 0.00%	2 1.40%	0 0.00%	2 1.96%	0 0.00%	2 2.63%
p value *			0.742			0.761		0.244		0.522		0.239		0.11
MMR														
Wild type	161 93.60%	67 97.10%	33 84.62%	61 95.31%	95 91.35%	66 97.06%	65 94.20%	96 93.20%	24 82.76%	137 95.80%	66 94.29%	95 93.14%	91 94.79%	70 92.11%
Mutation	11 6.40%	2 2.90%	6 15.38%	3 4.69%	9 8.65%	2 2.94%	4 5.80%	7 6.80%	5 17.24%	6 4.20%	4 5.71%	7 6.86%	5 5.21%	6 7.89%
p value *			0.03			0.134		0.793		0.009		0.762		0.475
BER														
Wild type	160 93.02%	65 94.20%	37 94.87%	58 90.63%	96 92.31%	64 94.12%	65 94.20%	95 92.23%	27 93.10%	133 93.01%	66 94.29%	94 92.16%	91 94.79%	69 90.79%
Mutation	12 6.98%	4 5.80%	2 5.13%	6 9.38%	8 7.69%	4 5.88%	4 5.80%	8 7.77%	2 6.90%	10 6.99%	4 5.71%	8 7.84%	5 5.21%	7 9.21%
p value *			0.631			0.649		0.619		0.985		0.59		0.306

Table 4. Cont.

Genes	Histology			Type			FIGO Stage		Tumor Grade		Recurrence		Death	
	OSA	OEA	OCCA	I	II	Early	Advanced	Low	High	No	Yes	No	Yes
NER														
Wild type	66 95.65%	39 100.00%	62 96.88%	102 98.08%	65 95.59%	67 97.10%	100 97.09%	29 100.00%	138 96.50%	67 95.71%	100 98.04%	93 96.88%	74 97.37%
Mutation	3 4.35%	0 0.00%	2 3.13%	2 1.92%	3 4.41%	2 2.90%	3 2.91%	0 0.00%	5 3.50%	3 4.29%	2 1.96%	3 3.13%	2 2.63%
p value *			0.43		0.342		0.996		0.307		0.373		0.848
TLS														
Wild type	69 100.00%	39 100.00%	63 98.44%	103 99.04%	68 100.00%	69 100.00%	102 99.03%	29 100.00%	142 99.30%	70 100.00%	101 99.02%	96 100.00%	75 98.68%
Mutation	0 0.00%	0 0.00%	1 1.56%	1 0.96%	0 0.00%	0 0.00%	1 0.97%	0 0.00%	1 0.70%	0 0.00%	1 0.98%	0 0.00%	1 1.32%
p value *			0.428		0.417		0.412		0.652		0.406		0.26
DSBR														
Wild type	57 82.61%	36 92.31%	60 93.75%	97 93.27%	56 82.35%	64 92.75%	89 86.41%	26 89.66%	127 88.81%	64 91.43%	89 87.25%	89 92.71%	64 84.21%
Mutation	12 17.39%	3 7.69%	4 6.25%	7 6.73%	12 17.65%	5 7.25%	14 13.59%	3 10.34%	16 11.19%	6 8.57%	13 12.75%	7 7.29%	12 15.79%
p value *			0.092		0.026		0.193		0.895		0.391		0.077
SSBR														
Wild type	60 86.96%	31 79.49%	54 84.38%	86 82.69%	59 86.76%	59 85.51%	86 83.50%	22 75.86%	123 86.01%	59 84.29%	86 84.31%	83 86.46%	62 81.58%
Mutation	9 13.04%	8 20.51%	10 15.63%	18 17.31%	9 13.24%	10 14.49%	17 16.50%	7 24.14%	20 13.99%	11 15.71%	16 15.69%	13 13.54%	14 18.42%
p value *			0.591		0.473		0.722		0.171		0.996		0.382
CCR														
Wild type	29 42.03%	30 76.92%	60 93.75%	91 87.50%	28 41.18%	60 86.96%	59 57.28%	24 82.76%	95 66.43%	57 81.43%	62 60.78%	74 77.08%	45 59.21%
Mutation	40 57.97%	9 23.08%	4 6.25%	13 12.50%	40 58.82%	9 13.04%	44 42.72%	5 17.24%	48 33.57%	13 18.57%	40 39.22%	22 22.92%	31 40.79%
p value *			<0.001		<0.001		<0.001		0.083		0.004		0.012

Table 4. Cont.

Genes		Histology			Type		FIGO Stage		Tumor Grade		Recurrence		Death	
		OSA	OEA	OCCA	I	II	Early	Advanced	Low	High	No	Yes	No	Yes
DDR														
Wild type	94 54.65%	21 30.43%	26 66.67%	47 73.44%	74 71.15%	20 29.41%	50 72.46%	44 42.72%	20 68.97%	74 51.75%	47 67.14%	47 46.08%	63 65.63%	31 40.79%
1 gene mutation	57 33.14%	35 50.72%	7 17.95%	15 23.44%	22 21.15%	35 51.47%	14 20.29%	43 41.75%	5 17.24%	52 36.36%	16 22.86%	41 40.20%	24 25.00%	33 43.42%
2 gene mutations	15 8.72%	12 17.39%	2 5.13%	1 1.56%	3 2.88%	12 17.65%	2 2.90%	13 12.62%	0 0.00%	15 10.49%	4 5.71%	11 10.78%	6 6.25%	9 11.84%
3 gene mutations	2 1.16%	1 1.45%	1 2.56%	0 0.00%	1 0.96%	1 1.47%	1 1.45%	1 0.97%	1 3.45%	1 0.70%	1 1.43%	1 0.98%	1 1.04%	1 1.32%
4 gene mutations	2 1.16%	0 0.00%	2 5.13%	0 0.00%	2 1.92%	0 0.00%	2 2.90%	0 0.00%	2 6.90%	0 0.00%	2 2.86%	0 0.00%	2 2.08%	0 0.00%
5 gene Mutations	1 0.58%	0 0.00%	1 2.56%	0 0.00%	1 0.96%	0 0.00%	0 0.00%	1 0.97%	1 3.45%	0 0.00%	0 0.00%	1 0.98%	0 0.00%	1 1.32%
6 gene mutations	1 0.58%	0 0.00%	0 0.00%	1 1.56%	1 0.96%	0 0.00%	0 0.00%	1 0.97%	0 0.00%	1 0.70%	0 0.00%	1 0.98%	0 0.00%	1 1.32%
Total mutations	78 45.35%	48 69.57%	13 33.33%	17 26.56%	30 28.85%	48 70.59%	19 27.54%	59 57.28%	9 31.03%	69 48.25%	23 32.86%	55 53.92%	33 34.38%	45 59.21%
p value *		<0.001			<0.001		<0.001		0.089		0.006		0.001	

Note: BER: base excision repair; CCR: cell cycle regulation; DDR: DNA damage response; DSBR: double-strand break repair; HR: homologous recombination; MMR: mismatch repair; NER: nucleotide excision repair; NHEJ: nonhomologous DNA end joining; OSA: ovarian serous carcinoma; OEA: ovarian endometrioid carcinoma; OCCA: ovarian clear cell carcinoma; SSBR: single-strand break repair; TLS: translesion synthesis. * Pearson's chi-squared test

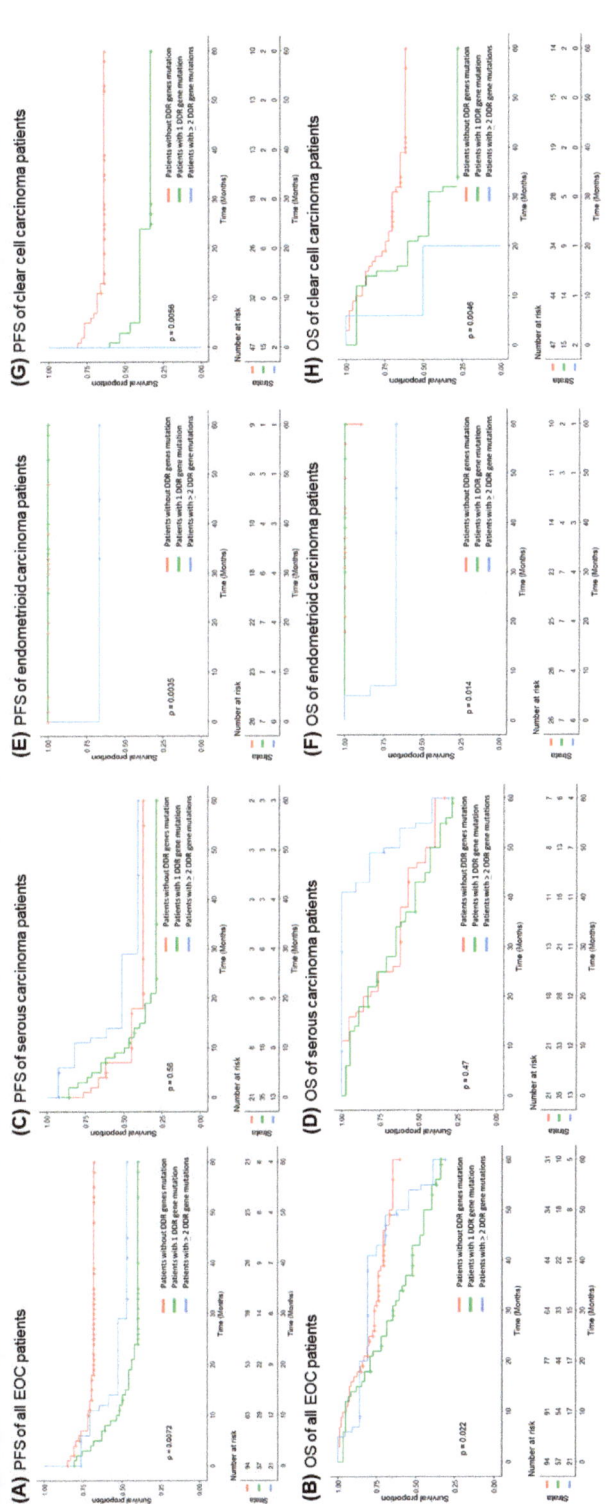

Figure 2. Kaplan–Meier analysis of progression-free survival (PFS) and overall survival (OS) in 172 epithelial ovarian carcinoma (EOC) patients. (**A**) PFS of 172 EOC patients. Note: EOC patients with DDR gene mutation(s) had shorter PFS ($p = 0.0072$, log-rank test). (**B**) OS of 172 EOC patients. Note: EOC patients with DDR gene mutation(s) had shorter OS ($p = 0.022$, log-rank test) (**C**) PFS of 69 serous carcinoma patients. Note: Serous carcinoma patients with ≥2 DDR gene mutations had a trend of better PFS although no statistical significance. (**D**) OS of 69 serous carcinoma patients. Note: Serous carcinoma patients with ≥2 DDR gene mutations had a trend of better OS although no statistical significance. (**E**) PFS of 39 endometrioid carcinoma patients. Note: Endometrioid carcinoma patients with ≥2 DDR gene mutations had poor PFS ($p = 0.0035$, log-rank test). (**F**) OS of 39 endometrioid carcinoma patients. Note: Endometrioid carcinoma patients with ≥2 DDR gene mutations had poor OS ($p = 0.014$, log-rank test). (**G**) PFS of 64 clear cell carcinoma patients. Note: Clear cell carcinoma patients with ≥2 DDR gene mutations had significantly shorter PFS ($p = 0.0056$, log-rank test). (**H**) OS of 64 clear cell carcinoma patients. Note: Clear cell carcinoma patients with ≥2 DDR gene mutations had significantly shorter OS ($p = 0.0046$, log-rank test).

Table 5. Cox regression model for the risk factors for recurrence and death in all patients (n = 172).

Factors	n	Recurrence				Death			
		Univariate		Multivariate		Univariate		Multivariate	
		Hazard Ratio (95% CI)	p	Hazard Ratio (95% CI)	p	Hazard Ratio (95% CI)	p	Hazard Ratio (95% CI)	p
Histology									
OSA	69	1 (reference)		1 (reference)		1 (reference)		1 (reference)	
OEA	39	0.17 (0.08–0.37)	<0.001	0.42 (0.16–1.12)	0.082	0.12 (0.04–0.38)	<0.001	0.45 (0.13–1.55)	0.205
OCCA	64	0.96 (0.64–1.44)	0.835			1.37 (0.86–2.18)	0.188		
Type									
I	104	1 (reference)		1 (reference)		1 (reference)		1 (reference)	
II	68	2.69 (1.81–4.00)	<0.001	0.77 (0.46–1.28)	0.311	1.88 (1.19–2.96)	0.007	0.35 (0.20–0.60)	<0.001
FIGO stage									
Early	69	1 (reference)		1 (reference)		1 (reference)		1 (reference)	
Advanced	103	5.29 (3.16–8.85)	<0.001	3.08 (1.63–5.80)	0.001	6.84 (3.28–14.25)	<0.001	4.82 (2.09–11.09)	<0.001
Tumor grade									
Low	29	1 (reference)		1 (reference)		1 (reference)		1 (reference)	
High	143	5.57 (2.26–13.70)	<0.001	1.68 (0.55–5.15)	0.366	17.97 (2.50–129.29)	0.004	7.38 (0.93–58.28)	0.058
Debulking surgery									
Suboptimal	60	1 (reference)		1 (reference)		1 (reference)		1 (reference)	
Optimal	112	0.28 (0.18–0.41)	<0.001	0.51 (0.32–0.80)	0.004	0.26 (0.16–0.41)	<0.001	0.38 (0.22–0.64)	<0.001
HR									
Wild type	154	1 (reference)				1 (reference)			
Mutation	18	1.22 (0.67–2.23)	0.516			1.15 (0.59–2.25)	0.674		
NHEJ									
Wild type	170	1 (reference)				1 (reference)			
Mutation	2	2.04 (0.50–8.28)	0.319			2.52 (0.62–10.32)	0.197		
MMR									
Wild type	161	1 (reference)				1 (reference)			
Mutation	11	1.31 (0.61–2.83)	0.487			1.88 (0.81–4.33)	0.139		

Table 5. Cont.

Factors		n	Recurrence				Death			
			Univariate		Multivariate		Univariate		Multivariate	
			Hazard Ratio (95% CI)	p	Hazard Ratio (95% CI)	p	Hazard Ratio (95% CI)	p	Hazard Ratio (95% CI)	p
BER	Wild type	160	1 (reference)				1 (reference)			
	Mutation	12	1.32 (0.64–2.71)	0.454			1.70 (0.78–3.72)	0.185		
NER	Wild type	167	1 (reference)				1 (reference)			
	Mutation	5	0.58 (0.14–2.36)	0.449			0.71 (0.18–2.91)	0.639		
TLS	Wild type	171	1 (reference)				1 (reference)		1 (reference)	
	Mutation	1	5.19 (0.71–37.89)	0.104			33.76 (3.95–289.00)	0.001	9.57 (1.08–84.83)	0.042
DSBR	Wild type	153	1 (reference)				1 (reference)			
	Mutation	19	1.23 (0.69–2.20)	0.488			1.20 (0.63–2.27)	0.584		
SSBR	Wild type	145	1 (reference)				1 (reference)			
	Mutation	27	1.10 (0.64–1.87)	0.736			1.46 (0.82–2.61)	0.202		
CCR	Wild type	119	1 (reference)		1 (reference)		1 (reference)			
	Mutation	53	1.68 (1.12–2.50)	0.011	0.98 (0.58–1.66)	0.939	1.54 (0.97–2.45)	0.066		
DDR	Wild type	94	1 (reference)		1 (reference)		1 (reference)		1 (reference)	
	1 gene mutation	57	1.71 (1.12–2.60)	0.013	1.18 (0.73–1.91)	0.496	1.96 (1.20–3.20)	0.007	1.57 (0.97–2.54)	0.062
	≥2 gene mutations	21	1.52 (0.84–2.76)	0.171			1.56 (0.78–3.11)	0.207		

Note: BER: base excision repair; CCR: cell cycle regulation; DDR: DNA damage response; DSBR: double-strand break repair; HR: homologous recombination; MMR: mismatch repair; NER: nucleotide excision repair; NHEJ: nonhomologous DNA end joining; OSA: ovarian serous carcinoma; OEA: ovarian endometrioid carcinoma; OCCA: ovarian clear cell carcinoma; SSBR: single-strand break repair; TLS: translesion synthesis.

4. Discussion

Our study showed that nearly half of the epithelial ovarian cancer (EOC) patients had DNA damage response (DDR) gene mutations with varied proportions of histological subtypes. Two-thirds of serous adenocarcinoma patients, one-third of endometrioid adenocarcinoma patients and one-fourth of clear cell carcinoma patients had DDR gene mutations. Our DDR gene panel consisted of the genes involved in single-strand break repair, double-strand break repair and cell cycle regulation, including the genes recommended by National Comprehensive Cancer Network (NCCN) guidelines as cost-effective tools for assessing the lifetime risk of EOC, such as *ATM, BRCA1/2, BRIP1, MLH1, MSH2, MSH6, PALB2, RAD51C* and *RAD51D* [32]. The major components of DDR gene mutations were CCR in serous, CCR and SSBR in endometrioid and SSBR in clear cell carcinomas; CCR and DSBR in type II tumors (high-grade serous carcinoma in the cohort); and SSBR in type I tumors. A multiple DDR gene panel increased the detection rate of somatic mutation of genes involved in DNA damage repair pathway in comparison with a *BRCA* test alone. The percentage of *BRCA 1/2* somatic mutation in serous carcinoma was 7.2, which was compatible with the 6–7% in previous studies [33–37]. The non-*BRCA* HR somatic mutation of our study was more than 10% in serous and endometrioid carcinomas, and the MMR somatic mutation was around 15% in endometrioid carcinomas, which was compatible with the previous study [38].

Our study showed that ovarian clear cell carcinoma patients with DDR gene mutations had an unfavorable survival prognosis. Those who had somatic DDR mutations were significantly associated with advanced-stage carcinomas, tumor recurrence and tumor-related death. The trend was different in histological subtypes as serous carcinomas or type II tumors with DDR mutation showed a better survival trend. Non-serous or type I EOC patients with DDR mutations had a poor prognosis, especially in clear cell carcinoma. Ovarian clear cell carcinoma is an aggressive drug-resistant subtype of EOC in association with endometriosis and glycogen accumulation. It accounts for about 5–13% of all EOCs in Western populations, but up to 20–25% in East Asia, including Taiwan [2,3]. Previous studies showed that the somatic mutations of ovarian clear cell carcinoma (mainly in *ARID1A, PIK3CA, KRAS* and *PPP2R1A*) might be related to chromatin remodeling, cell proliferation, cell cycle checkpointing and cytoskeletal organization [39–49]. However, the frequent mutations of *ARID1A, PIK3CA, PPP2R1A* or *TP53* in ovarian clear cell carcinoma did not correlate well with the prognosis [45]. Other infrequent gene mutations of clear cell carcinoma included *ARID1B, ARID3A, CREBBP, CSMD3, CTNNB1, LPHN3, LRP1B, MAGEE1, MLH1, MLL3, MUC4, PIK3R1, PTEN* and *TP53* [41,43,46,48,49]. DDR gene mutations in ovarian clear cell carcinoma was unclear in the literature, and our finding of an unfavorable prognosis in clear cell carcinoma patients with DDR gene mutations could provide useful information.

Our DDR gene panel could provide a scientific rationale for patient selection in future clinical trials that target DNA damage repair response pathways, especially in clear cell carcinoma. *BRCA* gene tests or companion HRD assays are currently suggested for PARPi, but there are unmet problems that need to be resolved [11–15,20]. The most important one is that the HRD assays cannot consistently identify patients who do not benefit from PARPi therapy. The consensus for the cut-off value was indeterminate because the thresholds of HRD assays were developed from retrospective exploratory analyses [11,50,51]. Generally, advance-stage, high-grade serous carcinoma patients with tumor *BRCA* (t*BRCA*) mutations, including germline (g*BRCA*) or somatic (s*BRCA*), derived the greatest benefit from PARPi maintenance therapy [11–15]. Approximately 11–18% of patients had a g*BRCA* mutation, and another 6–7% patients had an s*BRCA* mutation with a negative g*BRCA* test [33–37]. However, about 5% of g*BRCA* mutated patients tested negative for t*BRCA* [52–54]. The non-*BRCA* HR gene mutations were usually pooled together to interpret the association with clinical outcomes in previous studies because of their relatively low prevalence [35,55–57]. Twenty-one platinum-sensitive recurrent patients with non-*BRCA* somatic mutations (*BRIP1, CDK12, RAD54L* and *RAD51B*) derived benefit from olaparib in study 19 [58]. In ARIEL2, there were 20 patients with non-*BRCA* HR gene mutations (*ATM, BRIP1, CHEK2, FANCA, FANCI, FANCM, NBN, RAD51B, RAD51C* and *RAD54L*), but the sensitivity in discriminating a rucaparib response was only 11% [59]. However, *BRCA* wild type EOC patients still benefitted from PARPi, which indicated that a *BRCA* test by itself was inadequate for selecting EOC patients for PARPi [13–15]. It needs to be determined which individual or panel of non-*BRCA* HR genes could be used to predict a PARPi response, especially in non-serous EOC patients.

There were limitations to our study. First, germline gene mutations were not investigated. These not only inform the patients but also identify family members of the possible risk of malignancy [52–54]. The NCCN suggested germline gene tests of *ATM, BRCA1/2, BRIP1, MLH1, MSH2, MSH6, PALB2, RAD51C, RAD51D* and *STK11* to assess the lifetime risk of EOC [32], but how many genes should be included in the panel is inconclusive. Second, the numerous variants of uncertain significance (VUSs) identified by multiple gene panels would cause controversy in risk assessment and management [60–62]. The biological functions and clinical impacts of most individual mutations in the genomic loci have not been well characterized, especially for VUSs [63]. Even in the well-studied *BRCA* gene, there is a difference among laboratories in the VUS reporting rate (3–50%), detection protocols and management strategies [64]. Further sharing and integration of gene sequencing data in an open database might decrease VUSs. Third, the cohort sample was not large enough; only the trends of clinical prognosis that correlated with each DDR pathway were found. Further large-scale investigations are needed.

5. Conclusions

Our study found that nearly half of the EOC patients had DDR gene mutations of varying proportions in the histological subtypes. Patients with somatic DDR mutations were significantly associated with advanced-stage carcinoma, tumor recurrence and tumor-related death. Type I EOC patients with DDR mutations had an unfavorable prognosis, especially for clear cell carcinoma. A broad multiple-gene DDR panel would provide not only comprehensive information of gene mutations but also a rationale for a future study of a novel therapy target for DNA damage response pathways.

Supplementary Materials: The following are available online at https://www.mdpi.com/article/10.3390/biomedicines9101384/s1, Figure S1: Variants of uncertain significance (VUS) with the potential of being deleterious mutations, Figure S2: The distribution of all 114 deleterious DDR gene mutations, Table S1: Variants of uncertain significance (VUSs) with the potential of being deleterious mutations in the cohort, Table S2: The percentages of DDR gene mutations in all patients.

Author Contributions: Conceptualization, Y.-C.C., P.-H.L., W.-F.C. and C.-A.C.; methodology, Y.-C.C. and P.-H.L.; software, P.-H.L. and T.-P.L.; validation, Y.-C.C., P.-H.L. and T.-P.L.; formal analysis, Y.-C.C., P.-H.L. and T.-P.L.; investigation, Y.-C.C., Y.-J.T., H.-C.H., C.-Y.W., C.-Y.L., H.S.; resources, Y.-C.C., K.-T.K., Y.-J.T., H.-C.H., C.-Y.W., C.-Y.L., H.S., C.-A.C. and W.-F.C.; data curation, Y.-C.C., P.-H.L. and T.-P.L.; writing—original draft preparation, Y.-C.C. and P.-H.L.; writing—review and editing, C.-A.C. and W.-F.C.; visualization, Y.-C.C. and P.-H.L.; supervision, C.-A.C. and W.-F.C.; funding acquisition, Y.-C.C., C.-A.C. and W.-F.C. All authors have read and agreed to the published version of the manuscript.

Funding: This work was supported by research grants from the National Taiwan University Hospital (NTUH. 105-N02, UN105-059, 108-S4230 and 109-S4570).

Institutional Review Board Statement: The study was conducted according to the guidelines of the Declaration of Helsinki, and approved by the Ethics Committee of National Taiwan University Hospital (201509042RINA, approved on 24 November 2015 and 201608025RINA, approved on 07 October 2016).

Informed Consent Statement: Informed consent was obtained from all subjects involved in the study.

Data Availability Statement: The datasets generated and/or analyzed during the current study are available from the corresponding author on reasonable request.

Acknowledgments: The authors thank the A1 laboratory of the National Taiwan University Hospital for the Illumina Miseq NGS platform, the National Applied Research Laboratories for providing access of high-performance computer to analyze NGS data, and the 7th Core Laboratory Facility of the Department of Medical Research of National Taiwan University Hospital for supporting the work.

Conflicts of Interest: The authors declare no conflict of interest.

References

1. Siegel, R.L.; Miller, K.D.; Fuchs, H.E.; Jemal, A. Cancer Statistics, 2021. *CA Cancer J. Clin* **2021**, *71*, 7–33. [CrossRef]
2. Torre, L.A.; Trabert, B.; DeSantis, C.E.; Miller, K.D.; Samimi, G.; Runowicz, C.D.; Gaudet, M.M.; Jemal, A.; Siegel, R.L. Ovarian cancer statistics, 2018. *CA Cancer J. Clin.* **2018**, *68*, 284–296. [CrossRef]
3. Chiang, Y.C.; Chen, C.A.; Chiang, C.J.; Hsu, T.H.; Lin, M.C.; You, S.L.; Cheng, W.F.; Lai, M.S. Trends in incidence and survival outcome of epithelial ovarian cancer: 30-year national population-based registry in Taiwan. *J. Gynecol. Oncol.* **2013**, *24*, 342–351. [CrossRef]
4. Jayson, G.C.; Kohn, E.C.; Kitchener, H.C.; Ledermann, J.A. Ovarian cancer. *Lancet* **2014**, *384*, 1376–1388. [CrossRef]
5. Coleman, R.L.; Monk, B.J.; Sood, A.K.; Herzog, T.J. Latest research and treatment of advanced-stage epithelial ovarian cancer. *Nat. Rev. Clin. Oncol.* **2013**, *10*, 211–224. [CrossRef] [PubMed]
6. Gurung, A.; Hung, T.; Morin, J.; Gilks, C.B. Molecular abnormalities in ovarian carcinoma: Clinical, morphological and therapeutic correlates. *Histopathology* **2013**, *62*, 59–70. [CrossRef] [PubMed]
7. Colombo, P.E.; Fabbro, M.; Theillet, C.; Bibeau, F.; Rouanet, P.; Ray-Coquard, I. Sensitivity and resistance to treatment in the primary management of epithelial ovarian cancer. *Crit. Rev. Oncol./Hematol.* **2014**, *89*, 207–216. [CrossRef]
8. Perren, T.J.; Swart, A.M.; Pfisterer, J.; Ledermann, J.A.; Pujade-Lauraine, E.; Kristensen, G.; Carey, M.S.; Beale, P.; Cervantes, A.; Kurzeder, C.; et al. A phase 3 trial of bevacizumab in ovarian cancer. *N. Engl. J. Med.* **2011**, *365*, 2484–2496. [CrossRef]
9. Oza, A.M.; Cook, A.D.; Pfisterer, J.; Embleton, A.; Ledermann, J.A.; Pujade-Lauraine, E.; Kristensen, G.; Carey, M.S.; Beale, P.; Cervantes, A.; et al. Standard chemotherapy with or without bevacizumab for women with newly diagnosed ovarian cancer (ICON7): Overall survival results of a phase 3 randomised trial. *Lancet Oncol.* **2015**, *16*, 928–936. [CrossRef]
10. Burger, R.A.; Brady, M.F.; Bookman, M.A.; Fleming, G.F.; Monk, B.J.; Huang, H.; Mannel, R.S.; Homesley, H.D.; Fowler, J.; Greer, B.E.; et al. Incorporation of bevacizumab in the primary treatment of ovarian cancer. *N. Engl. J. Med.* **2011**, *365*, 2473–2483. [CrossRef]
11. González-Martín, A.; Pothuri, B.; Vergote, I.; DePont Christensen, R.; Graybill, W.; Mirza, M.R.; McCormick, C.; Lorusso, D.; Hoskins, P.; Freyer, G.; et al. Niraparib in Patients with Newly Diagnosed Advanced Ovarian Cancer. *N. Engl. J. Med.* **2019**, *381*, 2391–2402. [CrossRef] [PubMed]
12. Moore, K.; Colombo, N.; Scambia, G.; Kim, B.G.; Oaknin, A.; Friedlander, M.; Lisyanskaya, A.; Floquet, A.; Leary, A.; Sonke, G.S.; et al. Maintenance Olaparib in Patients with Newly Diagnosed Advanced Ovarian Cancer. *N. Engl. J. Med.* **2018**, *379*, 2495–2505. [CrossRef] [PubMed]
13. Mirza, M.R.; Monk, B.J.; Herrstedt, J.; Oza, A.M.; Mahner, S.; Redondo, A.; Fabbro, M.; Ledermann, J.A.; Lorusso, D.; Vergote, I.; et al. Niraparib Maintenance Therapy in Platinum-Sensitive, Recurrent Ovarian Cancer. *N. Engl. J. Med.* **2016**, *375*, 2154–2164. [CrossRef] [PubMed]
14. Coleman, R.L.; Oza, A.M.; Lorusso, D.; Aghajanian, C.; Oaknin, A.; Dean, A.; Colombo, N.; Weberpals, J.I.; Clamp, A.; Scambia, G.; et al. Rucaparib maintenance treatment for recurrent ovarian carcinoma after response to platinum therapy (ARIEL3): A randomised, double-blind, placebo-controlled, phase 3 trial. *Lancet* **2017**, *390*, 1949–1961. [CrossRef]
15. Pujade-Lauraine, E.; Ledermann, J.A.; Selle, F.; Gebski, V.; Penson, R.T.; Oza, A.M.; Korach, J.; Huzarski, T.; Poveda, A.; Pignata, S.; et al. Olaparib tablets as maintenance therapy in patients with platinum-sensitive, relapsed ovarian cancer and a BRCA1/2 mutation (SOLO2/ENGOT-Ov21): A double-blind, randomised, placebo-controlled, phase 3 trial. *Lancet Oncol.* **2017**, *18*, 1274–1284. [CrossRef]
16. Brown, J.S.; O'Carrigan, B.; Jackson, S.P.; Yap, T.A. Targeting DNA Repair in Cancer: Beyond PARP Inhibitors. *Cancer Discov.* **2017**, *7*, 20–37. [CrossRef]
17. Pearl, L.H.; Schierz, A.C.; Ward, S.E.; Al-Lazikani, B.; Pearl, F.M. Therapeutic opportunities within the DNA damage response. *Nat. Rev. Cancer* **2015**, *15*, 166–180. [CrossRef]
18. Hanahan, D.; Weinberg, R.A. Hallmarks of cancer: The next generation. *Cell* **2011**, *144*, 646–674. [CrossRef]
19. Vilenchik, M.M.; Knudson, A.G. Endogenous DNA double-strand breaks: Production, fidelity of repair, and induction of cancer. *Proc. Natl. Acad. Sci. USA* **2003**, *100*, 12871–12876. [CrossRef]
20. Miller, R.E.; Leary, A.; Scott, C.L.; Serra, V.; Lord, C.J.; Bowtell, D.; Chang, D.K.; Garsed, D.W.; Jonkers, J.; Ledermann, J.A.; et al. ESMO recommendations on predictive biomarker testing for homologous recombination deficiency and PARP inhibitor benefit in ovarian cancer. *Ann. Oncol.* **2020**, *31*, 1606–1622. [CrossRef]

21. Prat, J. Staging classification for cancer of the ovary, fallopian tube, and peritoneum. *Int. J. Gynaecol. Obstet.* **2014**, *124*, 1–5. [CrossRef] [PubMed]
22. Lin, P.H.; Kuo, W.H.; Huang, A.C.; Lu, Y.S.; Lin, C.H.; Kuo, S.H.; Wang, M.Y.; Liu, C.Y.; Cheng, F.T.; Yeh, M.H.; et al. Multiple gene sequencing for risk assessment in patients with early-onset or familial breast cancer. *Oncotarget* **2016**. [CrossRef] [PubMed]
23. Li, H.; Durbin, R. Fast and accurate short read alignment with Burrows-Wheeler transform. *Bioinformatics* **2009**, *25*, 1754–1760. [CrossRef]
24. Li, H.; Handsaker, B.; Wysoker, A.; Fennell, T.; Ruan, J.; Homer, N.; Marth, G.; Abecasis, G.; Durbin, R. The Sequence Alignment/Map format and SAMtools. *Bioinformatics* **2009**, *25*, 2078–2079. [CrossRef]
25. Mimori, T.; Nariai, N.; Kojima, K.; Takahashi, M.; Ono, A.; Sato, Y.; Yamaguchi-Kabata, Y.; Nagasaki, M. iSVP: An integrated structural variant calling pipeline from high-throughput sequencing data. *BMC Syst. Biol.* **2013**, *7* (Suppl. S6), S8. [CrossRef] [PubMed]
26. McKenna, A.; Hanna, M.; Banks, E.; Sivachenko, A.; Cibulskis, K.; Kernytsky, A.; Garimella, K.; Altshuler, D.; Gabriel, S.; Daly, M.; et al. The Genome Analysis Toolkit: A MapReduce framework for analyzing next-generation DNA sequencing data. *Genome Res.* **2010**, *20*, 1297–1303. [CrossRef]
27. Wang, K.; Li, M.; Hakonarson, H. ANNOVAR: Functional annotation of genetic variants from high-throughput sequencing data. *Nucleic Acids Res.* **2010**, *38*, e164. [CrossRef]
28. Plon, S.E.; Eccles, D.M.; Easton, D.; Foulkes, W.D.; Genuardi, M.; Greenblatt, M.S.; Hogervorst, F.B.; Hoogerbrugge, N.; Spurdle, A.B.; Tavtigian, S.V. Sequence variant classification and reporting: Recommendations for improving the interpretation of cancer susceptibility genetic test results. *Hum. Mutat.* **2008**, *29*, 1282–1291. [CrossRef]
29. Adzhubei, I.A.; Schmidt, S.; Peshkin, L.; Ramensky, V.E.; Gerasimova, A.; Bork, P.; Kondrashov, A.S.; Sunyaev, S.R. A method and server for predicting damaging missense mutations. *Nat. Methods* **2010**, *7*, 248–249. [CrossRef]
30. Kumar, P.; Henikoff, S.; Ng, P.C. Predicting the effects of coding non-synonymous variants on protein function using the SIFT algorithm. *Nat. Protoc.* **2009**, *4*, 1073–1081. [CrossRef]
31. Mathe, E.; Olivier, M.; Kato, S.; Ishioka, C.; Hainaut, P.; Tavtigian, S.V. Computational approaches for predicting the biological effect of p53 missense mutations: A comparison of three sequence analysis based methods. *Nucleic Acids Res.* **2006**, *34*, 1317–1325. [CrossRef] [PubMed]
32. Daly, M.B.; Pal, T.; Berry, M.P.; Buys, S.S.; Dickson, P.; Domchek, S.M.; Elkhanany, A.; Friedman, S.; Goggins, M.; Hutton, M.L.; et al. Genetic/Familial High-Risk Assessment: Breast, Ovarian, and Pancreatic, Version 2.2021, NCCN Clinical Practice Guidelines in Oncology. *J. Natl. Compr. Canc. Netw.* **2021**, *19*, 77–102. [CrossRef] [PubMed]
33. Hennessy, B.T.; Timms, K.M.; Carey, M.S.; Gutin, A.; Meyer, L.A.; Flake, D.D., 2nd; Abkevich, V.; Potter, J.; Pruss, D.; Glenn, P.; et al. Somatic mutations in BRCA1 and BRCA2 could expand the number of patients that benefit from poly (ADP ribose) polymerase inhibitors in ovarian cancer. *J. Clin. Oncol.* **2010**, *28*, 3570–3576. [CrossRef] [PubMed]
34. Cancer Genome Atlas Research Network. Integrated genomic analyses of ovarian carcinoma. *Nature* **2011**, *474*, 609–615. [CrossRef] [PubMed]
35. Pennington, K.P.; Walsh, T.; Harrell, M.I.; Lee, M.K.; Pennil, C.C.; Rendi, M.H.; Thornton, A.; Norquist, B.M.; Casadei, S.; Nord, A.S.; et al. Germline and somatic mutations in homologous recombination genes predict platinum response and survival in ovarian, fallopian tube, and peritoneal carcinomas. *Clin. Cancer Res.* **2014**, *20*, 764–775. [CrossRef]
36. Walsh, T.; Casadei, S.; Lee, M.K.; Pennil, C.C.; Nord, A.S.; Thornton, A.M.; Roeb, W.; Agnew, K.J.; Stray, S.M.; Wickramanayake, A.; et al. Mutations in 12 genes for inherited ovarian, fallopian tube, and peritoneal carcinoma identified by massively parallel sequencing. *Proc. Natl. Acad. Sci. USA* **2011**, *108*, 18032–18037. [CrossRef]
37. Alsop, K.; Fereday, S.; Meldrum, C.; deFazio, A.; Emmanuel, C.; George, J.; Dobrovic, A.; Birrer, M.J.; Webb, P.M.; Stewart, C.; et al. BRCA mutation frequency and patterns of treatment response in BRCA mutation-positive women with ovarian cancer: A report from the Australian Ovarian Cancer Study Group. *J. Clin. Oncol.* **2012**, *30*, 2654–2663. [CrossRef]
38. Leskela, S.; Romero, I.; Cristobal, E.; Pérez-Mies, B.; Rosa-Rosa, J.M.; Gutierrez-Pecharroman, A.; Caniego-Casas, T.; Santón, A.; Ojeda, B.; López-Reig, R.; et al. Mismatch Repair Deficiency in Ovarian Carcinoma: Frequency, Causes, and Consequences. *Am. J. Surg. Pathol.* **2020**, *44*, 649–656. [CrossRef]
39. Tan, D.S.; Miller, R.E.; Kaye, S.B. New perspectives on molecular targeted therapy in ovarian clear cell carcinoma. *Br. J. Cancer* **2013**, *108*, 1553–1559. [CrossRef]
40. Jones, S.; Wang, T.L.; Shih Ie, M.; Mao, T.L.; Nakayama, K.; Roden, R.; Glas, R.; Slamon, D.; Diaz, L.A., Jr.; Vogelstein, B.; et al. Frequent mutations of chromatin remodeling gene ARID1A in ovarian clear cell carcinoma. *Science* **2010**, *330*, 228–231. [CrossRef]
41. Yang, Q.; Zhang, C.; Ren, Y.; Yi, H.; Luo, T.; Xing, F.; Bai, X.; Cui, L.; Zhu, L.; Ouyang, J.; et al. Genomic characterization of Chinese ovarian clear cell carcinoma identifies driver genes by whole exome sequencing. *Neoplasia* **2020**, *22*, 399–430. [CrossRef]
42. Kim, S.I.; Lee, J.W.; Lee, M.; Kim, H.S.; Chung, H.H.; Kim, J.W.; Park, N.H.; Song, Y.S.; Seo, J.S. Genomic landscape of ovarian clear cell carcinoma via whole exome sequencing. *Gynecol. Oncol.* **2018**, *148*, 375–382. [CrossRef]
43. Murakami, R.; Matsumura, N.; Brown, J.B.; Higasa, K.; Tsutsumi, T.; Kamada, M.; Abou-Taleb, H.; Hosoe, Y.; Kitamura, S.; Yamaguchi, K.; et al. Exome Sequencing Landscape Analysis in Ovarian Clear Cell Carcinoma Shed Light on Key Chromosomal Regions and Mutation Gene Networks. *Am. J. Pathol.* **2017**, *187*, 2246–2258. [CrossRef]
44. Gounaris, I.; Brenton, J.D. Molecular pathogenesis of ovarian clear cell carcinoma. *Future Oncol. (Lond. Engl.)* **2015**, *11*, 1389–1405. [CrossRef] [PubMed]

45. Takenaka, M.; Köbel, M.; Garsed, D.W.; Fereday, S.; Pandey, A.; Etemadmoghadam, D.; Hendley, J.; Kawabata, A.; Noguchi, D.; Yanaihara, N.; et al. Survival Following Chemotherapy in Ovarian Clear Cell Carcinoma Is Not Associated with Pathological Misclassification of Tumor Histotype. *Clin. Cancer Res.* **2019**, *25*, 3962–3973. [CrossRef] [PubMed]
46. Su, Y.F.; Tsai, E.M.; Chen, C.C.; Wu, C.C.; Er, T.K. Targeted sequencing of a specific gene panel detects a high frequency of ARID1A and PIK3CA mutations in ovarian clear cell carcinoma. *Clin. Chim. Acta Int. J. Clin. Chem.* **2019**, *494*, 1–7. [CrossRef] [PubMed]
47. Shibuya, Y.; Tokunaga, H.; Saito, S.; Shimokawa, K.; Katsuoka, F.; Bin, L.; Kojima, K.; Nagasaki, M.; Yamamoto, M.; Yaegashi, N.; et al. Identification of somatic genetic alterations in ovarian clear cell carcinoma with next generation sequencing. *Genes Chromosomes Cancer* **2018**, *57*, 51–60. [CrossRef] [PubMed]
48. Maru, Y.; Tanaka, N.; Ohira, M.; Itami, M.; Hippo, Y.; Nagase, H. Identification of novel mutations in Japanese ovarian clear cell carcinoma patients using optimized targeted NGS for clinical diagnosis. *Gynecol. Oncol.* **2017**, *144*, 377–383. [CrossRef]
49. Friedlander, M.L.; Russell, K.; Millis, S.; Gatalica, Z.; Bender, R.; Voss, A. Molecular Profiling of Clear Cell Ovarian Cancers: Identifying Potential Treatment Targets for Clinical Trials. *Int. J. Gynecol. Cancer* **2016**, *26*, 648–654. [CrossRef]
50. Coleman, R.L.; Fleming, G.F.; Brady, M.F.; Swisher, E.M.; Steffensen, K.D.; Friedlander, M.; Okamoto, A.; Moore, K.N.; Efrat Ben-Baruch, N.; Werner, T.L.; et al. Veliparib with First-Line Chemotherapy and as Maintenance Therapy in Ovarian Cancer. *N. Engl. J. Med.* **2019**, *381*, 2403–2415. [CrossRef]
51. Ray-Coquard, I.; Pautier, P.; Pignata, S.; Pérol, D.; González-Martín, A.; Berger, R.; Fujiwara, K.; Vergote, I.; Colombo, N.; Mäenpää, J.; et al. Olaparib plus Bevacizumab as First-Line Maintenance in Ovarian Cancer. *N. Engl. J. Med.* **2019**, *381*, 2416–2428. [CrossRef] [PubMed]
52. Konstantinopoulos, P.A.; Norquist, B.; Lacchetti, C.; Armstrong, D.; Grisham, R.N.; Goodfellow, P.J.; Kohn, E.C.; Levine, D.A.; Liu, J.F.; Lu, K.H.; et al. Germline and Somatic Tumor Testing in Epithelial Ovarian Cancer: ASCO Guideline. *J. Clin. Oncol.* **2020**, *38*, 1222–1245. [CrossRef]
53. Vergote, I.; Banerjee, S.; Gerdes, A.M.; van Asperen, C.; Marth, C.; Vaz, F.; Ray-Coquard, I.; Stoppa-Lyonnet, D.; Gonzalez-Martin, A.; Sehouli, J.; et al. Current perspectives on recommendations for BRCA genetic testing in ovarian cancer patients. *Eur. J. Cancer* **2016**, *69*, 127–134. [CrossRef]
54. Lancaster, J.M.; Powell, C.B.; Chen, L.M.; Richardson, D.L. Society of Gynecologic Oncology statement on risk assessment for inherited gynecologic cancer predispositions. *Gynecol. Oncol.* **2015**, *136*, 3–7. [CrossRef]
55. Norquist, B.M.; Brady, M.F.; Harrell, M.I.; Walsh, T.; Lee, M.K.; Gulsuner, S.; Bernards, S.S.; Casadei, S.; Burger, R.A.; Tewari, K.S.; et al. Mutations in Homologous Recombination Genes and Outcomes in Ovarian Carcinoma Patients in GOG 218: An NRG Oncology/Gynecologic Oncology Group Study. *Clin. Cancer Res.* **2018**, *24*, 777–783. [CrossRef]
56. Loveday, C.; Turnbull, C.; Ramsay, E.; Hughes, D.; Ruark, E.; Frankum, J.R.; Bowden, G.; Kalmyrzaev, B.; Warren-Perry, M.; Snape, K.; et al. Germline mutations in RAD51D confer susceptibility to ovarian cancer. *Nat. Genet.* **2011**, *43*, 879–882. [CrossRef]
57. McCabe, N.; Turner, N.C.; Lord, C.J.; Kluzek, K.; Bialkowska, A.; Swift, S.; Giavara, S.; O'Connor, M.J.; Tutt, A.N.; Zdzienicka, M.Z.; et al. Deficiency in the repair of DNA damage by homologous recombination and sensitivity to poly(ADP-ribose) polymerase inhibition. *Cancer Res.* **2006**, *66*, 8109–8115. [CrossRef]
58. Hodgson, D.R.; Dougherty, B.A.; Lai, Z.; Fielding, A.; Grinsted, L.; Spencer, S.; O'Connor, M.J.; Ho, T.W.; Robertson, J.D.; Lanchbury, J.S.; et al. Candidate biomarkers of PARP inhibitor sensitivity in ovarian cancer beyond the BRCA genes. *Br. J. Cancer* **2018**, *119*, 1401–1409. [CrossRef]
59. Swisher, E.M.; Lin, K.K.; Oza, A.M.; Scott, C.L.; Giordano, H.; Sun, J.; Konecny, G.E.; Coleman, R.L.; Tinker, A.V.; O'Malley, D.M.; et al. Rucaparib in relapsed, platinum-sensitive high-grade ovarian carcinoma (ARIEL2 Part 1): An international, multicentre, open-label, phase 2 trial. *Lancet Oncol.* **2017**, *18*, 75–87. [CrossRef]
60. Bonnet, C.; Krieger, S.; Vezain, M.; Rousselin, A.; Tournier, I.; Martins, A.; Berthet, P.; Chevrier, A.; Dugast, C.; Layet, V.; et al. Screening BRCA1 and BRCA2 unclassified variants for splicing mutations using reverse transcription PCR on patient RNA and an ex vivo assay based on a splicing reporter minigene. *J. Med. Genet.* **2008**, *45*, 438–446. [CrossRef]
61. Cartegni, L.; Chew, S.L.; Krainer, A.R. Listening to silence and understanding nonsense: Exonic mutations that affect splicing. *Nat. Rev. Genet.* **2002**, *3*, 285–298. [CrossRef]
62. Li, H.; LaDuca, H.; Pesaran, T.; Chao, E.C.; Dolinsky, J.S.; Parsons, M.; Spurdle, A.B.; Polley, E.C.; Shimelis, H.; Hart, S.N.; et al. Classification of variants of uncertain significance in BRCA1 and BRCA2 using personal and family history of cancer from individuals in a large hereditary cancer multigene panel testing cohort. *Genet. Med.* **2020**, *22*, 701–708. [CrossRef]
63. Alexandrov, L.B.; Kim, J.; Haradhvala, N.J.; Huang, M.N.; Tian Ng, A.W.; Wu, Y.; Boot, A.; Covington, K.R.; Gordenin, D.A.; Bergstrom, E.N.; et al. The repertoire of mutational signatures in human cancer. *Nature* **2020**, *578*, 94–101. [CrossRef]
64. Toland, A.E.; Forman, A.; Couch, F.J.; Culver, J.O.; Eccles, D.M.; Foulkes, W.D.; Hogervorst, F.B.L.; Houdayer, C.; Levy-Lahad, E.; Monteiro, A.N.; et al. Clinical testing of BRCA1 and BRCA2: A worldwide snapshot of technological practices. *NPJ Genom. Med.* **2018**, *3*, 7. [CrossRef]

Article

Long-Term Survival and Clinicopathological Implications of DNA Mismatch Repair Status in Endometrioid Endometrial Cancers in Hong Kong Chinese Women

Jacqueline Ho Sze Lee [1,*], Joshua Jing Xi Li [2], Chit Chow [2], Ronald Cheong Kin Chan [2], Johnny Sheung Him Kwan [2], Tat San Lau [1], Ka Fai To [2], So Fan Yim [1], Suet Ying Yeung [1] and Joseph Kwong [1,3]

1. Department of Obstetrics and Gynaecology, Faculty of Medicine, The Chinese University of Hong Kong, Hong Kong 999077, China; lautatsan@cuhk.edu.hk (T.S.L.); sfyim@cuhk.edu.hk (S.F.Y.); carolyeung@cuhk.edu.hk (S.Y.Y.); j.kwong@keele.ac.uk (J.K.)
2. Department of Anatomical and Cellular Pathology, Faculty of Medicine, The Chinese University of Hong Kong, Hong Kong 999077, China; joshuali@cuhk.edu.hk (J.J.X.L.); chit@cuhk.edu.hk (C.C.); ronaldckchan@cuhk.edu.hk (R.C.K.C.); shkwan@cuhk.edu.hk (J.S.H.K.); kfto@cuhk.edu.hk (K.F.T.)
3. School of Medicine, Faculty of Medicine and Health Sciences, Keele University, Newcastle-under-Lyme ST5 5BG, UK
* Correspondence: jaclee@cuhk.edu.hk; Tel.: +852-3505-2748

Abstract: To investigate the role of DNA mismatch repair status (MMR) in survival of endometrioid endometrial cancer in Hong Kong Chinese women and its correlation to clinical prognostic factors, 238 patients with endometrioid endometrial cancer were included. Tumor MMR status was evaluated by immunohistochemistry. Clinical characteristics and survival were determined. Association of MMR with survival and clinicopathological parameters were assessed. MMR deficiency (dMMR) was found in 43 cases (16.5%). dMMR was associated with poor prognostic factors including older age, higher stage, higher grade, larger tumor size and more radiotherapy usage. Long-term survival was worse in dMMR compared to the MMR proficient group. The dMMR group had more deaths, shorter disease-specific survival (DSS), shorter disease-free survival (DFS), less 10-year DSS, less 10-year DFS, and more recurrence. The 5-year DSS and 5-year DFS in the dMMR group only showed a trend of worse survival but did not reach statistical significance. In conclusion, dMMR is present in a significant number of endometrioid endometrial cancers patients and is associated with poorer clinicopathological factors and survival parameters in the long run. dMMR should be considered in the risk stratification of endometrial cancer to guide adjuvant therapy and individualisation for longer follow up plan.

Keywords: endometrioid endometrial cancer; DNA mismatch repair (MMR); MMR deficient (dMMR); long-term survival

1. Introduction

Endometrial cancer is the most common gynaecological cancer in the developed world and its incidence is on a continual rise. Endometrial carcinogenesis is driven by defects in signal transduction pathways such as the DNA mismatch repair (MMR) pathway, p53 pathway [1], phosphatidylinositol 3 kinase (PI3K)–AKT pathway, and WNT/ β-catenin signalling pathway [2]. Microsatellite instability (MSI) and phosphatase and tensin homolog (*PTEN*) mutation are the commonest genetic alterations in endometrial cancer [3].

The MMR system is a strand-specific DNA repair system which maintains genomic stability. MMR proteins, including MutL Homolog 1 (MLH1), MutS Homolog 2 (MSH2), MutS Homolog 6 (MSH6) and PMS1 Homolog 2, Mismatch Repair System Component (PMS2), are responsible for repairing base-base mismatch during DNA replication. MMR system also promotes cell cycle arrest and programmed cell deaths in response to DNA damage [4]. Microsatellites are short repetitive nucleotide sequences of DNA, which are prone to slippage and replication errors due to its repetitive structure. Therefore, when the MMR system is inactivated, it could lead to accumulation of DNA replication errors and MSI (in which the number of repeated DNA bases in a microsatellite is different from what it was when the microsatellite was inherited. In addition, inactivation of MMR system increases spontaneous mutations in the cells and is associated with cancers [4].

Deficiencies in MMR proteins were reported in 20% to 30% of endometrial cancers [5,6]. MMR deficiency can be somatic or germline. The majority of deficient mismatch repair deficiency in endometrial cancers is sporadic resulting from somatic mutations [3]. The presence of a germline mutation is suggestive of Lynch syndrome, a hereditary cancer syndrome associated with multiple cancers including colorectal and endometrial cancer [7]. Lynch syndrome is caused by an autosomal dominant germline mutation of one of the MMR genes, *MLH1*, *MSH2*, *MSH6* and *PMS2* [7].

There are three ways to detect defects in MMR system: immunohistochemistry (IHC), polymerase chain reaction (PCR)-based assays and next-generation sequencing (NGS) [8]. IHC can identify defects in MMR protein expression, classifying tumors as MMR proficient (pMMR) or MMR deficient (dMMR) [9,10]. PCR and NGS can evaluate for MSI, classifying tumors into high (MSI-H) or low (MSI-L) or stable levels (MSS) of MSI [8–11]. A study found a high correlation of IHC and PCR, with a concordance rate of 96% [9], while another study showed that IHC alone missed 17% of MSI cases identified by PCR [12]. The 2020 ESGO/ESTRO/ ESP guideline on endometrial cancer had recommended IHC as the preferred approach to identify defects in MMR gene because of its wide availability and cost-effectiveness [13].

Endometrial cancer patients generally have good prognosis with a 5-year survival rate of around 80% [14]. However, some cases (~20%) do recur [15] and prognostic markers are needed to select high-risk patients for adjuvant treatment and close monitoring [16]. Traditionally, endometrial cancers are classified into type 1 and type 2. Type 1 endometrial cancers are characterized by being estrogen-related, of endometrioid histology, occurring in pre-menopausal obese women and have more favourable prognosis. Type 2 endometrial cancers are characterised by being non-estrogen related, developing from atrophic endometrium, of non-endometrioid histology, occurring in post-menopausal women and have poorer prognosis [17]. Clinicopathological factors associated with worse survival include older age, higher tumor stage, higher grade, non-endometrioid histology and the presence of lymphovascular space invasion (LVSI) [14].

dMMR is an established carcinogenesis mechanism in endometrial cancer. However, its clinical significance remains controversial. Some studies had showed that dMMR was associated with older age, higher grade, higher stage disease, larger tumor, more LVSI and deeper myometrial invasion [5,18]. By contrast, some studies found no difference in stage, grade or LVSI [16]. dMMR tumors were more often of endometrioid than non-endometrioid histology with dMMR found in 51.4% of endometrioid tumors but only 20% of serous/clear cell tumors [19]. The relationship between dMMR and endometrial cancer survival is still unclear. A recent study involving 728 cases found that in endometrioid endometrial cancer, somatic dMMR was associated with worse disease specific survival (DSS) when compared to pMMR tumors (hazard ratio HR = 2.18) [14]. The worse prognosis was particularly evident in early-stage cancer [3,20] of endometrioid histology [5,14]. A decrease recurrence free survival had also been reported in a small number of studies [5]. Opposing findings were reported in another study involving 473 cases of endometrial cancer, showing that dMMR were associated with improved DSS (HR = 0.3) [6]. No difference in survival was found in some other studies [16]. A meta-analysis failed to find any association between survival and MMR status [21].

In additional to prognostic implications, MMR analysis is useful in the development of precision medicine in endometrial cancer [1]. It can guide the delivery of adjuvant therapy [22] and act as a biomarker to predict a response to immunotherapy [23]. Immunotherapy with immune checkpoint inhibitor such as anti-programmed death (PD)-1 and anti-PD-ligand 1 (PD-L1) antibodies is a rapidly emerging anti-cancer therapy [24].

The study's primary objective is to investigate the role of MMR status in the long-term survival of endometrial cancer patients of endometrioid histology. The secondary objectives include determining the prevalence of dMMR in Chinese endometrial cancer patients and its correlation to known prognostic factors such as lymph node involvement, disease grade, disease stage and presence of LVSI. Ninety percent of endometrial cancer is of endometrioid histology and its behavior is very different from non-endometrioid tumors, with the latter having poorer prognosis [16]. In view of the high prevalence of endometrioid tumors, the difference in clinical behavior from non-endometrioid tumors, more dMMR being reported in endometrioid tumors compared to non-endometrioid tumors (51.4% vs. 20%) [3,18,19,25], and the detrimental effect of dMMR being more reported in endometrioid tumors, our study focused on endometrioid tumors.

2. Materials and Methods

2.1. Patients

This is a retrospective study including 238 cases. Endometrial cancer of endometrioid histology was identified from the electronic database of Prince of Wales Hospital, a Hong Kong public hospital. Patients with hysterectomy performed and histology of surgical specimen analyzed from February 2001 to June 2010 were included. Baseline demographics were collected from the hospital electronic medical record system. Treatment data including operation performed, radiotherapy and chemotherapy were collected. The standard surgical treatments for endometrial cancer include total hysterectomy and bilateral salpingoophorectomy. Pelvic and/or para-aortic lymphadenectomy may be performed depending on the surgical risk, tumor grade, histology, cervical involvement, enlargement of lymph node and depth of myometrial invasion (as assessed by pre-operative endometrial sampling), MRI and intra-operative examination. In general, lymphadenectomy will be performed for cases of stage IB or above or high-grade disease whereas a radical hysterectomy will be performed if cervical invasion is suspected. The need for adjuvant therapy will be discussed in a multi-disciplinary meeting including gynaecologists, clinical oncologists and pathologists.

Pathological data including tumor size (maximum tumor dimension), grade, LVSI, myometrial invasion, cervical invasion, pelvic and para-aortic lymph node involvement, survival data (including 5-year and 10-year disease free survival (DFS), disease specific survival (DSS), overall survival (OS)), and recurrence were collected. Endometrial cancer staging and grading were based on the publication from the International Federation of Gynecology and Obstetrics in 2009. The OS was determined from the date of treatment to date of last contact or death from any cause. The DSS was determined from the date of treatment to date of last contact or death resulting from endometrial cancer. The DFS was determined from the date of treatment to the date of recurrence diagnosis. The study was approved by the local institutional ethics committee (CREC Ref. No. 2019.716).

2.2. Mismatch Repair (MMR) Status Analysis with Immunohistochemistry (IHC)

The tumor expression of MMR proteins including MLH1, MSH2, MSH6 and PMS2 were evaluated by IHC. Immunostaining was performed on 4 μm unstained formalin-fixed paraffin embedded slides with Ventana Optiview detection kit and 3,3'-Diaminobenzidine as chromogen. The list of antibodies used, and protocols adopted are listed in Table S1. Intensity of immunohistochemical staining was characterized into levels 0, 1, 2, 3 with level ≥ 1 regarded as a positive stain. MMR protein expression was considered as retained when there was $\geq 10\%$ positive staining in tumor cell nuclei, whereas staining in <10% was considered as indeterminate and 0% staining was considered as loss of expression provided that the internal control was positive [26,27]. If the internal control was negative, the result would be interpreted as non-informative. The tumor was regarded as dMMR if there was a loss of one or more of the four MMR protein expressions [16]. A paired loss of MLH1/PMS2 or MSH2/MSH6 will indicate a defect in the dominant partner (MLH1 or MSH2). The MMR results were interpreted separately by two pathologists.

2.3. Statistical Analysis

Sample size calculation was performed with the online survival curve sample size calculation tool provided by the Centre for Clinical Research and Biostatistics of the Chinese University of Hong Kong [28]. The significance level and power of test were set at 0.05. Median OS was set at 225 months, hazard ratio as 0.42 and rate of dMMR as 20% based on previously published studies [19,29]. The follow-up duration was set at 120 months. A required sample size of 214 was obtained. The data were analysed with software Statistical Package for Social Science Statistics Version 22. Survival was evaluated with Kaplan–Meier survival analysis and compared statistically using a log rank test. Cox regression analysis was used to assess the hazard ratio of MMR status on survival. The association of MMR protein status with clinicopathological parameters was assessed by the Chi square test, Fisher's exact test and t-test. Statistical significance was set at two-sided $p < 0.05$.

3. Results

3.1. MMR Protein Expression

Protein expression of MLH1, MSH2, MSH6 and PMS2 was evaluated in a total of 238 cases of endometrial cancer of endometrioid histology by IHC. Representative results of immunohistochemical staining of MLH1, MSH2, MSH6 and PMS2 are shown in Figure 1a–e. Cases were considered as MLH1 loss, MSH2 loss, MSH6 loss, and PMS2 loss are shown in Figure 1a, 1b, 1c and 1d, respectively. A representative case with all MMR proteins retained is shown in Figure 1e.

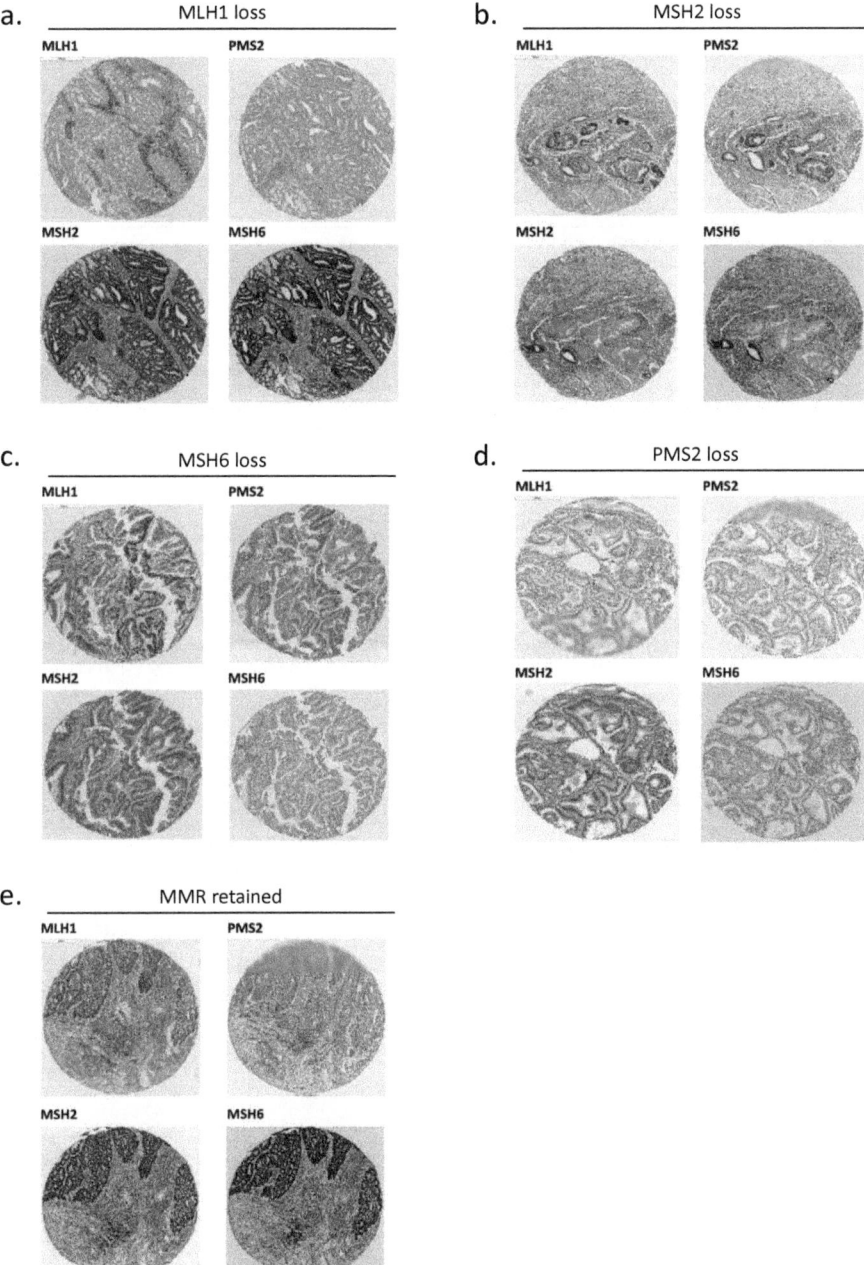

Figure 1. Expression of mismatch repair (MMR) proteins in endometrioid endometrial cancer tissues. (**a**) A representative case of MLH1 loss, immunohistochemistry (IHC) staining showed loss of MLH1 protein expression in tumor cells. (**b**) A representative case of MSH2 loss, IHC staining showed loss of MSH2 protein expression in tumor cells. (**c**) A representative case of MSH6 loss, IHC staining showed loss of MSH6 protein expression in tumor cells. (**d**) A representative case of PMS2 loss, IHC staining showed loss of PMS2 protein expression in tumor cells. (**e**) A representative case of MMR retained, IHC staining showed all four of the MMR proteins (MLH1, MSH2, MSH6 and PMS2) retained in tumor cells.

Loss of one or more of the four MMR protein expressions was seen in 43 cases (16.5%), which were regarded as dMMR. Among these cases, 62.8% (27/43) with MLH1 loss, 14% (6/43) with MSH2 loss, 2.3% (1/43) with MSH6 loss, and 20.9% (9/43) with PMS2 loss (Table 1). Therefore, the most common type of deficient MMR protein was MLH1, followed by PMS2. All MMR proteins were retained in 162 cases (62.1%), which were regarded as pMMR. The result was indeterminate in 33 cases (12.6%) (Table 1).

Table 1. MMR expression in endometrioid endometrial cancer.

MMR Status	Number [Percentage]
MMR Retained	162/238 [62.1%]
MMR Loss	43/238 [16.5%]
- MLH1 Loss	- 27/43 [62.8%]
- PMS2 Loss	- 9/43 [20.9%]
- MSH2 Loss	- 6/43 [14%]
- MSH6 Loss	- 1/43 [2.3%]
MMR Indeterminate	33/238 [12.6%]
- PMS2 Indeterminate	- 27/33 [81.8%]
- MSH6 Indeterminate	- 4/33 [12%]
- MLH2 Indeterminate	- 2/33 [6%]

3.2. Clinical Characteristics

Two hundred and five cases with deficient MMR (dMMR) or proficient MMR (pMMR) were included in the analysis. The clinical parameters are shown in Table 2. The mean age was larger in the dMMR compared to the pMMR group (57.9 vs. 53.6, $p = 0.04$). Adjuvant pelvic radiotherapy was more frequently given to the dMMR group ($p = 0.03$), while adjuvant vault radiotherapy and chemotherapy were similar. Stage IA endometrial cancer was more common in the pMMR than dMMR group (71% vs. 48.8%, $p = 0.01$), while stage II endometrial cancer was more common in the dMMR than pMMR group (18.6% vs. 8%, $p = 0.05$). The number of early-stage cases (stages I and II) and late-stage cases (stages III and IV) were not different ($p = 0.18$).

Table 2. MMR status in association with clinical parameters.

Clinical Parameters	MMR Deficient ($n = 43$)	MMR Proficient ($n = 162$)	p-Value
Age	Mean 57.9 (SD 11.29)	Mean 53.6 (SD 12.29)	0.04
Parity (missing $n = 62$)	Mean 2.33 (SD 2.19)	Mean 1.82 (SD 1.49)	0.14
Parity	(missing $n = 13$)	(missing $n = 49$)	
- 0	- 9/30 ((30%)	- 30/113 (26.5%)	
- 1	- 2/30 (6.75)	- 17/113 (15%)	
- 2	- 7/30 (23.3%)	- 30/113 (26.5%)	
- 3	- 5/30 (16.7%)	- 22/113 (19.5%)	
- ≥4	- 7/30 (23.3%)	- 14/113 (12.4%)	
Menopause	22/40 (55%)	76/152 (50%)	0.7
Colorectal cancer	3/43 (7%)	4/162 (2.5%)	0.16
Operation			
- Total hysterectomy	- 38/43 (88.4%)	- 156/162 (96.3%)	0.08
- Radical Hysterectomy	- 5/43 (11.6%)	- 6/162 (3.7%)	
- Pelvic lymphadenectomy	- 12/43 (27.9%)	- 46/162 (28.4%)	
- Para-aortic lymphadenectomy	- 10/43 (23.3%)	- 26/162 (16%)	
Bilateral salpingoophorectomy	43/43 (100%)	153/162 (94.4%)	0.25

Table 2. Cont.

Clinical Parameters	MMR Deficient (n = 43)	MMR Proficient (n = 162)	p-Value
Adjuvant vault radiotherapy	10/43 (23.3%)	24/162 (14.8%)	0.28
Adjuvant pelvic radiotherapy	18/43 (41.9%)	38/162 (23.5%)	0.03
Adjuvant chemotherapy	3/43 (7%)	12/162 (7.4%)	0.61
Stage			
- IA	- 21/43 (48.8%)	- 115/162 (71%)	0.01
- IB	- 8/43 (18.6%)	- 21/162 (13%)	
- II	- 8/43 (18.6%)	- 13/162 (8%)	0.05
- IIIA	- 2/43 (4.7%)	- 7/162 (4.3%)	
- IIIB	- 1/43 (2.3%)	- 2/162 (1.2%)	
- IIIC1	- 1/43 (2.3%)	- 1/162 (0.6%)	
- IIIC2	- 2/43 (4.7%)	- 3/162 (1.9%)	

3.3. Pathological Characteristics

The association of pathological parameters with MMR status is shown in Table 3. Uterine tumors were larger in the dMMR than pMMR group ($p = 0.01$) and dMMR were associated with higher grade disease ($p = 0.01$). Pathological findings in deep myometrial invasion, cervical invasion, LVSI, pelvic and para-aortic lymph node involvement were not different between pMMR and dMMR tumors. Although the difference did not reach statistical significance, there was a trend towards more deep myometrial invasion, cervical invasion and LVSI in the dMMR group (Table 3).

Table 3. MMR status associated with pathological parameters.

Pathological Parameters	MMR Deficient (n = 43)	MMR Proficient (n = 162)	p-Value
Uterine tumour size (cm)	Mean 3.39 (SD 2.26)	Mean 2.46 (SD 1.89)	0.01
Grade			
- 1	- 24/43 (55.8%)	- 131/162 (80.9%)	0.01
- 2	- 14/43 (32.6%)	- 26/162 (16%)	
- 3	- 5/43 (11.6%)	- 5/162 (3.1%)	
Deep myometrial invasion	13/43 (30.2%)	28/162 (17.3%)	0.09
Cervical invasion	11/43 (25.6%)	20/162 (12.3%)	0.06
Lymphovascular space invasion (LVSI) (missing n = 88)	10/26 (38.5%)	17/91 (18.7%)	0.07
Pelvic lymph node involved	2/12 (16.7%) (Not performed n = 31)	3/46 (6.5%) (Not performed n = 116)	0.59
Para-aortic lymph node involved	2/10 (20%) (Not performed n = 33)	3/26 (11.5%) (Not performed n =136)	0.43

3.4. Survival and Prognosis

The prognostic impact of MMR status was examined in our survival analysis. Throughout the entire cohort, the median follow up was 138 months (range 5 to 223 months). There were 33 deaths (16.1%), median OS was 137 months (range: 5 to 223 months), median DSS was 141 months (range: 14 to 223 months) and median DFS was 137 months (range: 2 to 217 months). For the pMMR group, median follow up was 140 months (range 5 to 223 months). There were 23 deaths (14.2%). For the dMMR group, the median follow up was 122 months (range 17 to 207 months). There were 10 deaths (23.3%), a percentage higher than the pMMR group. The median OS, DSS and DFS are lower than in the dMMR group than the pMMR group, with a median OS of 122 months (range: 17 to 207 months) vs. 139 months (range: 5 to 223 months), median DSS of 123 months (range: 17 to 207 months) vs. 146 months (range: 14 to 223 months) and median DFS of 121 months (range: 2 to 207 months) vs. 139 months (range: 5 to 217 months) respectively. The Kaplan–Meier curves for the OS, DSS and DFS are shown in Figure 2a-c. The rate of 5-year OS/ DSS/ DFS, 10-year OS/ DSS/ DFS and recurrence are shown in Table 4. Ten-year DSS and DFS were significantly higher in the pMMR than dMMR group (94.8% vs. 80%, p = 0.02; 87.3% vs. 73.5%, p = 0.05) (Table 4). However, the 5-year DSS and DFS only showed a trend of better survival in the pMMR than dMMR group but did not reach statistical significance (Table 4). DFS was longer in the pMMR than dMMR group (p = 0.01), with a hazard ratio of 0.25 (95% CI 0.09 to 0.71) (Figure 2b). The DSS was also longer in the pMMR than dMMR group (p = 0.01), with a HR of 0.22 (95% CI 0.07 to 0.71) (Figure 2b). However, OS was similar between the two groups (p = 0.14) (Figure 2a). The recurrence rate was lower in the pMMR than dMMR group (4.3% vs. 16.3%, p = 0.01) (Table 4).

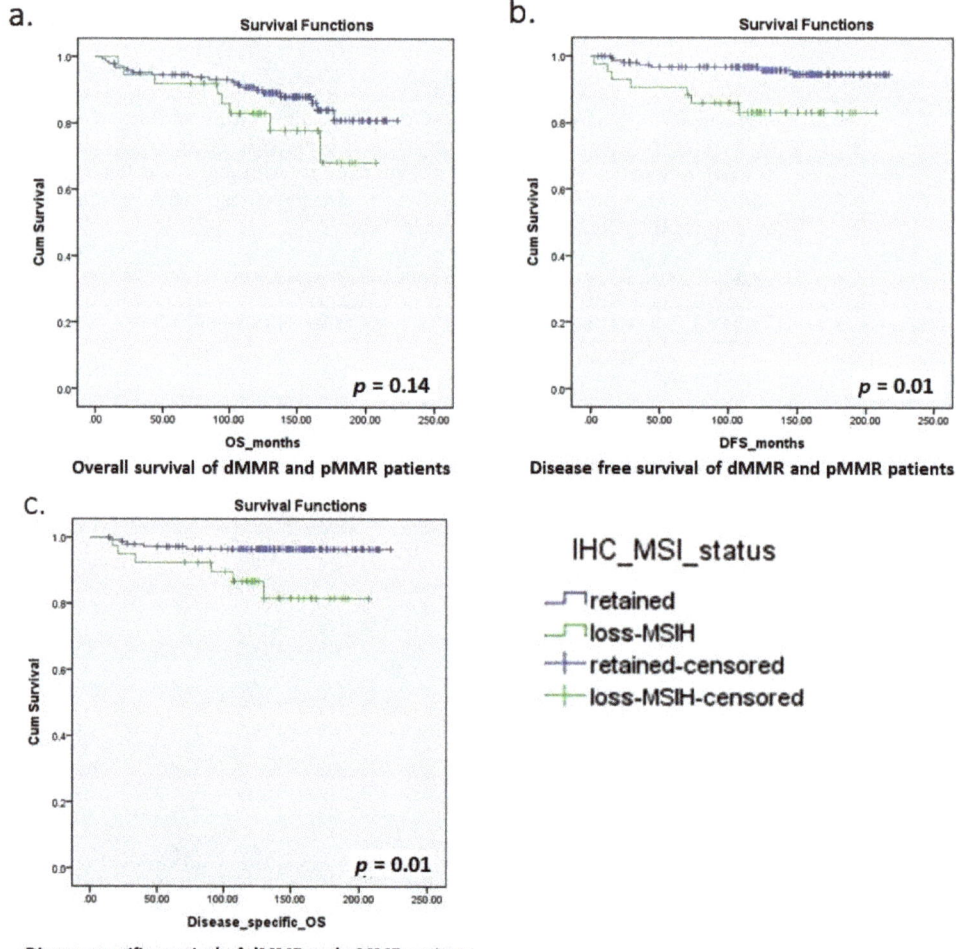

Figure 2. Kaplan–Meier curves for overall survival (OS), disease-free survival (DFS) and disease-specific survival (DSS) of dMMR and pMMR patients. (**a**) overall survival, (**b**) disease-free survival, and (**c**) disease-specific survival of dMMR and pMMR patients.

Table 4. MMR status in association with survival parameters.

Survival Parameters	MMR Deficient (n = 43)	MMR Proficient (n = 162)	p-Value
5 years overall survival	39/43 (90.7%) (Loss to follow up n = 0)	145/157 (92.4%) (Loss to follow up n = 5)	0.46
10 years overall survival	26/34 (76.5%) (Loss to follow up n = 9)	117/134 (87.3%) (Loss to follow up n = 28)	0.19
5 years disease-specific overall survival	36/39 (92.3%) (Loss to follow up n = 0)	134/139 (96.4%) (Loss to follow up n = 5)	0.38
10 years disease-specific overall survival	24/30 (80%) (Loss to follow up n = 9)	110/116 (94.8%) (Loss to follow up n = 28)	0.02
5 years disease-free survival	39/43 (90.7%) (Loss to follow up n = 0)	144/157 (91.7%) (Loss to follow up n = 5)	0.52
10 years disease-free survival	25/34 (73.5%) (Loss to follow up n = 9)	117/134 (87.3%) (Loss to follow up n = 28)	0.05
Disease recurrence	7/43 (16.3%)	1/162 (4.3%)	0.01

4. Discussion

MMR status has been intensively studied in recent years as a prognostic indicator in endometrial cancer. In colorectal cancer, MSI-H has been shown in multiple studies to be strongly associated with better prognosis [30]; however, results have been contradictory in endometrial cancer. In a meta-analysis including 23 studies [21], no definite evidence between MMR status and detrimental survival in endometrial cancer was found [21]. However, only one out of 23 studies showed an improved overall survival [6] in that meta-analysis and this outlier led to the insignificant conclusion [6]. In that particular study, 20% of cases were of non-endometrioid histology [6]. A study involving 728 cases found a worse DSS in only endometrioid tumors with somatic MMR deficiency (HR 2.18), while no difference was found for germline mutation or when both endometrioid and non-endometrioid tumors were included [14]. The detrimental effect of dMMR on endometrial cancer survival was also seen in another study with a HR of 3.25 for DFS and HR of 4.2 for DSS [20]. Other studies only detected poorer survival in early stage endometrioid tumor [3]. These findings reflected the different clinical implication dMMR has on various endometrial cancer subtypes and somatic or germline mutation.

The contradictory results of different studies may be due to lack of stratification of cases into (1) somatic or germline mutation and (2) endometrioid or non-endometrioid cancer. Our study, being the first to focus only on endometrioid tumors, had showed that somatic dMMR in endometrioid endometrial cancer was associated with worse clinico-pathological factors including older patient age, larger tumor size, more advanced-stage disease, higher-grade disease and increased need of adjuvant radiotherapy. The poor prognostic implications were reflected in the survival analysis, with more recurrence noticed in the dMMR group and a shorter DFS observed, despite more adjuvant therapy being used in the dMMR group. The poor prognostic implication was particularly profound in the long term, with the 10 years DSS and DFS being significantly higher in the pMMR than dMMR group (94.8% vs. 80%, $p = 0.02$; 87.3% vs. 73.5%, $p = 0.05$) but five-year DSS and DFS only showing a trend of better survival in the pMMR group (96.4% vs. 92.3%, $p = 0.38$; 91.7% vs. 90.7%, $p = 0.52$). The findings of our study further indicated that in a specific group of patients (endometrioid histology), somatic dMMR may be a prognostic indicator.

Early-stage endometrioid histology accounts for >60% of endometrial cancers [31], therefore, our findings are relevant to the majority of endometrial cancer patients. The addition of MMR status in the risk stratification process can potentially identify a proportion of poor prognostic patients in this originally low risk group for individualized treatment and follow up plan. The poor long-term survival in the dMMR group indicated the need of an individualized follow up plan based on risk assessment. Currently, most international guidelines recommend 5-year follow up for endometrial cancer patients [32,33]. However, our results showed that the 5-year survival of dMMR and pMMR group were not very much different and the obvious difference occurs at 5 to 10 years follow up. In the dMMR group, longer follow up to 10 years should be considered. Moreover, more aggressive adjuvant treatment plan may be appropriate for this higher-risk group.

4.1. Personalized Medicine in Endometrial Cancer

Traditionally, endometrial cancer had been classified by clinical characteristics such as grade of disease. Recently, there is emerging evidence on the utility of genetic and epigenetic characteristics as prognostic markers for endometrial cancer [34]. The latest 2020 ESGO/ESTRO/ ESP guideline on endometrial cancer recommended encouraging molecular classification in all endometrial cancers [13]. Knowledge of the genetic and epigenetic characteristics of individuals can allow personalized medicine tailored to the individual's genetic profile. The Cancer Genome Atlas Research Network had classified endometrial cancer into four categories: *POLE* hypermutated, MSI hypermutated, copy number low (*p53* abnormal) and copy number high [35]. Molecular testing is relevant in the risk stratification for prognosis and adjuvant therapy usage, guidance for immunotherapy and pre-screening for Lynch syndrome [13].

4.2. Personalized Medicine in Endometrial Cancer—Adjuvant Treatment

Molecular markers are increasingly being incorporated into traditional risk stratification model to identify high risk patients, especially in high-risk endometrial cancers where evidence has shown that molecular biomarkers can serve as better prognostic markers. For example, *POLE* hypermutated high risk endometrial cancer was found to have excellent prognosis, while *p53* abnormal tumours had poor prognosis [13]. Molecular classification can further guide the usage of adjuvant therapy and individualise a follow-up plan based on patients' molecular characteristics. MMR status has been well demonstrated in colorectal cancer to be an effective predictor for treatment efficacy in adjuvant setting [30], allowing a more tailored adjuvant therapy. In endometrial cancer, there is limited evidence showing a better response rate of dMMR tumors to platinum-based chemotherapy than pMMR tumors (67% vs. 44%) [31]. In a study with 158 endometrial cancer patients receiving chemotherapy and 66 patients receiving radiotherapy, there was a significant increase in OS and PFS in dMMR, non-endometrioid tumors treated with radiotherapy and pMMR stage III/IV patients treated with adjuvant chemotherapy [22]. The majority of endometrial cancers are stage IA disease which is considered as low risk, and adjuvant therapy is not recommended based on current recommendations which utilize clinicopathological factors [36]. With emerging evidence of the adverse effect of dMMR, adjuvant therapy can be considered to improve survival in dMMR early-stage endometrioid endometrial cancer patients. This risk stratification with molecular markers may be a superior model than the existing clinicopathological model or could be an adjunct to formulation of adjuvant treatment.

4.3. Personalized Medicine in Endometrial Cancer—Immunotherapy

Molecular characteristics can predict response to new therapeutic agents such as immunotherapy. For example, MSI analysis has been proven in colorectal cancer to be an effective biomarker to predict response to pembrolizumab, a PD-1 immune checkpoint inhibitors that targets and block PD-1 [37]. The objective response to Pembrolizumab is 40% in the dMMR group compared to 0% in the pMMR group [37]. The evidence with endometrial cancer is not as robust. Nonetheless, pembrolizumab has been approved by the FDA for use in recurrent or metastatic endometrial cancer together with all other types of dMMR tumours [38]. The overall response rate to Pembrolizumab was 39.6%, while the response rate in endometrial cancer alone was 36% [39]. Immunotherapy is very expensive and not without adverse effects. Therefore, the selection of patients who will benefit is important. MMR status can potentially be a biomarker to predict treatment efficacy of PD-1 immune checkpoint inhibitor in endometrial cancer patients [40]. This molecular approach is promising, especially in metastatic recurrent disease where patients would otherwise, be incurable.

4.4. Personalized Medicine in Endometrial Cancer—Lynch Syndrome Screening

Approximately 3% of endometrial cancer patients carry germline MMR gene mutations [13]. A germline mutation in MMR genes results in Lynch syndrome, an inherited cancer syndrome predisposing patients to multiple cancer development, including colorectal and endometrial cancers [41]. Lynch syndrome was found to be present in 5.4% of Chinese endometrial cancer patients [10]. Traditionally, screening of Lynch syndrome has been based on clinical parameters, such as the personal and family history of Lynch-associated malignancies. Somatic loss of MMR expression may be associated with a presence of germline mutation. MSI is a well-established and effective genetic marker for detection of Lynch syndrome [9]. Expanding a universal screening program for Lynch syndrome to include patients with endometrial cancer has been shown to identify 50% more Lynch syndrome patients [42], who would largely be missed by screening based on clinical parameters. The latest guideline from ESGO/ESTRO/ESP and International Society of Gynaecological Pathology recommended testing of MMR with IHC to screen for Lynch syndrome [13]. An early detection can allow appropriate cancer risk reducing intervention to be undertaken in the patients and their relatives, potentially improving their survival.

The strength of our study includes a large sample size of 238 cases focusing on somatic dMMR of endometrioid histology endometrial cancers. The long follow up with a median follow up of more than 10 years is also longer than most of the published studies [3,14,22]. Furthermore, all four MMR protein expressions were evaluated in our study whereas only one to two MMR protein expressions were evaluated in some previous studies [21]. However, the rate of dMMR of 16.5% in our study is less than that reported in other studies [5,6]. This is because we adopted a strict criteria defining dMMR with <1% staining, while staining in <10% was considered as indeterminate, leading to a high proportion of cases being reported as indeterminate (12.6%). If the indeterminate cases were also considered potentially negative, most of the dMMR rates reported in other studies [5,6] would fall into the possible range of dMMR in our cohort (16.5–29.1%). On the other hand, the survival analysis may be affected by the imbalance of age, stage of disease and adjuvant therapy received between the dMMR and pMMR groups. Furthermore, information on other somatic tumour markers such as *p53* and *POLE* status which also affects survival was not available. Lymph node dissection was performed on only 58 cases which is too low to draw any definite conclusion.

5. Conclusions

MMR deficiency is present in 16.5% of Hong Kong Chinese women with endometroid endometrial cancers. dMMR is associated with poor clinicopathological factors, worse DFS, DSS and more recurrence. The worse prognosis is particularly evident in the long term at 5 to 10 years follow up.

Supplementary Materials: The following are available online at https://www.mdpi.com/article/10.3390/biomedicines9101385/s1, Table S1: Antibodies and conditions used in immunohistochemistry of MMR proteins.

Author Contributions: Conceptualization, J.H.S.L., J.J.X.L. and J.K.; methodology, J.H.S.L., J.J.X.L., C.C., R.C.K.C., J.S.H.K. and T.S.L.; formal analysis, J.H.S.L.; investigation, J.H.S.L. and J.J.X.L.; writing—original draft preparation, J.H.S.L., J.J.X.L. C.C. and T.S.L.; writing—review and editing, J.H.S.L., J.J.X.L., C.C., R.C.K.C., J.S.H.K., T.S.L., K.F.T., S.F.Y., S.Y.Y. and J.K. All authors have read and agreed to the published version of the manuscript.

Funding: The research was supported by Health and Medical Research Fund (HMRF) Hong Kong (07183826) to J.H.S.L. and J.K.

Institutional Review Board Statement: The study was conducted according to the guidelines of the Declaration of Helsinki, and approved by the Clinical Research Ethics Committee of The Chinese University of Hong Kong (CREC Ref. No. 2019.716).

Informed Consent Statement: Informed consent was obtained from all subjects involved in the study. Written informed consent has been obtained from the patient(s) to publish this paper.

Data Availability Statement: The data presented in this study are available on request from the corresponding author. The data are not publicly available due to privacy.

Conflicts of Interest: The authors declare no conflict of interest.

References

1. Shikama, A.; Minaguchi, T.; Matsumoto, K.; Akiyama-Abe, A.; Nakamura, Y.; Michikami, H.; Nakao, S.; Sakurai, M.; Ochi, H.; Onuki, M.; et al. Clinicopathologic implications of DNA mismatch repair status in endometrial carcinomas. *Gynecol. Oncol.* **2016**, *140*, 226–233. [CrossRef]
2. Nout, R.A.; Bosse, T.; Creutzberg, C.L.; Jürgenliemk-Schulz, I.M.; Jobsen, J.J.; Lutgens, L.C.; van der Steen-Banasik, E.M.; van Eijk, R.; ter Haar, N.T.; Smit, V.T. Improved risk assessment of endometrial cancer by combined analysis of MSI, PI3K–AKT, Wnt/β-catenin and P53 pathway activation. *Gynecol. Oncol.* **2012**, *126*, 466–473. [CrossRef]
3. Mackay, H.J.; Gallinger, S.; Tsao, M.S.; McLachlin, C.M.; Tu, D.; Keiser, K.; Eisenhauer, E.A.; Oza, A. Prognostic value of microsatellite instability (MSI) and PTEN expression in women with endometrial cancer: Results from studies of the NCIC Clinical Trials Group (NCIC CTG). *Eur. J. Cancer* **2010**, *46*, 1365–1373. [CrossRef]
4. Li, G.-M. Mechanisms and functions of DNA mismatch repair. *Cell Res.* **2008**, *18*, 85–98. [CrossRef]
5. Cosgrove, C.M.; Cohn, D.; Hampel, H.; Frankel, W.L.; Jones, D.; McElroy, J.P.; Suarez, A.A.; Zhao, W.; Chen, W.; Salani, R.; et al. Epigenetic silencing of MLH1 in endometrial cancers is associated with larger tumor volume, increased rate of lymph node positivity and reduced recurrence-free survival. *Gynecol. Oncol.* **2017**, *146*, 588–595. [CrossRef] [PubMed]
6. Black, D.; Soslow, R.A.; Levine, D.A.; Tornos, C.; Chen, S.C.; Hummer, A.J.; Bogomolniy, F.; Olvera, N.; Barakat, R.R.; Boyd, J. Clinicopathologic Significance of Defective DNA Mismatch Repair in Endometrial Carcinoma. *J. Clin. Oncol.* **2006**, *24*, 1745–1753. [CrossRef] [PubMed]
7. Hampel, H.; Frankel, W.; Panescu, J.; Lockman, J.; Sotamaa, K.; Fix, D.; Comeras, I.; La Jeunesse, J.; Nakagawa, H.; Westman, J.A.; et al. Screening for Lynch Syndrome (Hereditary Nonpolyposis Colorectal Cancer) among Endometrial Cancer Patients. *Cancer Res.* **2006**, *66*, 7810–7817. [CrossRef] [PubMed]
8. Middha, S.; Zhang, L.; Nafa, K.; Jayakumaran, G.; Wong, D.; Kim, H.R.; Sadowska, J.; Berger, M.F.; Delair, D.F.; Shia, J.; et al. Reliable Pan-Cancer Microsatellite Instability Assessment by Using Targeted Next-Generation Sequencing Data. *JCO Precis. Oncol.* **2017**, *2017*, 1–17. [CrossRef]
9. Bartley, A.N.; Luthra, R.; Saraiya, D.S.; Urbauer, D.L.; Broaddus, R.R. Identification of Cancer Patients with Lynch Syndrome: Clinically Significant Discordances and Problems in Tissue-Based Mismatch Repair Testing. *Cancer Prev. Res.* **2012**, *5*, 320–327. [CrossRef]
10. Chao, X.; Li, L.; Wu, M.; Ma, S.; Tan, X.; Zhong, S.; Bi, Y.; Lang, J. Comparison of screening strategies for Lynch syndrome in patients with newly diagnosed endometrial cancer: A prospective cohort study in China. *Cancer Commun.* **2019**, *39*, 42. [CrossRef]
11. Bruegl, A.S.; Ring, K.L.; Daniels, M.; Fellman, B.M.; Urbauer, D.L.; Broaddus, R.R. Clinical Challenges Associated with Universal Screening for Lynch Syndrome–Associated Endometrial Cancer. *Cancer Prev. Res.* **2016**, *10*, 108–115. [CrossRef]
12. Wadee, W.G.R. Immunohistochemical mismatch repair deficiency versus PCR microsatellite instability: A tale of two methodologies in endometrial carcinomas. *Eur. J. Gynaecol. Oncol.* **2020**, *41*, 952–959. [CrossRef]
13. Concin, N.; Matias-Guiu, X.; Vergote, I.; Cibula, D.; Mirza, M.R.; Marnitz, S.; Ledermann, J.; Bosse, T.; Chargari, C.; Fagotti, A.; et al. ESGO/ESTRO/ESP guidelines for the management of patients with endometrial carcinoma. *Radiother. Oncol.* **2021**, *154*, 327–353. [CrossRef] [PubMed]
14. Nagle, C.M.; O'Mara, T.A.; Tan, Y.; Buchanan, D.D.; Obermair, A.; Blomfield, P.; Quinn, M.A.; Webb, P.M.; Spurdle, A.B.; on behalf of the Australian Endometrial Cancer Study Group. Endometrial cancer risk and survival by tumor MMR status. *J. Gynecol. Oncol.* **2018**, *29*, e39. [CrossRef] [PubMed]
15. Salvesen, H.B.; Haldorsen, I.S.; Trovik, J. Markers for individualised therapy in endometrial carcinoma. *Lancet Oncol.* **2012**, *13*, e353–e361. [CrossRef]

16. Ruiz, I.; Martín-Arruti, M.; Lopez-Lopez, E.; Garcia-Orad, A. Lack of association between deficient mismatch repair expression and outcome in endometrial carcinomas of the endometrioid type. *Gynecol. Oncol.* **2014**, *134*, 20–23. [CrossRef]
17. Bokhman, J.V. Two pathogenetic types of endometrial carcinoma. *Gynecol. Oncol.* **1983**, *15*, 10–17. [CrossRef]
18. An, H.J.; Kim, K.I.; Kim, J.Y.; Shim, J.Y.; Kang, H.; Kim, T.H.; Kim, J.K.; Jeong, J.K.; Lee, S.Y.; Kim, S.J. Microsatellite instability in endometrioid type endometrial adenocarcinoma is associated with poor prognostic indicators. *Am. J. Surg. Pathol.* **2007**, *31*, 846–853. [CrossRef]
19. Fountzilas, E.; Kotoula, V.; Pentheroudakis, G.; Manousou, K.; Polychronidou, G.; Vrettou, E.; Poulios, C.; Papadopoulou, E.; Raptou, G.; Pectasides, E.; et al. Prognostic implications of mismatch repair deficiency in patients with nonmetastatic colorectal and endometrial cancer. *ESMO Open* **2019**, *4*, e000474. [CrossRef]
20. Bilbao, C.; Lara, P.C.; Ramírez, R.; Henríquez-Hernández, L.A.; Rodríguez, G.; Falcón, O.; León, L.; Perucho, M.; Díaz-Chico, B.N.; Díaz-Chico, J.C. Microsatellite Instability Predicts Clinical Outcome in Radiation-Treated Endometrioid Endometrial Cancer. *Int. J. Radiat. Oncol.* **2010**, *76*, 9–13. [CrossRef] [PubMed]
21. Diaz-Padilla, I.; Romero, N.; Amir, E.; Matias-Guiu, X.; Vilar, E.; Muggia, F.; Garcia-Donas, J. Mismatch repair status and clinical outcome in endometrial cancer: A systematic review and meta-analysis. *Crit. Rev. Oncol.* **2013**, *88*, 154–167. [CrossRef]
22. Resnick, K.E.; Frankel, W.L.; Morrison, C.D.; Fowler, J.M.; Copeland, L.J.; Stephens, J.; Kim, K.H.; Cohn, D.E. Mismatch repair status and outcomes after adjuvant therapy in patients with surgically staged endometrial cancer. *Gynecol. Oncol.* **2010**, *117*, 234–238. [CrossRef] [PubMed]
23. Le, D.T.; Durham, J.N.; Smith, K.N.; Wang, H.; Bartlett, B.R.; Aulakh, L.K.; Lu, S.; Kemberling, H.; Wilt, C.; Luber, B.S.; et al. Mismatch repair deficiency predicts response of solid tumors to PD-1 blockade. *Science* **2017**, *357*, 409–413. [CrossRef]
24. Di Tucci, C.; Capone, C.; Galati, G.; Iacobelli, V.; Schiavi, M.C.; Di Donato, V.; Muzii, L.; Panici, P.B. Immunotherapy in endometrial cancer: New scenarios on the horizon. *J. Gynecol. Oncol.* **2019**, *30*, e46. [CrossRef] [PubMed]
25. Nelson, G.S.; Pink, A.; Lee, S.; Han, G.; Morris, D.; Ogilvie, T.; Duggan, M.A.; Köbel, M. MMR deficiency is common in high-grade endometrioid carcinomas and is associated with an unfavorable outcome. *Gynecol. Oncol.* **2013**, *131*, 309–314. [CrossRef]
26. Powell, M. Immunohistochemistry to determine mismatch repair-deficiency in endometrial cancer: The appropriate standard. *Ann. Oncol.* **2017**, *28*, 9–10. [CrossRef] [PubMed]
27. Sarode, V.R.; Robinson, L. Screening for Lynch Syndrome by Immunohistochemistry of Mismatch Repair Proteins: Significance of Indeterminate Result and Correlation With Mutational Studies. *Arch. Pathol. Lab. Med.* **2019**, *143*, 1225–1233. [CrossRef]
28. Centre for Clinical Research and Biostatistics. Survival Analysis: Comparison of Two Survival Curves—Lachin. Available online: https://www2.ccrb.cuhk.edu.hk/stat/survival/Lachin1981 (accessed on 3 September 2021).
29. Schröer, A.; Köster, F.; Fischer, D.; Dubitscher, R.M.; Woll-Hermann, A.; Diedrich, K.; Friedrich, M.; Salehin, D. Immunohistochemistry of DNA mismatch repair enzyme MSH2 is not correlated with prognostic data from endometrial carcinomas. *Anticancer. Res.* **2009**, *29*, 4833–4837.
30. Ribic, C.M.; Sargent, D.; Moore, M.J.; Thibodeau, S.N.; French, A.J.; Goldberg, R.M.; Hamilton, S.R.; Laurent-Puig, P.; Gryfe, R.; Shepherd, L.E.; et al. Tumor Microsatellite-Instability Status as a Predictor of Benefit from Fluorouracil-Based Adjuvant Chemotherapy for Colon Cancer. *New Engl. J. Med.* **2003**, *349*, 247–257. [CrossRef]
31. Kato, M.; Takano, M.; Miyamoto, M.; Sasaki, N.; Goto, T.; Tsuda, H.; Furuya, K. DNA mismatch repair-related protein loss as a prognostic factor in endometrial cancers. *J. Gynecol. Oncol.* **2015**, *26*, 40–45. [CrossRef]
32. Colombo, N.; Preti, E.; Landoni, F.; Carinelli, S.; Colombo, A.; Marini, C.; Sessa, C. Endometrial cancer: ESMO Clinical Practice Guidelines for diagnosis, treatment and follow-up. *Ann. Oncol.* **2013**, *24*, vi33–vi38. [CrossRef]
33. Sundar, S.; Balega, J.; Crosbie, E.; Drake, A.; Edmondson, R.; Fotopoulou, C.; Gallos, I.; Ganesan, R.; Gupta, J.; Johnson, N.; et al. BGCS uterine cancer guidelines: Recommendations for practice. *Eur. J. Obstet. Gynecol. Reprod. Biol.* **2017**, *213*, 71–97. [CrossRef]
34. Cavaliere, A.; Perelli, F.; Zaami, S.; Piergentili, R.; Mattei, A.; Vizzielli, G.; Scambia, G.; Straface, G.; Restaino, S.; Signore, F. Towards Personalized Medicine: Non-Coding RNAs and Endometrial Cancer. *Heal.* **2021**, *9*, 965. [CrossRef]
35. The Cancer Genome Atlas Research Network; Kandoth, C.; Schultz, N.; Cherniack, A.D.; Akbani, R.; Liu, Y.; Shen, H.; Robertson, A.G.; Pashtan, I.; Shen, R.; et al. Integrated genomic characterization of endometrial carcinoma. *Nature* **2013**, *497*, 67–73. [CrossRef]
36. Koh, W.-J.; Abu-Rustum, N.R.; Bean, S.; Bradley, K.; Campos, S.M.; Cho, K.; Chon, H.S.; Chu, C.; Cohn, D.; Crispens, M.A.; et al. Uterine Neoplasms, Version 1.2018, NCCN Clinical Practice Guidelines in Oncology. *J. Natl. Compr. Cancer Netw.* **2018**, *16*, 170–199. [CrossRef] [PubMed]
37. Le, D.T.; Uram, J.N.; Wang, H.; Bartlett, B.R.; Kemberling, H.; Eyring, A.D.; Skora, A.D.; Luber, B.S.; Azad, N.S.; Laheru, D.; et al. PD-1 Blockade in Tumors with Mismatch-Repair Deficiency. *N. Engl. J. Med.* **2015**, *372*, 2509–2520. [CrossRef] [PubMed]
38. Food and Drug Administration. FDA Grants Accelerated Approval to Pembrolizumab for First Tissue/Site Agnostic Indication. Available online: https://www.fda.gov/drugs/resources-information-approved-drugs/fda-grants-accelerated-approval-pembrolizumab-first-tissuesite-agnostic-indication (accessed on 4 April 2021).
39. Marcus, L.; Lemery, S.J.; Keegan, P.; Pazdur, R. FDA Approval Summary: Pembrolizumab for the Treatment of Microsatellite Instability-High Solid Tumors. *Clin. Cancer Res.* **2019**, *25*, 3753–3758. [CrossRef] [PubMed]
40. Ono, R.; Nakayama, K.; Nakamura, K.; Yamashita, H.; Ishibashi, T.; Ishikawa, M.; Minamoto, T.; Razia, S.; Ishikawa, N.; Otsuki, Y.; et al. Dedifferentiated Endometrial Carcinoma Could be A Target for Immune Checkpoint Inhibitors (Anti PD-1/PD-L1 Antibodies). *Int. J. Mol. Sci.* **2019**, *20*, 3744. [CrossRef]

41. Kastrinos, F.; Uno, H.; Ukaegbu, C.; Alvero, C.; McFarland, A.; Yurgelun, M.B.; Kulke, M.H.; Schrag, D.; Meyerhardt, J.A.; Fuchs, C.S.; et al. Development and Validation of the PREMM5 Model for Comprehensive Risk Assessment of Lynch Syndrome. *J. Clin. Oncol.* **2017**, *35*, 2165–2172. [CrossRef] [PubMed]
42. Adar, T.; Rodgers, L.H.; Shannon, K.M.; Yoshida, M.; Ma, T.; Mattia, A.; Lauwers, G.Y.; Iafrate, A.J.; Hartford, N.M.; Oliva, E.; et al. Universal screening of both endometrial and colon cancers increases the detection of Lynch syndrome. *Cancer* **2018**, *124*, 3145–3153. [CrossRef]

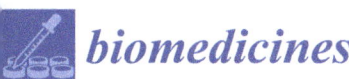

Article

Biological Planning of Radiation Dose Based on In Vivo Dosimetry for Postoperative Vaginal-Cuff HDR Interventional Radiotherapy (Brachytherapy)

Tamer Soror [1,2,*,†], Ramin Chafii [1,†], Valentina Lancellotta [3], Luca Tagliaferri [3] and György Kovács [4]

1. Radiation Oncology Department, University of Lübeck/UKSH-CL, 23562 Lübeck, Germany; r.chafii@gmail.com
2. National Cancer Institute (NCI), Radiation Oncology Department, Cairo University, Giza 12613, Egypt
3. UOC Radioterapia Oncologica, Dipartimento di Diagnostica per Immagini, Radioterapia Oncologica ed Ematologia, Fondazione Policlinico Universitario A. Gemelli, IRCCS, 00168 Roma, Italy; valentina.lancellotta@policlinicogemelli.it (V.L.); luca.tagliaferri@policlinicogemelli.it (L.T.)
4. Gemelli-INTERACTS, Università Cattolica del Sacro Cuore, 00168 Roma, Italy; gyorgy.kovacs@unicatt.it
* Correspondence: tamer.soror@nci.cu.edu.eg; Tel.: +49-17623-695626
† Equal contribution.

Abstract: (1) Background: Postoperative vaginal-cuff HDR interventional radiotherapy (brachytherapy) is a standard treatment in early-stage endometrial cancer. This study reports the effect of in vivo dosimetry-based biological planning for two different fractionation schedules on the treatment-related toxicities. (2) Methods: 121 patients were treated. Group A (82) received 21 Gy in three fractions. Group B (39) received 20 Gy in four fractions. The dose was prescribed at a 5 mm depth or to the applicator surface according to the distance between the applicator and the rectum. In vivo dosimetry measured the dose of the rectum and/or urinary bladder. With a high measured dose, the dose prescription was changed from a 5 mm depth to the applicator surface. (3) Results: The median age was 66 years with 58.8 months mean follow-up. The dose prescription was changed in 20.7% of group A and in 41% of group B. Most toxicities were grade 1–2. Acute urinary toxicities were significantly higher in group A. The rates of acute and late urinary toxicities were significantly higher with a mean bladder dose/fraction of >2.5 Gy and a total bladder dose of >7.5 Gy. One patient had a vaginal recurrence. (4) Conclusions: Both schedules have excellent local control and acceptable rates of toxicities. Using in vivo dosimetry-based biological planning yielded an acceptable dose to the bladder and rectum.

Keywords: interventional radiotherapy; vaginal-cuff brachytherapy; HDR brachytherapy; in vivo dosimetry; endometrial cancer; biological planning

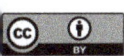

1. Introduction

In developed countries, endometrial cancer is the most common gynecological malignancy. In 2018, 382,069 new cases were estimated worldwide [1]. Most of the patients presented with an early-stage disease, where postoperative vaginal-cuff interventional radiotherapy (brachytherapy, VBT) was found to be non-inferior to postoperative external beam radiation treatment (EBRT) with equivalent rates of local vaginal recurrences as well as distant metastases [2,3].

Compared with EBRT or EBRT combined with VBT, VBT has better late toxicity sequences and offers a better quality of life. In addition to global health status, patients treated with VBT alone had a better social function [4–8]. Furthermore, the use of EBRT or EBRT combined with HDR-VBT resulted in higher treatment costs and higher toxicity without the survival benefit as compared to BT alone [9–11].

HDR-VBT as the sole adjuvant post-operative radiation technique is currently considered the standard care for many subgroups of patients with early-stage disease [12–14].

The American Brachytherapy Society (ABS) recommends treating the proximal 3–5 cm of the vaginal cuff with HDR-VBT postoperatively [3]. Different fractionation schedules are endorsed with the fraction size ranging between 2.5 and 7 Gy. The dose could be prescribed to the vaginal/applicator surface or at depth (3–5 mm). There is no optimal schedule, and the selection of fractionation schedules is usually dependent on the institutional experience and workload [3]. However, pathologic examination of the vaginal wall found that 95% of the lymphatic channels are located within a 3 mm depth of the vaginal surface. Subsequently, dose prescription to depth may provide adequate coverage of such lymphatics [15].

Nevertheless, prescribing the dose at a depth of 5 mm might subsequently result in increasing the dose to the nearby organs at risk (OAR), particularly the rectum and the urinary bladder, which in turn may increase the rates of treatment-related toxicities. Furthermore, changes in the patient's anatomy and the applicator positioning differences between treatment fractions can lead to a change in the dose calculated to OAR [10].

In vivo dosimetry (IVD) measures the actual absorbed radiation dose in the patient while being treated. IVD is able to detect dose variation due to errors in dose calculation, applicator positioning errors, or changes in the patient's anatomy [16].

At our institution, IVD is routinely used to measure the dose to OAR for the patients receiving postoperative HDR-VBT. The depth of dose prescription could be changed subsequently, hence biological planning. This retrospective study reports the effect of IVD-based biological planning for two different fractionation schedules on treatment-related toxicities.

2. Materials and Methods

2.1. Patients

Medical records of the patients with endometrial cancer who received postoperative adjuvant vaginal-cuff HDR-BT using IVD-based biological planning without EBRT from January 2006 to December 2014 were retrospectively reviewed. Only patients with a follow-up of at least 6 months were included in the analysis.

2.2. Vaginal Brachytherapy

From January 2006 to July 2010, the patients were treated with 21 Gy in 3 fractions over 3 weeks (group A). The active treatment length was the upper two-thirds of the rest-vaginal length. Afterwards, the treatment scheme was changed to 20 Gy in 4 fractions over 4 weeks (group B). Only the proximal 3 cm of the vaginal cuff was treated.

All the patients were treated using a vaginal cylinder applicator with the maximum diameter that could be introduced into the vagina (25, 30, and 35 mm). The applicator was introduced parallel to the treatment table and fixed using a fixing tray, Figure 1.

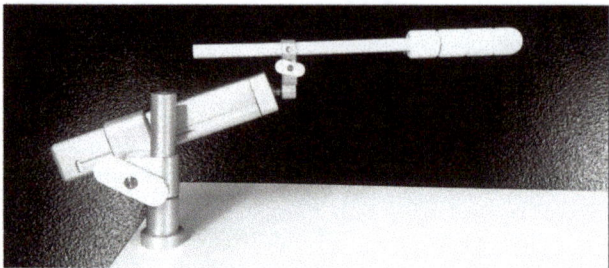

Figure 1. Cylinder vaginal applicator fixed using the fixing tray (Elekta Brachytherapy, Veenendaal, The Netherlands).

Two orthogonal X-ray images were then acquired to verify the applicator position as well as the rectal and bladder points according to the international commission on reporting radiation units and measurements (ICRU), report number 38 [17]. Correction of the applicator position was performed when needed, Figure 2.

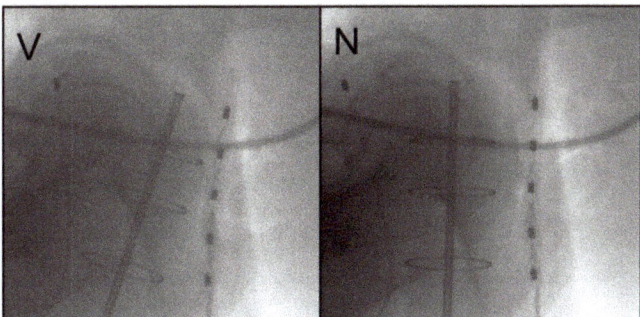

Figure 2. Lateral pre-interventional X-ray, before (V) and after (N) correction of the applicator position with consecutive reduction in the applied rectal dose.

Generally, the dose was prescribed to a 5 mm depth of the applicator surface or to the applicator/vaginal surface. This was decided for each individual patient according to the measured distance between the applicator and the rectal probe on the pre-interventional orthogonal X-ray images. If the distance was below 0.5 cm, the dose was prescribed to the applicator/vaginal surface. Otherwise, the dose was prescribed to a 5 mm depth of the applicator surface.

2.3. In Vivo Dosimetry

A semiconductor-probes system was used to measure the dose to the rectum and/or urinary bladder (Multidos T10004; PTW, Freiburg, Germany). The rectal probe has five ionization chamber detectors; the highest measured dose of the five chambers was documented, while the bladder probe has only one measuring chamber.

IVD was used to measure the rectal and/or urinary bladder radiation dose. When the measured radiation dose during the first fraction was considered high, the dose prescription of the further fractions was changed from a 5 mm depth to the surface applicator. This led to a subsequent decrease in the measured rectal and/or urinary bladder radiation dose.

2.4. Follow-Up

Patients were regularly examined by a gynecologist every 3 months in the first 3 years, then every 6 months for 2 years. Pelvic and intravaginal ultrasound examinations were performed by the gynecologist, and additional investigations were carried out only if needed. A radiation oncologist documented the treatment-related acute toxicities under treatment as well as 6 weeks after treatment, and late toxicities were documented yearly. The grading of recorded toxicities was performed according to the Common Terminology Criteria for Adverse Events 4.0.

2.5. Statistical Analysis

Results are reported as the absolute value with the corresponding percentage, as the median with range, or as the mean with standard deviation (SD). A chi-square (χ^2) test was used to compare categorical data and an independent T-test was used to compare continuous data. Follow-up duration was calculated starting from the date of HDR-BT to the date of death or last available visit. The statistical significance level was established at $p < 0.05$. Statistical analyses were performed using IBM SPSS Statistics for Windows, Version 20.0. (Armonk, NY, USA: IBM Corp).

3. Results

One hundred twenty-one patients were identified. The median age for the whole cohort was 66 years (44–87), and the mean follow-up period was 58.8 months (±33.4). The median interval between surgery and the start of brachytherapy was 6 weeks (range: 5–8). All patients had an early-stage disease (Stage I–II) except for only one patient who had a positive iliac lymph node where the EBRT was contraindicated due to wound complications. Patients and disease characteristics are summarized in Table 1.

Table 1. Patients and disease characteristics.

Characteristics		
Age	Median (range)	66 (44–87)
BMI	Mean (±SD)	29.9 (±7.8)
Menopause	Premenopause	8 (6.6%)
	Postmenopause	113 (93.4%)
Histology	Endometrioid adenocarcinoma	114 (94.3%)
	Serous adenocarcinoma	5 (4.1%)
	Clear cell carcinoma	1 (0.8%)
	Undifferentiated carcinoma	1 (0.8%)
Grading	Grade 1	47
	Grade 2	44
	Grade 3	30
Lymphovascular space invasion	No	105 (86.8%)
	Focal	16 (13.2%)
	Substantial	0 (0%)
Lymphadenectomy	Yes	100 (82.7%)
	No	21 (17.3%)
Myometrial invasion	No	24 (19.8%)
	Less than 50%	45 (37.2%)
	More than 50%	52 (43%)
T-stage	pT1a	69 (57%)
	pT1b	40 (33.1%)
	pT2	12 (9.9%)
N-stage	Nx	17 (14%)
	cN0	4 (3.3%)
	pN0	99 (81.8%)
	N1	1 (0.8%)
FIGO clinical stage	Stage IA	69 (57%)
	Stage IB	39 (32.2%)
	Stage II	12 (9.9%)
	Stage IIIc	1 (0.8%)

SD = standard deviation; FIGO = Fédération Internationale de Gynécologie et d'Obstétrique.

Group A included 82 patients, while group B included 39 patients. In group A, the dose prescription was changed from 0.5 mm to the applicator/vaginal surface with a recorded mean rectal and/or bladder dose of 5.5 Gy (±0.9) in 20.7% of the patients. In group B, the dose prescription was changed with a mean dose of 2.6 Gy (±0.8) in 41% of the patients, Table 2.

In group A, the dose prescription was changed in 17 patients after the first fraction. In the second fraction, the mean rectal dose was reduced by a mean of 1.2 Gy (±1), and the mean urinary bladder dose was reduced by a mean of 1.3 Gy (±1). In group B, the change in prescription was documented in 16 patients. Subsequently, the mean rectal dose was reduced by a mean of 0.6 Gy (±0.2) and the mean urinary bladder dose was reduced by a mean of 0.4 Gy (±0.2) in the following fraction.

Table 3 shows the rectal and bladder mean doses per fraction as well as the mean total dose for three subgroups of patients according to the dose prescription; to the vaginal surface, to a 5 mm depth, and when the prescription was changed following IVD.

Table 2. Brachytherapy dose prescription among treatment groups.

	Group A (No. 82)	Group B (No. 39)	All Patients (No.121)
Dose prescribed to vaginal surface	54 (65.9%)	16 (41%)	70 (57.9%)
Dose prescribed to 5 mm depth	11 (13.4%)	7 (17.9%)	18 (14.9%)
Dose prescription changed	17 (20.7%)	16 (41%)	33 (27.3%)

Table 3. Mean rectal and bladder doses between treatment groups.

	Group A (No. 82)		Group B (No. 39)	
	Mean rectal dose/fraction	Mean rectal total dose	Mean rectal dose/fraction	Mean rectal total dose
Dose prescribed to vaginal surface	3.9 Gy (±0.5)	11.5 Gy (±1.6)	2.7 Gy (±0.5)	10.6 Gy (±2.1)
Dose prescribed to 5 mm depth	4.1 Gy (±0.4)	12.4 Gy (±1.1)	3.2 Gy (±0.5)	12.8 Gy (±2.1)
Dose prescription changed	4.3 Gy (±0.5)	12.9 Gy (±1.4)	2.2 Gy (±0.6)	9.7 Gy (±2.2)
	Mean bladder dose/fraction	Mean bladder total dose	Mean bladder dose/fraction	Mean bladder total dose
Dose prescribed to vaginal surface	2.6 Gy (±0.5)	7.6 Gy (±1.6)	1.9 Gy (±0.4)	7.9 Gy (±2.1)
Dose prescribed to 5 mm depth	2.9 Gy (±0.6)	8.8 Gy (±1.9)	2.3 Gy (±0.4)	9.2 Gy (±1.4)
Dose prescription changed	2.7 Gy (±0.6)	8.1 Gy (±1.6)	2.1 Gy (±0.5)	8.2 Gy (±1.9)

3.1. Acute and Late Radiation Toxicities

All recorded acute toxicities were grade 1–2. There was no significant difference in the rates of GIT or vaginal toxicities between the two treatment groups. Acute urinary reactions were significantly higher in group A patients, 31.7% versus 12.8% ($p = 0.02$). There was no difference in the distribution of late radiation reactions between both treatment groups, Table 4. Nearly all chronic toxicities were grade 1–2 except for one patient who had grade 3 chronic radiation cystitis and three patients who had grade 3 vaginal dryness; all grade 3 toxicities were among group A patients.

Table 4. Acute and late radiation toxicity between treatment groups.

		Group A (No. 82)	Group B (No. 39)	p
Acute	GIT	10 (12.2%)	4 (10.3%)	0.6
	Urinary	26 (31.7%)	5 (12.8%)	0.02
	Vaginal	15 (18.3%)	6 (15.4%)	0.8
Late	GIT	5 (6.1%)	2 (5.1%)	0.4
	Urinary	14 (17.1%)	2 (5.1%)	0.7
	Vaginal	15 (18.3%)	8 (20.5%)	0.6

Further analyses were performed considering the mean dose per fraction as well as the mean total dose to the rectum for the whole cohort and its impact on the rates of GIT and urinary toxicities. No significant difference could be proved in the rates of acute as well as late GIT toxicities for patients with a mean rectal dose per fraction of >3 Gy versus ≤3 Gy. Likewise, with a mean total rectal dose of >12 Gy versus ≤12 Gy. However, most of the recorded toxicities were found in patients with higher doses, Table 5.

On the contrary, the rates of acute and late urinary toxicities were significantly higher with a mean bladder dose per fraction of ≤2.5 Gy versus >2.5 Gy (19.6% versus 33.3%, $p = 0.04$, and 6.5% versus 15.6%, $p = 0.04$ respectively). Moreover, there were more late urinary toxicities with a total bladder dose of ≤7.5 Gy versus >7.5 Gy (6.6% versus 15.2, $p = 0.04$), Table 5.

Table 5. Rectal and bladder doses in relation to GIT and urinary toxicities.

	Mean Rectal Dose/Fraction			Mean Rectal Total Dose		
	≤3 Gy (no. = 28)	>3 Gy (no. = 84)	p	≤12 Gy (no. = 65)	>12 Gy (no. = 47)	p
Acute GIT toxicities	2 (7.1%)	10 (13.1%)	0.6	8 (12.3%)	7 (12.8%)	0.9
Late GIT toxicities	1 (3.5%)	6 (7.1)	NA	1 (4.6%)	4 (8.5%)	NA
	Mean bladder dose/fraction			Mean bladder total dose		
	≤2.5 Gy (no. = 46)	>2.5 Gy (no. = 45)	p	≤7.5 Gy (no. = 45)	>7.5 Gy (no. = 46)	p
Acute urinary toxicities	9 (19.6%)	15 (33.3%)	0.04	11 (24.4%)	13 (28.3%)	0.9
Late urinary toxicities	3 (6.5%)	7 (15.6%)	0.04	3 (6.6%)	7 (15.2%)	0.04

3.2. Treatment Outcomes

Only one patient in the whole cohort had vaginal vault recurrence (Stage Ib endometrioid adenocarcinoma). Distant and/or pelvic metastases were diagnosed in four patients (two endometrioid adenocarcinoma, one undifferentiated carcinoma, one serous adenocarcinoma). The mean time for metastases was 16.7 months (±7.1). Death was recorded in six patients with a mean survival of 46.2 months (±30.8). There was no difference in mean survival between patients in group A versus group B (44.7 months versus 47.8 months, $p = 0.9$).

4. Discussion

This study reports the clinical outcomes and the treatment-related toxicity following postoperative adjuvant VBT for early-stage endometrial cancer in two fractionation schedules using IVD-based biological planning. Both treatment groups showed acceptable rates of treatment-related toxicities and were mostly grade 1–2, which is in agreement with the results of randomized studies that compared VBT to EBRT [2,4–6,18,19]. Sorbe and Smeds evaluated four different fractionation schedules for HDR-VBT with fraction size ranging from 4.5 to 9 Gy, with dose prescription at 1 cm. Their results show that increasing the fraction size or the treatment length was associated with treatment-related toxicities [20]. Another report of 157 patients adopted a fraction size of 4 Gy for six treatments and prescribed the dose to the vaginal surface; no ≥ grade 2 treatment-related toxicities were found [21]. Furthermore, due to the excellent rates of local control as well as the low toxicities associated with the VBT, studies have focused on reducing the number of fractions or the total treatment time [22–24]. In the present study, two fractionation schedules were compared. Only acute urinary reactions of grade 1–2 were associated with a larger fraction size of 7 Gy compared to 5 Gy. No difference was shown for other toxicities between the two schedules.

Two-dimensional (2D) dosimetry calculated from orthogonal X-ray films is still widely adopted, especially in large centers with high workloads. The introduction of three-dimensional (3D) planning based on computer tomography (CT) images is usually limited only to the first fraction. The quality assurance protocol for the international ongoing molecular-integrated risk-profile-guided adjuvant treatment of endometrial cancer (PORTEC-4a) necessitates 3D planning during at least one fraction [25]. The comparing of both planning techniques was performed, with a correlation of the ICRU rectal and bladder points with a dose to 2cc on 3D [26]. There were no significant bladder dose differences between both planning techniques. However, rectal doses were significantly variable [26]. Owing to logistic limitations, 3D planning cannot be performed with every VBT fraction. Therefore, biologic planning based on IVD offers the advantage of monitoring the dose to the OAR during every treatment fraction and plane changes may be applied when needed.

In order to reduce the toxicity following VBT, dose prescription should be individualized. Several factors were found to play a role: the thickness of the vaginal wall, the anatomical variations, and the size of the used vaginal cylinder applicator [27,28]. Furthermore, the vaginal surface dose was found to be variable along the treatment length. With a 5 mm depth dose prescription, it ranged from 81% to 172% versus a range from 90% to 106% with a surface dose prescription. Both ranges are comparable and offer an acceptable coverage of the target [28].

In the present study, the selection of prescription depth was dependent primarily on the distance between the applicator and the rectal probe. For a smaller distance, a dose prescription at the applicator/vaginal surface was selected. Otherwise, a 5 mm depth for the prescription was preferred. During the first fraction, the dose to rectum and/or bladder was monitored by IVD. When the monitored dose was considered high, the prescription was changed to the surface if it was originally prescribed to a 5 mm depth. This approach led to a subsequent decrease in the monitored doses during the following fractions. Through our innovative two-step protocol, comparable mean doses to the bladder and rectum were achieved within both fractionation schedules.

Cut-off values of the mean dose per fraction as well as the mean total dose to the rectum and bladder were analyzed. Higher rates of toxicities were observed with higher doses, and statistical significance was partially confirmed probably due to the limitation of there being a small number of events.

Few studies have used IVD during HDR-VBT. The aim of IVD was mostly for real-time dose-rate monitoring and dose verification for quality assurance purposes [29–31]. One study used IVD to measure the actual dose to the rectum during HDR-VBT and compared it to the rectal dose as determined by the treatment planning system (TPS); the mean dose discrepancy was 2.2 Gy [32]. Other studies compared the actual dose to the rectum with the dose from TPS during HDR brachytherapy for prostate and cervix cancers [33–35]. In the current study, we used the IVD exclusively for monitoring the doses to the OAR, and modification of the plan occurred accordingly.

Notably, there are considerable limitations to using such an IVD system. Firstly, there is interfractional variation in the positioning of the rectal probe, which may be reflected in the subsequent measured doses. Secondly, as the rectal probe has five measuring chambers, we had to consider only the highest measurement. If the highest measurement is at one of the end measuring chambers, there would be a possibility that a further higher dose is not measured and thus the maximum rectal dose is not recorded. The values used in this work refer to the highest measured doses within the available measurement chambers and are therefore not to be always considered as the absolute rectal maximum doses. However, as the relative differences are considered and evaluated, a directional trend could be achieved.

Both fractionation schedules offered an excellent local control, and only one patient (0.8%) had a vaginal vault recurrence. Other studies reported local recurrence rates ranging from 0% to 3% [2,3,7].

5. Conclusions

Based on our results, postoperative HDR-VBT is a safe adjuvant treatment for early-stage endometrial cancer with excellent local control and acceptable rates of treatment-related toxicities. Both fractionation schedules, 21 Gy in three fractions and 20 Gy in four fractions, are comparable. Considering the individual patient's anatomical variation together with IVD-based biological planning, an acceptable dose to the bladder and rectum could be achieved. Further studies are needed to validate the role of IVD during HDR-VBT.

Author Contributions: Conceptualization, G.K. and T.S.; methodology, R.C.; software validation, T.S., R.C. and T.S.; formal analysis, R.C. and T.S.; investigation, T.S.; resources, R.C.; data curation, T.S.; writing—original draft preparation, T.S.; writing—review and editing, T.S., G.K., R.C., L.T., V.L.; visualization, T.S.; supervision, G.K.; project administration, T.S.; funding acquisition, G.K. and T.S. All authors have read and agreed to the published version of the manuscript.

Funding: This research received no external funding.

Institutional Review Board Statement: The study was conducted according to the guidelines of the Declaration of Helsinki, and approved by the Ethics Committee of the University of Lübeck (protocol code: 15-281A, date of approval: 29.09.2015). All patients signed an informed consent before treatment.

Informed Consent Statement: Informed consent was obtained from all subjects involved in the study.

Data Availability Statement: Data available on request due to restrictions, e.g., privacy or ethical. The data presented in this study are available on request from the corresponding author. The data are not publicly available due to institutional policy.

Conflicts of Interest: The authors declare no conflict of interest.

References

1. Bray, F.; Ferlay, J.; Soerjomataram, I.; Siegel, R.L.; Torre, L.A.; Jemal, A. Global Cancer Statistics 2018: GLOBOCAN Estimates of Incidence and Mortality Worldwide for 36 Cancers in 185 Countries. *CA Cancer J. Clin.* **2018**, *68*, 394–424. [CrossRef]
2. Nout, R.; Smit, V.; Putter, H.; Jürgenliemk-Schulz, I.; Jobsen, J.; Lutgens, L.; van der Steen-Banasik, E.; Mens, J.; Slot, A.; Kroese, M.S.; et al. Vaginal Brachytherapy versus Pelvic External Beam Radiotherapy for Patients with Endometrial Cancer of High-Intermediate Risk (PORTEC-2): An Open-Label, Non-Inferiority, Randomised Trial. *Lancet* **2010**, *375*, 816–823. [CrossRef]
3. Small, W.; Beriwal, S.; Demanes, D.J.; Dusenbery, K.E.; Eifel, P.; Erickson, B.; Jones, E.; Rownd, J.J.; Santos, J.F.D.L.; Viswanathan, A.N.; et al. American Brachytherapy Society Consensus Guidelines for Adjuvant Vaginal Cuff Brachytherapy after Hysterectomy. *Brachytherapy* **2012**, *11*, 58–67. [CrossRef]
4. Jin, M.; Hou, X.; Sun, X.; Zhang, Y.; Hu, K.; Zhang, F. Impact of Different Adjuvant Radiotherapy Modalities on Women with Early-Stage Intermediate- to High-Risk Endometrial Cancer. *Int. J. Gynecol. Cancer* **2019**, *29*, 1264–1270. [CrossRef]
5. Nout, R.A.; Putter, H.; Jürgenliemk-Schulz, I.M.; Jobsen, J.J.; Lutgens, L.C.H.W.; van der Steen-Banasik, E.M.; Mens, J.W.M.; Slot, A.; Kroese, M.C.S.; van Bunningen, B.N.F.M.; et al. Quality of Life After Pelvic Radiotherapy or Vaginal Brachytherapy for Endometrial Cancer: First Results of the Randomized PORTEC-2 Trial. *J. Clin. Oncol.* **2009**, *27*, 3547–3556. [CrossRef] [PubMed]
6. Sorbe, B.G.; Horvath, G.; Andersson, H.; Boman, K.; Lundgren, C.; Pettersson, B. External Pelvic and Vaginal Irradiation Versus Vaginal Irradiation Alone as Postoperative Therapy in Medium-Risk Endometrial Carcinoma: A Prospective, Randomized Study—Quality-of-Life Analysis. *Int. J. Gynecol. Cancer* **2012**, *22*, 1281–1288. [CrossRef]
7. Lancellotta, V.; de Felice, F.; Vicenzi, L.; Antonacci, A.; Cerboneschi, V.; Costantini, S.; di Cristino, D.; Tagliaferri, L.; Cerrotta, A.; Vavassori, A.; et al. The Role of Vaginal Brachytherapy in Stage I Endometrial Serous Cancer: A Systematic Review. *J. Contemp. Brachytherapy* **2020**, *12*, 61. [CrossRef] [PubMed]
8. de Felice, F.; Lancellotta, V.; Vicenzi, L.; Costantini, S.; Antonacci, A.; Cerboneschi, V.; di Cristino, D.; Tagliaferri, L.; Cerrotta, A.; Vavassori, A.; et al. Adjuvant Vaginal Interventional Radiotherapy in Early-Stage Non-Endometrioid Carcinoma of Corpus Uteri: A Systematic Review. *J. Contemp. Brachytherapy* **2021**, *13*, 231. [CrossRef] [PubMed]
9. Lachance, J.A.; Stukenborg, G.J.; Schneider, B.F.; Rice, L.W.; Jazaeri, A.A. A Cost-Effective Analysis of Adjuvant Therapies for the Treatment of Stage I Endometrial Adenocarcinoma. *Gynecol. Oncol.* **2008**, *108*, 77–83. [CrossRef] [PubMed]
10. Suidan, R.S.; He, W.; Sun, C.C.; Zhao, H.; Smith, G.L.; Klopp, A.H.; Fleming, N.D.; Lu, K.H.; Giordano, S.H.; Meyer, L.A. National Trends, Outcomes, and Costs of Radiation Therapy in the Management of Low- and High-Intermediate Risk Endometrial Cancer. *Gynecol. Oncol.* **2019**, *152*, 439. [CrossRef]
11. Autorino, R.; Tagliaferri, L.; Campitelli, M.; Smaniotto, D.; Nardangeli, A.; Mattiucci, G.C.; Macchia, G.; Gui, B.; Miccò, M.; Mascilini, F.; et al. EROS Study: Evaluation between High-Dose-Rate and Low-Dose-Rate Vaginal Interventional Radiotherapy (Brachytherapy) in Terms of Overall Survival and Rate of Stenosis. *J. Contemp. Brachytherapy* **2018**, *10*, 315. [CrossRef] [PubMed]
12. Concin, N.; Matias-Guiu, X.; Vergote, I.; Cibula, D.; Mirza, M.R.; Marnitz, S.; Ledermann, J.; Bosse, T.; Chargari, C.; Fagotti, A.; et al. ESGO/ESTRO/ESP Guidelines for the Management of Patients with Endometrial Carcinoma. *Int. J. Gynecol. Cancer* **2021**, *31*, 12–39. [CrossRef]
13. Abu-Rustum, N.R.; Yashar, C.M.; Bradley, K.; Campos, S.M.; Chino, J.; Chon, H.S.; Chu, C.; Cohn, D.; Crispens, M.A.; Damast, S.; et al. NCCN Guidelines® Insights: Uterine Neoplasms, Version 3.2021: Featured Updates to the NCCN Guidelines. *J. Natl. Compr. Cancer Netw.* **2021**, *19*, 888–895. [CrossRef]
14. Emons, G.; Steiner, E.; Vordermark, D.; Uleer, C.; Bock, N.; Paradies, K.; Ortmann, O.; Aretz, S.; Mallmann, P.; Kurzeder, C.; et al. Interdisciplinary Diagnosis, Therapy and Follow-up of Patients with Endometrial Cancer. Guideline (S3-Level, AWMF Registry Number 032/034-OL, April 2018)—Part 2 with Recommendations on the Therapy and Follow-up of Endometrial Cancer, Palliative Care, Psycho-Oncological/Psychosocial Care/Rehabilitation/Patient Information and Healthcare Facilities. *Geburtshilfe Frauenheilkd.* **2018**, *78*, 1089. [CrossRef]
15. Choo, J.J.; Scudiere, J.; Bitterman, P.; Dickler, A.; Gown, A.M.; Zusag, T.W. Vaginal Lymphatic Channel Location and Its Implication for Intracavitary Brachytherapy Radiation Treatment. *Brachytherapy* **2005**, *4*, 236–240. [CrossRef]

16. Fonseca, G.P.; Johansen, J.G.; Smith, R.L.; Beaulieu, L.; Beddar, S.; Kertzscher, G.; Verhaegen, F.; Tanderup, K. In Vivo Dosimetry in Brachytherapy: Requirements and Future Directions for Research, Development, and Clinical Practice. *Phys. Imaging Radiat. Oncol.* **2020**, *16*, 1. [CrossRef]
17. Chassagne, D.; Dutreix, A.; Almond, P.; Burgers, J.M.V.; Busch, M.; Joslin, C.A. 3. Recommendations for Reporting Absorbed Doses and Volumes in Intracavitary Therapy. *Rep. Int. Comm. Radiat. Units Meas.* **2019**, *os-20*, 9–14. [CrossRef]
18. Aalders, J.; Abeler, V.; Kolstad, P.; Onsrud, M. Postoperative External Irradiation and Prognostic Parameters in Stage I Endometrial Carcinoma: Clinical and Histopathologic Study of 540 Patients—PubMed. Available online: https://pubmed.ncbi.nlm.nih.gov/6999399/ (accessed on 22 September 2021).
19. Sorbe, B.G.; Horvath, G.; Andersson, H.; Boman, K.; Lundgren, C.; Pettersson, B. External Pelvic and Vaginal Irradiation Versus Vaginal Irradiation Alone as Postoperative Therapy in Medium-Risk Endometrial Carcinoma—A Prospective Randomized Study. *Int. J. Radiat. Oncol. Biol. Phys.* **2012**, *82*, 1249–1255. [CrossRef] [PubMed]
20. Sorbe, B.G.; Smeds, A.-C. Postoperative Vaginal Irradiation with High Dose Rate Afterloading Technique in Endometrial Carcinoma Stage I. *Int. J. Radiat. Oncol. Biol. Phys.* **1990**, *18*, 305–314. [CrossRef]
21. Townamchai, K.; Lee, L.; Viswanathan, A.N. A Novel Low Dose Fractionation Regimen for Adjuvant Vaginal Brachytherapy in Early Stage Endometrial Cancer. *Gynecol. Oncol.* **2012**, *127*, 351. [CrossRef]
22. Rovirosa, Á.; Ascaso, C.; Herreros, A.; Sánchez, J.; Holub, K.; Camarasa, A.; Sabater, S.; Oses, G.; García-Miguel, J.; Rivera, Y.; et al. A New Short Daily Brachytherapy Schedule in Postoperative Endometrial Carcinoma. Preliminary Results. *Brachytherapy* **2017**, *16*, 147–152. [CrossRef]
23. Rovirosa, A.; Ascaso, C.; Arenas, M.; Sabater, S.; Herreros, A.; Camarasa, A.; Rios, I.; Holub, K.; Pahisa, J.; Biete, A. Can We Shorten the Overall Treatment Time in Postoperative Brachytherapy of Endometrial Carcinoma? Comparison of Two Brachytherapy Schedules. *Radiother. Oncol.* **2015**, *116*, 143–148. [CrossRef]
24. Ríos, I.; Rovirosa, A.; Ascaso, C.; Valduvieco, I.; Herreros, A.; Castilla, L.; Sabater, S.; Holub, K.; Pahisa, J.; Biete, A.; et al. Vaginal-Cuff Control and Toxicity Results of a Daily HDR Brachytherapy Schedule in Endometrial Cancer Patients. *Clin. Transl. Oncol.* **2015**, *18*, 925–930. [CrossRef]
25. Wortman, B.G.; Astreinidou, E.; Laman, M.S.; van der Steen-Banasik, E.M.; Lutgens, L.C.H.W.; Westerveld, H.; Koppe, F.; Slot, A.; van den Berg, H.A.; Nowee, M.E.; et al. Brachytherapy Quality Assurance in the PORTEC-4a Trial for Molecular-Integrated Risk Profile Guided Adjuvant Treatment of Endometrial Cancer. *Radiother. Oncol.* **2021**, *155*, 160–166. [CrossRef]
26. Russo, J.K.; Armeson, K.E.; Richardson, S. Comparison of 2D and 3D Imaging and Treatment Planning for Postoperative Vaginal Apex High-Dose Rate Brachytherapy for Endometrial Cancer. *Int. J. Radiat. Oncol. Biol. Phys.* **2012**, *83*, e75–e80. [CrossRef]
27. Sabater, S.; Andres, I.; Lopez-Honrubia, V.; Berenguer, R.; Sevillano, M.; Jimenez-Jimenez, E.; Rovirosa, A.; Arenas, M. Vaginal Cuff Brachytherapy in Endometrial Cancer—A Technically Easy Treatment? *Cancer Manag. Res.* **2017**, *9*, 351. [CrossRef] [PubMed]
28. Li, S.; Aref, I.; Walker, E.; Movsas, B. Effects of Prescription Depth, Cylinder Size, Treatment Length, Tip Space, and Curved End on Doses in High-Dose-Rate Vaginal Brachytherapy. *Int. J. Radiat. Oncol. Biol. Phys.* **2007**, *67*, 1268–1277. [CrossRef] [PubMed]
29. Belley, M.D.; Craciunescu, O.; Chang, Z.; Langloss, B.W.; Stanton, I.N.; Yoshizumi, T.T.; Therien, M.J.; Chino, J.P. Real-Time Dose-Rate Monitoring with Gynecologic Brachytherapy: Results of an Initial Clinical Trial. *Brachytherapy* **2018**, *17*, 1023–1029. [CrossRef] [PubMed]
30. Romanyukha, A.; Carrara, M.; Mazzeo, D.; Tenconi, C.; Al-Salmani, T.; Poder, J.; Cutajar, D.; Fuduli, I.; Petasecca, M.; Bucci, J.; et al. An Innovative Gynecological HDR Brachytherapy Applicator System for Treatment Delivery and Real-Time Verification. *Phys. Med.* **2019**, *59*, 151–157. [CrossRef]
31. Jamalludin, Z.; Jong, W.L.; Abdul Malik, R.; Rosenfeld, A.; Ung, N.M. Characterization of MOSkin Detector for in Vivo Dose Verification during Cobalt-60 High Dose-Rate Intracavitary Brachytherapy. *Phys. Med.* **2019**, *58*, 1–7. [CrossRef]
32. Carrara, M.; Romanyukha, A.; Tenconi, C.; Mazzeo, D.; Cerrotta, A.; Borroni, M.; Cutajar, D.; Petasecca, M.; Lerch, M.; Bucci, J.; et al. Clinical Application of MOSkin Dosimeters to Rectal Wall in Vivo Dosimetry in Gynecological HDR Brachytherapy. *Phys. Med.* **2017**, *41*, 5–12. [CrossRef] [PubMed]
33. Jamalludin, Z.; Malik, R.A.; Ung, N.M. Correlation Analysis of CT-Based Rectal Planning Dosimetric Parameters with in Vivo Dosimetry of MOSkin and PTW 9112 Detectors in Co-60 Source HDR Intracavitary Cervix Brachytherapy. *Phys. Eng. Sci. Med.* **2021**, *44*, 773–783. [CrossRef] [PubMed]
34. Jamalludin, Z.; Jong, W.L.; Malik, R.A.; Rosenfeld, A.B.; Ung, N.M. Evaluation of Rectal Dose Discrepancies between Planned and in Vivo Dosimetry Using MOSkin Detector and PTW 9112 Semiconductor Probe during 60Co HDR CT-Based Intracavitary Cervix Brachytherapy. *Phys. Med.* **2020**, *69*, 52–60. [CrossRef] [PubMed]
35. Poder, J.; Howie, A.; Brown, R.; Bucci, J.; Rosenfeld, A.; Enari, K.; Schreiber, K.; Carrara, M.; Bece, A.; Malouf, D.; et al. Towards Real Time In-Vivo Rectal Dosimetry during Trans-Rectal Ultrasound Based High Dose Rate Prostate Brachytherapy Using MOSkin Dosimeters. *Radiother. Oncol.* **2020**, *151*, 273–279. [CrossRef] [PubMed]

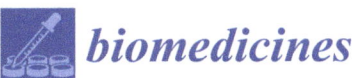

Review

Potential Impact of Human Cytomegalovirus Infection on Immunity to Ovarian Tumours and Cancer Progression

Momodou Cox [1], Apriliana E. R. Kartikasari [1], Paul R. Gorry [1], Katie L. Flanagan [1,2,3] and Magdalena Plebanski [1,*]

[1] School of Health & Biomedical Sciences, RMIT University, Melbourne 3082, Australia; momodou.cox@student.rmit.edu.au (M.C.); april.kartikasari@rmit.edu.au (A.E.R.K.); paul.gorry@rmit.edu.au (P.R.G.); katie.flanagan@ths.tas.gov.au (K.L.F.)
[2] School of Medicine and School of Health Sciences, University of Tasmania, Launceston 7250, Australia
[3] Department of Immunology and Pathology, Monash University, Melbourne 3004, Australia
* Correspondence: magdalena.plebanski@rmit.edu.au

Abstract: Ovarian cancer (OC) is one of the most common, and life-threatening gynaecological cancer affecting females. Almost 75% of all OC cases are diagnosed at late stages, where the 5-year survival rate is less than 30%. The aetiology of the disease is still unclear, and there are currently no screening method nor effective treatment strategies for the advanced disease. A growing body of evidence shows that human cytomegalovirus (HCMV) infecting more than 50% of the world population, may play a role in inducing carcinogenesis through its immunomodulatory activities. In healthy subjects, the primary HCMV infection is essentially asymptomatic. The virus then establishes a life-long chronic latency primarily in the hematopoietic progenitor cells in the bone marrow, with periodic reactivation from latency that is often characterized by high levels of circulating pro-inflammatory cytokines. Currently, infection-induced chronic inflammation is considered as an essential process for OC progression and metastasis. In line with this observation, few recent studies have identified high expressions of HCMV proteins on OC tissue biopsies that were associated with poor survival outcomes. Active HCMV infection in the OC tumour microenvironment may thus directly contribute to OC progression. In this review, we highlight the potential impact of HCMV infection-induced immunomodulatory effects on host immune responses to OC that may promote OC progression.

Keywords: human cytomegalovirus; ovarian cancer; cancer progression; inflammation; immunosuppression

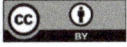

1. Background

Ovarian cancer (OC) is one of the most prevalent, aggressive, and life-threatening gynaecological malignancies affecting females. Ovarian tumours arise from either epithelial cells, stromal cells, or germ cells. Amongst them, epithelial OC constitutes more than 90% of malignant OC in developed countries [1,2]. About 75% of all OC cases are diagnosed at an advanced stage (stage 3–4) [3], where the 5-year survival rate is less than 30% [2]. The current standard of care for women diagnosed with OC is primary debulking surgery followed by platinum-based chemotherapy with paclitaxel and carboplatin. However, almost 66% of patients experience recurrence within two years of diagnosis and the majority of these recurrences are accounted for by patients diagnosed at late stages [4].

Presently, the early features of ovarian carcinogenesis remain unclear, and there is no effective early detection test or screening method to date [5]. Therefore, the identification of women with the disease is based on their clinical presentation, in combination with currently approved, albeit non-specific, tests including ultrasound and/or serum cancer antigen 125 (CA-125) and human epididymis 4 (HE4) levels, followed by histological confirmation with tissue biopsy [6]. Age, family history, as well as genetic mutations in *breast cancer (BRCA)1* or *BRCA2* genes are known risk factors for OC. *BRCA1* and *BRCA2* produce tumor suppressor proteins that help repair damaged DNA and their mutations are inherited in an autosomal dominant pattern [7–9]. Inheritance of such harmful mutations causes a compromised ability for cells to repair DNA damage, which leads to additional genetic alterations and ultimately cancer [10,11]. Additionally, women over the age of 45 years have a higher risk of developing OC partly due to an accumulation of somatic mutations during aging [12].

A combination of the classical OC risk factors highlighted above might create a tumour-favouring cellular environment, where some oncogenic viruses may reside and enhance their oncogenic capability. Even though the classification of human cytomegalovirus (HCMV) as an oncogenic virus remains controversial, there is strong emerging evidence showing a prevalence of HCMV infection in breast, colon, prostate, liver, cervical, and brain cancer patients [13]. In a study by Taher et al. [14], HCMV proteins and/or nucleic acids were detected in 98% of breast cancer derived metastatic brain tumours but not in healthy tissues surrounding HCMV-infected brain tumours, suggesting a potential association between HCMV infection and metastatic cancer. Despite the fact that infection with HCMV is rarely associated with OC, recent studies have shown that OC patients with high expression of HCMV-immediate early (IE) and HCMV-pp65 proteins by their ovarian tumours have shorter survival outcomes compared with those with little tumour expression of these proteins [15,16]. These data suggest that infection with HCMV could potentially promote cancer progression. Once HCMV infects host cells, it begins to counteract key anti-viral immune mechanisms needed to control the infection through secretion of immunosuppressive cytokines and impairment of cell-mediated immune responses that are also important in controlling tumour growth. Hence, the focus of this review is to highlight the potential impact of HCMV infection on immune responses to OC that may also promote cancer progression.

2. Human Cytomegalovirus (HCMV)

Human cytomegalovirus (HCMV), also known as human herpes virus 5 (HHV-5), infects about 83% of the world's population, approaching 100% in developing countries [17]. Following primary infection as shown in Figure 1, HCMV establishes a life-long chronic latency in humans [17], primarily in the cluster of differentiation (CD)34$^+$ hematopoietic progenitor cell population located in the bone marrow [18]. Latent infection is generally asymptomatic in immunocompetent individuals although symptomatic reactivation can occur, particularly in the immunocompromised or cancer patients [17]. High level circulating pro-inflammatory cytokines are the hallmark of latent HCMV reactivation, particularly when the CD34+ progenitor cells differentiate into inflammatory monocytes or infiltrating macrophages or dendritic cells, which then spread the virus to peripheral organs and body tissues thereby infecting and replicating in a broad number of cell types [18].

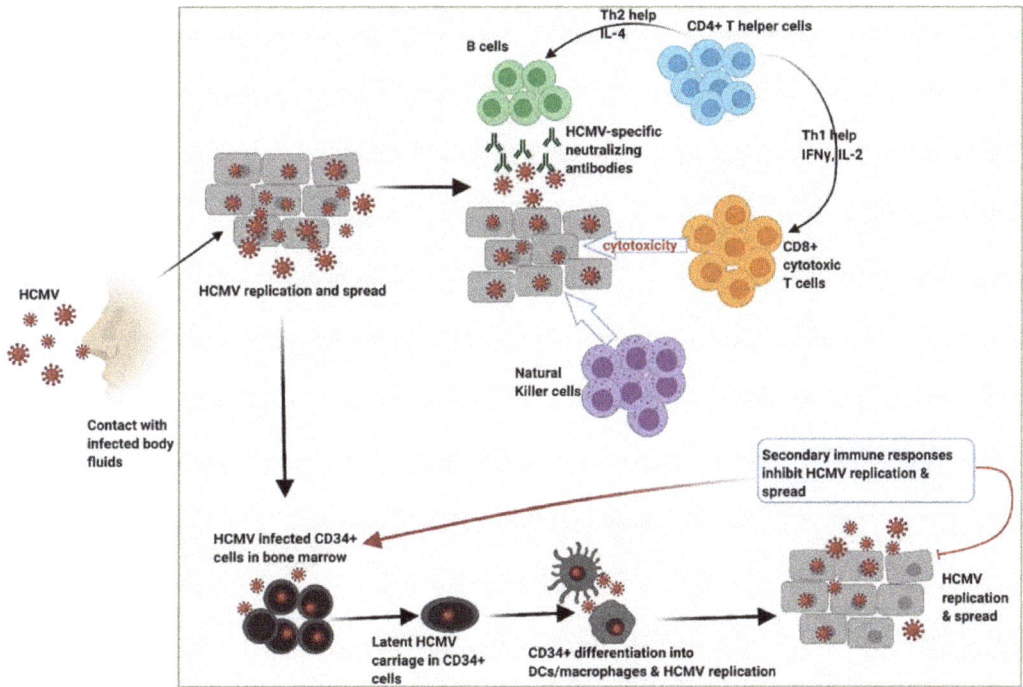

Figure 1. Following primary infection through contact with infected bodily fluids, HCMV replicates within host cells during which time robust immune responses are generated by the host that includes HCMV-specific neutralizing antibodies, natural killer cells and high frequencies of CD4$^+$ T helper cells and CD8$^+$ cytotoxic T cells. These responses subsequently control viral replication thereby resolving primary infection. However, HCMV has the potential to replicate and spread resulting in infection of CD34+ myeloid cells in the bone marrow and establishment of latency. Differentiation of HCMV-infected CD34+ cells into dendritic cells and macrophages contributes to new HCMV replication during which a secondary immune response induced that helps to inhibit HCMV replication spread. HCMV, human cytomegalovirus. Figure created with BioRender.com.

3. Effect of HCMV Infection on Innate and Adaptive Immune Response

Upon successful entry into host cells, HCMV begins to counteract various host immune response mechanisms needed to control the infection [19] as shown in Figure 2 below. Firstly, the tegument protein pp65 of HCMV represents the major component of mature virus particles that interferes with interferon regulatory factor 3 (IRF3) signalling that activates interferon-induced genes, by reducing IRF3 phosphorylation status and inhibiting its nuclear localisation. HCMV pp65 also downregulates nuclear factor kappa B (NF-κB) activation, further contributing to reduced type 1 interferon (IFN) production, the primary anti-viral cytokines [20]. Secondly, the recognition of HCMV's early viral proteins (such as intermediate early (IE) proteins 1 and 2) by CD8$^+$ T cells is nullified because the HCMV pp65 gene aids in the sequestration of HCMV- immediate early (IE)-1 proteins making them inaccessible to the CD8$^+$ T cell pool [20]. Thirdly, HCMV has unique short (US) gene regions within its genome encoding specific gene products (US2, US3, US6, US10, and US11) that contribute to HCMV-mediated the major histocompatibility complex (MHC)-I downregulation, thereby leading to the decreased presentation of HCMV-specific peptides to CD8$^+$ T cells [21,22]. Fourthly, to evade cytotoxicity-mediated by natural killer (NK) cells, HCMV expresses unique long (UL) proteins, such as pUL18 (MHC-I viral homolog) and pUL40, that help to inhibit NK cell cytotoxic responses via a "missing self" mechanism [20]. The viral protein pUL18 binds to β2-macroglobulin and then engages with leukocyte immunoglobulin-like receptor 1 (LIR-1), a class I MHC receptor related to killer inhibitory receptors (KIRs), to induce inhibitory signals preventing NK cell-mediated cytolysis. Additionally, pUL40 binds to MHC class I antigen/human leukocyte antigen (HLA)-E and stabilize its surface expression thus amplifying its interaction with NK cell inhibitory receptor, CD94/natural killer group (NKG)-2A (CD94/NKG2A). Fifthly, it is generally acknowledged that interleukin (IL)-10 produced by regulatory T cells (Tregs) plays an important role in suppressing immune responses during HCMV infection. HCMV also produces cmv-IL10 or pUL10, a homolog of human IL-10 that has immunosuppressive properties similar to human IL-10 [23]. Lastly, a study by Wagner et al. [24] has shown that HCMV-derived protein UL18 stimulates the development of an immature phenotype of dendritic cells (DC) by interfering with CD40 ligand-induced maturation of DCs, resulting in reduced MHC-class II expression on immature monocyte-derived DCs. This could potentially reduce the activation of CD4+ T-cell responses as well as decrease the elimination of virus-infected cells or tumours by CD8+ cytotoxic T cells.

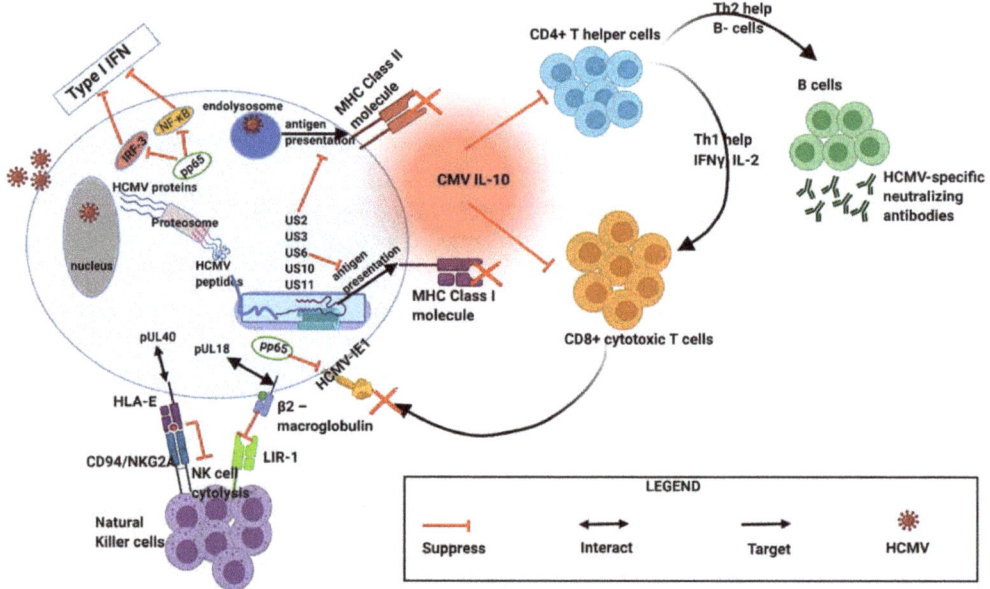

Figure 2. During primary infection, HCMV employs various mechanisms to mediate immune evasion. HCMV expresses viral genes and proteins that interfere with host interferon responses (pp65), inhibit natural killer cell recognition or activation (pUL40 and pUL18), inhibit CD4+ and CD8+ T-cell recognition by preventing MHC Class I and II antigen processing and presentation (e.g., US2, US3, US6, US10, US11). CMV IL-10 (viral IL-10 homologue) produced by infected cells further acts to suppress CD4+ and C8+ T cell responses. HCMV, human cytomegalovirus; MHC, major histocompatibility complex (MHC); US, unique short; UL, unique long. Figure created with BioRender.com.

Chronic infection with HCMV causes huge clonal expansion of the CD8+ T cell compartment, but a lesser expansion of CD4+ T cells, leading to inversion of the normal CD4:CD8 ratio to less than 1 [17]. The HCMV-driven expanded CD8+ T cell subset is usually terminally differentiated due to their high expression of CD57 (a marker of differentiation) and loss of expression of CD27 (a marker of activation) and CD28 (co-stimulatory molecule). The combination of chronic HCMV infection, terminally differentiated T cells and inverted CD4:CD8 T cell ratio results in an "immune risk profile" (IRP) that has been strongly associated with immunosenescence and early death in the elderly [25]. Moreover, Bennett et al. [26] also proposed that HCMV-driven inflammation is associated with aging, so called "inflammaging". Besides changes in CD4+ and CD8+ T cells, infection with HCMV also influences NK cell differentiation, activation, and receptor expression. Goodier et al. [27] have shown that HCMV infection is associated with rapid phenotypic and functional differentiation of NK cells (CD57+ NK cells), the majority of which express the activating CD94/NKG2C receptor. Expansion of NKG2C+ NK cells can also be achieved by co-culture with HCMV-infected fibroblasts [28].

4. Anti-Tumor Immunity in Ovarian Cancer

The human immune system employs various host-protective and anti-tumour mechanisms to prevent ovarian tumours from developing (Figure 3A). Of these, cell-mediated cytotoxicity is the most effective mechanism employed by the immune system to help prevent the establishment of OC and it involves two main cell types: CD8+ cytotoxic T cells (CTLs) and natural killer (NK) cells [29,30]. CTLs perform their effector mechanisms in two steps: MHC class I interaction with T cell receptor (TCR) followed by granule mediated killing. Upon MHC-I antigen recognition by TCR on CTLs, a polarisation of the CTL occurs that ensures a level of organization between the CTL and target cell. The CTL undergoes morphological changes and expresses lytic granules such as perforin and granzymes (granule enzymes), which are released to kill target cells [31,32]. Perforin polymerizes to form pores in the target cells, which allow granzymes such as granzyme B to gain entry into target cells [33]. Granzyme B has complex effects within the target cell and promotes apoptosis via BID (a BH3 domain-containing proapoptotic Bcl2 family member) and activation of caspase, a family of protease enzymes involved in programmed cell death [34]. Data from previous studies have shown that the immune system of OC patients is greatly impacted by the developing tumour (Figure 3B) due to the high presence of Tregs in the tumour microenvironment (TME) that classically inhibit CTL responses [35]. Recent studies have shown that the TME's immune status, including the presence of pro-inflammatory cytokines and Tregs, and the absence of tumour-infiltrating CD8+ T cells are all strongly correlated with OC recurrence [35–37]. Conversely, the presence of tumour-infiltrating CD8+ T cells and a high CD8+ T cell/Treg ratio is associated with substantially better survival outcomes, thus highlighting the importance of CTL-mediated immune responses in OC [38].

Conventionally, NK cells, comprising of about 5–10% of peripheral blood lymphocytes, are considered to be part of the innate immune system and have the capacity to kill tumor cells without the need for prior sensitization [39]. Previous studies have shown that NK-mediated effector functions are highly regulated by a balance between inhibitory and activation signals. NK cells express inhibitory receptors such as KIRs that recognize MHC class I on target cells and deliver inhibitory signals to suppress NK cells function [40–42]. As tumour cells express little or no MHC class I molecules, they become highly susceptible to NK-mediated cytolysis in what is referred to as the "missing self" hypothesis. Compared with CD8+ T cells, a study by Webb et al. [43] showed that infiltrating NK cells expressing the tissue-resident memory marker CD103 (CD103+ NK cells) are most often found with CD8+ T cells and these cells were the best predictor of positive survival outcomes in primary OC. Besides CD8+ T cells and NK cells, the presence of tumour-infiltrating mature and activated dendritic cells (DCs) have been shown to correlate with a better prognosis in OC. They express CD107a, a marker of activation, and help attract more anti-tumour cell such as CTLs and NK cells to the TME [44].

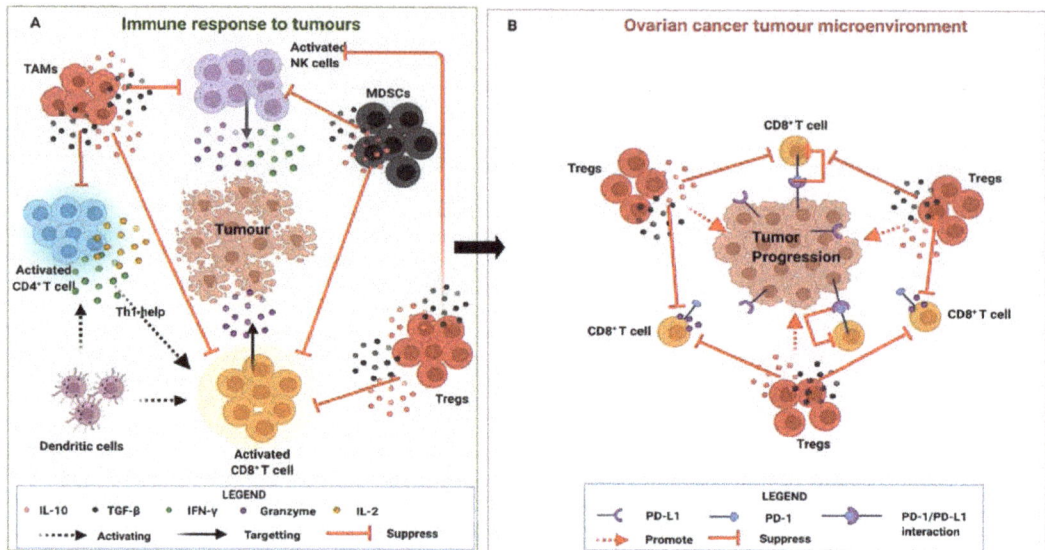

Figure 3. (**A**) The human immune system harbours various immune cells such as natural killer (NK) cells, CD8$^+$ T cells, CD4$^+$ T helper cells and dendritic cells (DCs) that play an important role in controlling the developing tumour. DCs and CD4$^+$ T cells via IL-2 and INF-γ secretion activate CD8$^+$ cytotoxic T cells (CTLs) and NK cells which then produce toxic molecules such as granzymes that target the developing tumour. However, pro-tumour cells such as regulatory T cells (Tregs), myeloid-derived suppressor cells (MDSCs) and tumour-associated macrophages (TAMs) produce immunosuppressive cytokines (IL-10 and TGF-β) that inhibit CDTLs and NK cells effector responses. (**B**). The ovarian cancer tumour microenvironment is commonly characterised by high frequencies of infiltrating Tregs and a high Tregs:CD8$^+$ T cell ratio that promotes tumour progression. Ovarian tumour also expresses PD-L1 that further inhibits CD8$^+$ T cell effector responses upon ligation with PD-1. Figure created with BioRender.com.

5. Immune Homeostasis

An overly reactive immune system is also detrimental as it could result in tissue damage if it fails to resolve. To minimize such damage, the immune system utilizes immune checkpoint inhibitory pathways that are essential for ensuring self-tolerance and moderating the extent and magnitude of effector responses of CTLs and NK cells. These inhibitory pathways involve surface inhibitory receptors such as cytotoxic T lymphocyte antigen-4 (CTLA-4) and programmed cell death protein 1 (PD-1; CD279). They are usually transiently expressed on activated T cells, B cells, macrophages, dendritic cells and Tregs under normal conditions but their increased and prolonged expression is a sign of T cell exhaustion [45]. PD-1 is more extensively expressed on activated cells than CTLA-4 and predominantly modulates effector CTL responses upon interaction with its ligand, programmed death-ligand 1 (PD-L1; B7-H1; CD274) and/or PD-L2 (B7-DC; CD273) on cancer cells (Figure 3B). Subsequently, their interaction generates potent inhibitory signals that inhibits kinases involved in T cell activation [46–50]. The CTLA-4 co-inhibitory receptor is constitutively expressed on T cells and competes with CD28 co-stimulatory receptor for binding to their cognate ligands CD80 (B7.1) and CD86 (B7.2) on cancer cells, for which it has a greater affinity, thereby effectively inhibiting CTL activation [51,52]. Other immune checkpoint inhibitory receptors such as lymphocyte activation gene-3 (LAG-3), T-cell immunoglobulin-3 (TIM-3), band T lymphocyte attenuator (BTLA) and T-cell immunoglobulin and ITIM domain (TIGIT) are also expressed on exhausted T cells and help regulate effector responses of CTLs [53].

6. HCMV Infection in Ovarian Cancer

Although HCMV infection is rarely associated with OC, a study by Shanmughapriya et al. [54] detected HCMV-gB by polymerase chain reaction (PCR) in approximately 50% of OC tissues, of which 80% were late stage invasive tumours, suggesting that HCMV infection in the TME may promote cancer progression or metastasis. More recently, another study assessed the presence of HCMV within OC tissue specimens obtained from diagnostic excisional biopsy pre-chemotherapy (DEBPC) and interval debulking surgery (IDS) after neoadjuvant chemotherapy (4–5 times Taxol/Paraplatin). In this study, OC patients with high levels of HCMV-IE and tegument pp65 proteins in their tumours had lower median overall survival compared to those with lower levels or no detectable HCMV proteins [15]. A second recent study by Radestad et al. [16] also investigated the prevalence of HCMV in ovarian cancer and its relation to clinical outcome. In their study, HCMV-IgG levels, HCMV-IE proteins, and pp65 proteins were all shown to be higher in OC patients with malignant or benign cystadenoma (benign ovarian epithelial tumour) compared with age-matched controls. Additionally, OC patients with focal HCMV-pp65 expression in their tumours accompanied with high IgG levels against HCMV were found to live longer when compared with patients showing high expression of HCMV-pp65 protein in their tumours [16]. These findings suggest a possible impact of HCMV infection on immune responses to ovarian tumours. It is important to highlight that the existence of an active HCMV infection with protein production is a rare occurrence in tissues of healthy individuals. Therefore, the presence of an active HCMV infection with HCMV-pp65 and HCMV-IE proteins on ovarian tumours is quite intriguing and needs further investigation in a larger cohorts of OC patients. This would help justify whether administering anti-HCMV treatment to OC patients experiencing active HCMV reactivation in their TME is needed in future personalised treatment approaches for such patients.

7. Significance of HCMV Infection in the OC TME

The OC tumour microenvironment (TME) harbors high numbers of pro-tumour cells such as myeloid derived suppressor cells (MDSCs), tumour-associated macrophages (TAMs) and Tregs compared to anti-tumour cells such as CTLs and NK cells. MDSCs and TAMs (M2 type) classically inhibit activation and cytotoxic functions of CTLs and NK cells through production of anti-inflammatory cytokines such as transforming growth factor-β (TGF-β) and interleukin (IL)-10 (Figure 3A). Indeed, TGF-β induces Treg development and activation, thus promoting an increased Treg presence in the OC TME [35,55]. As mentioned earlier, the presence of a higher ratio of Tregs to CTLs in the TME is known to be a poor prognostic indicator [56] and could be influenced by active HCMV infection in the TME.

HCMV infection is known to promote a cellular secretome that modulates its microenvironment by increasing the production of relevant immunosuppressive mediators, such as TGF-β-expressing Tregs and IL-10 [18]. These immunosuppressive mediators (Figure 4) may contribute to OC progression by inhibiting NK cell and CTL effector functions. HCMV viral protein cmvIL-10, a human IL-10 homologue further boosts this immunosuppressive activity by stimulating the maturation of immunosuppressive macrophages [57], and inhibiting DC maturation [58]. In breast cancer, cmvIL-10 was shown to directly promote growth and migration of breast cancer cells [59] and upregulate proto-oncogene Bcl-3 [57]. Together, these data suggest that active infection by HCMV promotes secretion of suppressive immunomodulatory mediators and the release of cmv-IL10 that may modulate T cell immune function and OC progression.

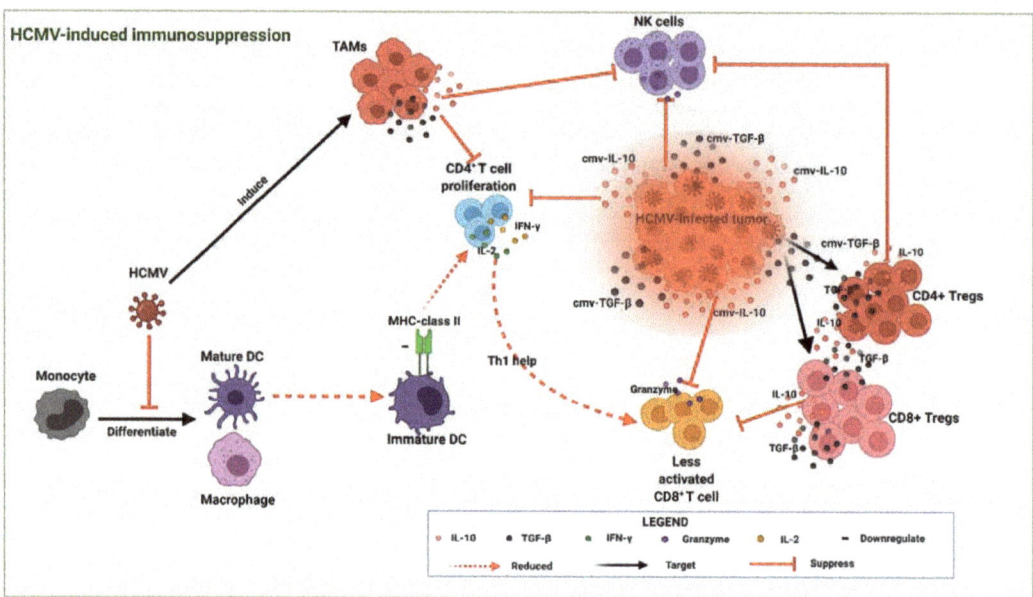

Figure 4. HCMV-infected tumour cells secrete viral cytokines (cIL-10 and c-TGF-β) that create an immunosuppressive environment (highlighted red zone) around the developing tumour thereby promoting tumour progression. cIL-10 and c-TGF-β also induce CD4$^+$ and CD8$^+$ Tregs that produce similar cytokines (IL-10 and TGF-β) further augmenting the immunosuppressive state by inhibiting cytotoxic CD8$^+$ T lymphocyte (CTL) and natural killer (NK) cell effector responses. HCMV also interferes with the differentiation of monocytes into mature dendritic cells (DCs) that leads to the establishment of immature DCs with reduced MHC-class II antigen presentation and subsequently less CD4$^+$ T cell proliferation and reduced Th1 help needed for enhanced CTL activation. Figure created with BioRender.com.

Since Tregs also recognise the same antigens as CD8$^+$ T cells, their increased presence in the TME could result in diminished immune responses to ovarian tumour antigens, and thus contribute to tumorigenic tolerance and immune evasion that may further promote OC progression. In context with current literature, Tregs consist of different subsets of immunosuppressive cells arising from CD4$^+$ and CD8$^+$ T cells [60]. While CD4$^+$ Tregs have been extensively studied, the lack of universal markers to distinguish CD8$^+$ Treg cells from conventional CD8$^+$ T cells means that the function of CD8$^+$ Tregs in cancer remains undefined [61]. Zhang et al. [62] identified the expression of Treg markers in CD8$^+$ T cells isolated from peripheral blood and fresh tumour tissues of OC patients. Their study found a higher percentage of CD8$^+$ Tregs (defined as CD8$^+$ CD25$^+$ FOXP3$^+$ CD28$^-$ CTLA-4$^+$) in OC patients compared with benign ovarian tumour patients and healthy controls. Furthermore, in the same study, high TGF-β1 levels also correlated positively with the percentage of CD8$^+$ Tregs and triggered the suppressive function of in vitro-induced CD8$^+$ Treg cells. The expression levels of FOXP3 in CD8$^+$ T cells were found to be positively associated with the stage of tumour in OC patients which implies that the OC TME may have the capacity to convert CD8$^+$ effector T cells into CD8$^+$FOXP3$^+$ suppressor cells in vivo [62]. These findings suggest that CD8$^+$FOXP3$^+$ Tregs may also contribute to antitumor immunity and OC progression, further highlighting their valuable role as potential predictors of clinical outcomes in OC patients. As stated earlier, HCMV-infected cells also secrete TGF-β to suppress effector T cell responses. Thus, HCMV-infected cells in TME might also augment the conversion of CD8$^+$ effector T cells into CD8$^+$FOXP3$^+$ suppressor cells, thereby shifting the immune balance within the TME from cytotoxic to an immunosuppressive state. Thus, a strategy to reverse the immunosuppressive HCMV-infected T cells could help enhance anti-tumour responses against HCMV-infected OC cells.

As mentioned earlier (Figure 2), some of the immune evasion mechanisms employed by HCMV to modulate host immune responses and establish latency can also exacerbate OC progression (Figure 5). A classic example is HCMV UL18 (MHC class I homologue) that helps to counteract NK cell cytotoxicity by binding to the NK cell inhibitory receptor NKG2A/CD94 [63]. In addition, the expression of HLA-E (a non-classical MHC class I protein) is upregulated on HCMV infected cells or tumours by HCMV UL40 that could further inhibit NK cell cytotoxicity against HCMV-infected ovarian tumours [20]. One of the key mechanisms by which NK cells perform their cytotoxic functions involves the interaction of TNF-related apoptosis-inducing ligand (TRAIL) with their cognate death receptors, TRAIL-R1 and TRAIL-R2. Clustering of the TRAIL-R1 and TRAIL-R2 through interaction with TRAIL results in their oligomerization, inducing development of the death-inducing signalling complex, and ultimately, caspase activation and cellular apoptosis [64]. However, HCMV glycoprotein UL141 has been shown to bind TRAIL death receptors directly [64] and thereby inhibiting the TRAIL-mediated killing of HCMV-infected ovarian tumours. Moreover, HCMV UL141 also downregulates the cell-surface expression of CD155, the ligand for the NK-cell-activating receptors DNAM1 and also targets the alternative DNAM1-activating ligand, CD112 [65].

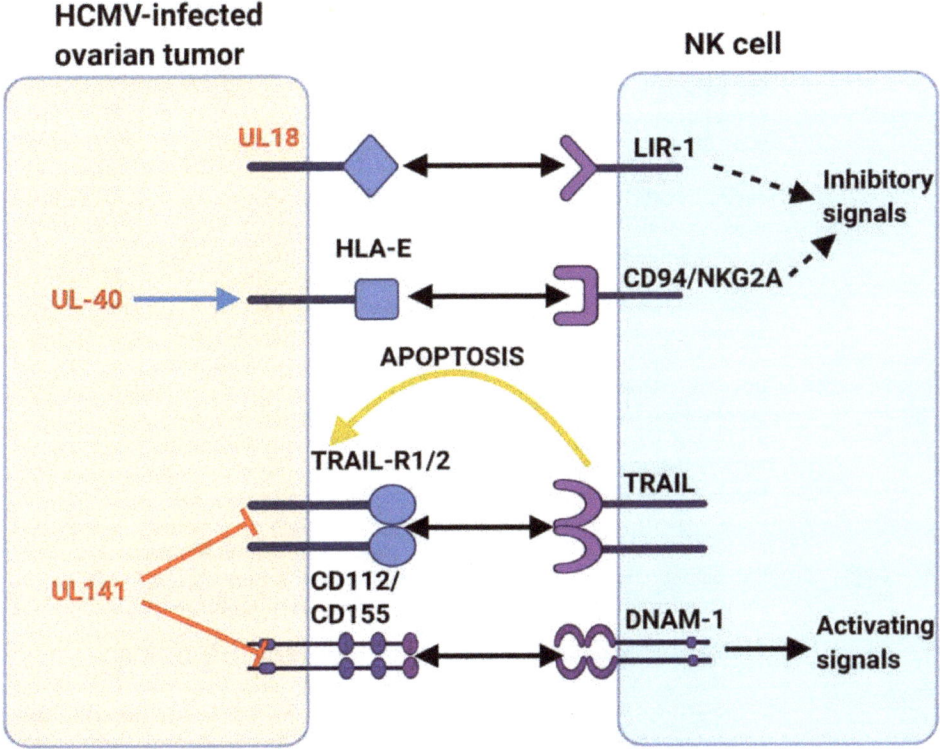

Figure 5. A summary of human cytomegalovirus (HCMV) modulation of natural killer (NK) cell cytotoxicity discussed in this review. Human proteins or receptors are labelled in black; HCMV proteins are labelled in red. The arrows represent actions. Two-pointed solid black arrow = interaction or ligation; one-pointed solid black arrow = intracellular NK cell activation signal; dotted black arrow = intracellular NK cell inhibition signal; yellow arrow = extracellular signal to target cell; red line = inhibits surface expression; blue arrow = increases surface expression. Figure created with BioRender.com.

8. Association between Human Leucocyte Antigens, γ Markers and Killer Immuno-Globulin-Like Receptors with Human Cytomegalovirus Infection

As described previously, NK cells help provide a major defence against primary HCMV infection through the interaction of their activating and inhibitory KIRs, and HLA class I molecules. Additionally, antibodies (humoral immunity) also play a key role in initiating NK cell responses to HCMV via antibody-dependent cell-mediated cytotoxicity (ADCC) that is known to be influenced by γ marker (GM) immunoglobulin allotypes [66]. GM allotypes are allelic hereditary variants encoded by autosomal codominant alleles that follows a Mendelian law of heredity, which are expressed on immunoglobulin constant region of γ1, γ2 and γ3 chains [66]. Several mechanisms have been suggested to account for the role GM allotypes play in the control of HCMV infections, which includes their ability to modulate the strength of ADCC and the avidity of the FcγR–IgG interaction thereby influencing the effectiveness of the immune responses [67]. A study by Pandey et al. [68] investigated the contribution of GM3/17 allotypes to the magnitude of antibody responses to HCMV glycoprotein B (gB), a component of the viral envelope that is required for HCMV infectivity to host cells. Their results showed GM3/17 allotypes at the γ1 locus, determined the level of HCMV-specific IgG antibodies to gB. However, the exact role of HCMV-specific antibodies in the control of HCMV infection in vivo remains unclear.

In order to provide further insight into the immune mechanisms controlling HCMV, a recent study investigated the interaction between HLA/KIR genes and GM allotypes in the control of HCMV infection within a Sicilian population. Di Bona et al. [69], assessed whether specific KIRs and HLA repertoire could influence the risk of developing symptomatic or asymptomatic disease upon primary HCMV infection. In their study, sixty immunocompetent patients with primary symptomatic HCMV infection were genotyped for KIR and their HLA ligands, along with sixty other individuals with a previous asymptomatic infection as controls. Their results showed that symptomatic patients had a significantly higher frequency of the homozygous A haplotype, which produces more of the inhibitory KIRs thus inhibitting NK cell function. Additionally, they also showed that symptomatic HCMV disease was associated with the HLABw4^T allele, whereby the gene product is the ligand of the inhibitory KIR. In a more recent study [67], the same immunocompetent patients with primary symptomatic HCMV infection were genotyped for GM3/17 and GM23 allotypes, along with the participants with a previous asymptomatic infection used as controls. The results of this study further revealed that the individuals carrying the GM23 allotypes (both homozygous and heterozygous), GM17/17, HLA-C2 and Bw4^T KIR-ligand groups were associated with the risk of developing symptomatic HCMV infection. Based on these findings, it is reasonable to speculate that OC patients that carry the same genotypic traits as mentioned above are at a higher risk of experiencing HCMV-induced OC progression. It further highlights the valuable role of HLA, KIRs and GM genotyping not only as potential predictors of clinical outcomes of HCMV-infected OC patients, but also in guiding our efforts to generate highly effective personalised immunotherapeutic strategies to improve OC survival outcomes.

9. Potential Modulation of Intrinsic Inhibitory Receptors by HCMV

The PD-1/PD-L1 pathway represents a mechanism employed by OC cells to evade endogenous anti-tumour adaptive immune responses. PD-L1 is commonly overexpressed on tumour cells in the TME and its ligation with PD-1 receptors on activated T cells leads to the inhibition of effector CTL responses [51], thus contributing to immune escape mechanisms associated with poor survival outcomes [53,70,71]. Therapeutic blockade of the PD-1/PD-L1 pathway has been shown to mediate tumour eradication with impressive clinical results [72]. A classic example in OC is durvalumab (anti-PD-L1), a human immunoglobulin G1 kappa monoclonal antibody that works by blocking the interaction of PD-L1 with PD-1 and CD80 thereby promoting antitumour immune responses [73]. Since it is an engineered monoclonal antibody (mAb), it does not induce antibody-dependent cellular cytotoxicity or complement-mediated cytotoxicity. To date, durvalumab has been given to many OC patients as part of ongoing studies, either as monotherapy or in combination with other anticancer agents. Combination therapy of durvalumab with olaparib (a drug that prevents DNA repair) induced objective responses in more than 70% of patients with relapsed, platinum-sensitive, *BRCA*-mutated OC [74].

In recent years, many studies have shown that PD-1 expression on the surface of CD4$^+$ and CD8$^+$ T cells is increased upon HCMV infection or reactivation [75–78]. A more recent study by Pesce et al. [79] identified a subset of fully mature NK cells expressing high PD-1 (PD-1^{bright}) in peripheral blood of HCMV-seropositive healthy individuals. The proportions of these PD-1^{bright} NK cells were also shown to be higher in the ascites of a cohort of OC patients, suggesting their possible expansion in TMEs. Functional analysis revealed a reduced proliferative capability and impaired antitumour activity that was partially restored by antibody (anti-PD-L1/2 mAb) mediated disruption of the PD-1/PD-L interaction [79]. Recently, many studies have reported elevated expression levels of PD-L1 on glioma cells in g lioblastoma (GBM) [80]. GBM is the most common adult primary brain tumour characterised by highly invasive infiltrative growth, no clear aetiology and poor overall survival. A more recent study by Qin et al. [81] showed that PD-L1 expression was higher in HCMV-infected glioma specimens compared to controls, and was mediated by activation of Toll-like receptor (TLR3), a molecule that plays a key role in antiviral recognition and the production of type I interferons. Furthermore, the expression levels of PD-L1 and TLR3 were significantly higher in HCVM-IE positive-gliomas compared with HCMV-IE negative-gliomas [81]. Currently, there are no data associating HCMV infection with increased PD-L1 expression in OC. Nonetheless, the above studies suggest increased PD-1 expression on T-cells and NK cells as well as PD-L1 on glioma cells driven by HCMV infection could negatively impact anti-PD-L1 based therapies such as durvalumab.

10. HCMV and Inflammation, a Possible Link for Ovarian Cancer Progression

HCMV infection in monocytes may leads to monocyte activation via activation of NF-κB, the transcription factor that controls cytokine production, and phosphoinositide-3-kinase (PI3K), an enzyme involved in cell differentiation pathways [82,83]. The polarisation and activation of monocytes due to HCMV infection or reactivation leads to high systemic levels of inflammatory cytokines, particularly tumour necrosis factor (TNF) and IL-6, as well as diminished immune function [84–88]. Such an augmented production of proinflammatory cytokines following HCMV infection or reactivation may induce cancer progression directly by promoting undesirable inflammatory conditions in the TME of OC leading to cancer development or suppressed immune function [15,89,90]. Indeed, previous studies have inferred a potential role of inflammatory factors in OC progression as observed in OC patients who have experienced pelvic inflammatory disease [3,91–93]. Although clinical HCMV disease is classically manifested only in immunocompromised individuals, there is substantial evidence also that HCMV reactivation occurs frequently in healthy seropositive individuals [88]. Such frequent HCMV reactivation may also exacerbate chronic conditions such as OC.

In OC, approximately one-third of patients present with ascites, a bulging accumulation of fluid in the peritoneal cavity, that is usually associated with resistance to platinum-based chemotherapy, disease recurrence, and poor survival outcomes [94,95]. Studies have shown that OC ascites suppresses the effector functions of both CTLs and NK cells, as it contains abundant immunosuppressive cells, soluble inflammatory mediators and growth factors, all of which helps to promote growth or proliferation of the ovarian tumour [96,97]. A study by Govindaraj et al. [98] showed that CD4$^+$ Tregs, particularly those expressing tumour necrosis factor (TNF) receptor 2 (TNFR2), from OC-associated ascites exert more suppressive capacity on effector CTLs than peripheral blood-derived TNFR2+ Tregs. Interestingly, the increased frequencies of TNFR2+ Tregs within the total CD4$^+$ T cell pool present in OC ascites was shown to be driven by the presence of pro-inflammatory IL-6 within the ascitic fluid as blockade of IL-6 resulted in reduced frequencies of CD4+TNFR2+ Tregs [97]. Since HCMV reactivation in the TME could lead to increased IL-6 production, these data suggest that active HCMV infection in the TME may also drive the expansion of highly suppressive CD4+TNFR2+ Tregs. Together, these data point towards a potential for an OC immunotherapy targeting IL-6 blockade or anti-HCMV for OC patients presenting with ascites or HCMV in order to improve survival outcomes.

11. Conclusions

Presently, there is an overwhelming research interest into personalised medicine, not only in OC but for many other cancers. Both HCMV and OC share similar disease mechanisms through impairment of CTL and NK cell responses thereby promoting their survival or progression. Previous studies have demonstrated that HCMV infects many cell types; promotes tumour growth and induces a pro-inflammatory environment. Furthermore, active HCMV infection creates an immunosuppressive TME that suppress tumour-specific immune responses. To-date, no clinical study has investigated the use of an anti-HCMV approach to treat OC patients infected with HCMV. In GBM patients, however, the use of anti-HCMV targeted T cell therapy has provided some beneficial treatment outcomes, especially in recurrent GBM patients. Therefore, it is reasonable to rationalise that personalised anti-HCMV treatment could potentially help improve the survival outcomes of OC, particularly in patients with active HCMV infection in their TME. Future studies are needed to evaluate the use of anti-HCMV therapy in combination with current established 1st line and 2nd line therapies and evaluate if this combination approach is efficient at improving the survival outcomes of patients with HCMV positive ovarian tumours.

Author Contributions: M.C. and M.P. designed and concepted the manuscript. M.C. drafted the whole manuscript. M.C., A.E.R.K., P.R.G., K.L.F. and M.P. wrote sections of the manuscript. All authors have read and agreed to the published version of the manuscript.

Funding: M.P. is an Australian National Health and Medical Research Council (NHMRC) Senior Research Fellow.

Institutional Review Board Statement: Not applicable.

Informed Consent Statement: Not applicable.

Data Availability Statement: Not applicable.

Conflicts of Interest: The authors declare no conflict of interest.

References

1. Sankaranarayanan, R.; Ferlay, J. Worldwide burden of gynaecological cancer: The size of the problem. *Best Pr. Res. Clin. Obstet. Gynaecol.* **2006**, *20*, 207–225. [CrossRef]
2. Reid, B.M.; Permuth, J.B.; Sellers, T.A. Epidemiology of ovarian cancer: A review. *Cancer Biol. Med.* **2017**, *14*, 9–32. [CrossRef]
3. Xie, X.; Yang, M.; Ding, Y.; Chen, J. Microbial infection, inflammation and epithelial ovarian cancer. *Oncol. Lett.* **2017**, *14*, 1911–1919. [CrossRef]
4. Kampan, N.C.; Madondo, M.T.; McNally, O.M.; A Quinn, M.; Plebanski, M. Paclitaxel and Its Evolving Role in the Management of Ovarian Cancer. *BioMed. Res. Int.* **2015**, *2015*, 1–21. [CrossRef] [PubMed]
5. Aust, S.; Seebacher-Shariat, V. Screening for ovarian cancer: Is there still hope? *MEMO Mag. Eur. Med. Oncol.* **2020**, *13*, 189–192. [CrossRef]
6. Kampan, N.C.; Madondo, M.T.; Reynolds, J.; Hallo, J.; McNally, O.M.; Jobling, T.W.; Stephens, A.N.; Quinn, M.A.; Plebanski, M. Pre-operative sera interleukin-6 in the diagnosis of high-grade serous ovarian cancer. *Sci. Rep.* **2020**, *10*, 1–15. [CrossRef] [PubMed]
7. Kuchenbaecker, K.B.; Hopper, J.L.; Barnes, D.R.; Phillips, K.-A.; Mooij, T.M.; Roos-Blom, M.-J.; Jervis, S.; Van Leeuwen, F.E.; Milne, R.L.; Andrieu, N.; et al. Risks of Breast, Ovarian, and Contralateral Breast Cancer for BRCA1 and BRCA2 Mutation Carriers. *JAMA* **2017**, *317*, 2402–2416. [CrossRef] [PubMed]
8. Neff, R.T.; Senter, L.; Salani, R. BRCA mutation in ovarian cancer: Testing, implications and treatment considerations. *Ther. Adv. Med. Oncol.* **2017**, *9*, 519–531. [CrossRef] [PubMed]
9. Alsop, K.; Fereday, S.; Meldrum, C.; DeFazio, A.; Emmanuel, C.; George, J.; Dobrovic, A.; Birrer, M.J.; Webb, P.M.; Stewart, C.; et al. BRCA Mutation Frequency and Patterns of Treatment Response in BRCA Mutation–Positive Women With Ovarian Cancer: A Report From the Australian Ovarian Cancer Study Group. *J. Clin. Oncol.* **2012**, *30*, 2654–2663. [CrossRef]
10. Roy, R.; Chun, J.; Powell, S.N. BRCA1 and BRCA2: Different roles in a common pathway of genome protection. *Nat. Rev. Cancer* **2011**, *12*, 68–78. [CrossRef]

11. Wu, J.; Lu, L.-Y.; Yu, X. The role of BRCA1 in DNA damage response. *Protein Cell* **2010**, *1*, 117–123. [CrossRef]
12. Risques, R.A.; Kennedy, S.R. Aging and the rise of somatic cancer-associated mutations in normal tissues. *PLoS Genet.* **2018**, *14*, e1007108. [CrossRef] [PubMed]
13. Luo, X.-H.; Meng, Q.; Rao, M.; Liu, Z.; Paraschoudi, G.; Dodoo, E.; Maeurer, M. The impact of inflationary cytomegalovirus-specific memory T cells on anti-tumour immune responses in patients with cancer. *Immunology* **2018**, *155*, 294–308. [CrossRef]
14. Taher, C.; Frisk, G.; Fuentes, S.; Religa, P.; Costa, H.; Assinger, A.; Vetvik, K.K.; Bukholm, I.R.; Yaiw, K.-C.; Smedby, K.E.; et al. High Prevalence of Human Cytomegalovirus in Brain Metastases of Patients with Primary Breast and Colorectal Cancers. *Transl. Oncol.* **2014**, *7*, 732–740. [CrossRef] [PubMed]
15. Carlson, J.W.; Rådestad, A.F.; Söderberg-Naucler, C.; Rahbar, A. Human cytomegalovirus in high grade serous ovarian cancer possible implications for patients survival. *Medicine* **2018**, *97*, e9685. [CrossRef] [PubMed]
16. Rådestad, A.F.; Estekizadeh, A.; Cui, H.L.; Kostopoulou, O.N.; Davoudi, B.; Hirschberg, A.L.; Carlson, J.; Rahbar, A.; Söderberg-Naucler, C. Impact of Human Cytomegalovirus Infection and its Immune Response on Survival of Patients with Ovarian Cancer. *Transl. Oncol.* **2018**, *11*, 1292–1300. [CrossRef] [PubMed]
17. Cox, M.; Adetifa, J.U.; Noho-Konteh, F.; Njie-Jobe, J.; Sanyang, L.C.; Drammeh, A.; Plebanski, M.; Whittle, H.C.; Rowland-Jones, S.L.; Robertson, I.; et al. Limited Impact of Human Cytomegalovirus Infection in African Infants on Vaccine-Specific Responses Following Diphtheria-Tetanus-Pertussis and Measles Vaccination. *Front. Immunol.* **2020**, *11*. [CrossRef] [PubMed]
18. Geisler, J.; Touma, J.; Rahbar, A.; Söderberg-Naucler, C.; Vetvik, K. A Review of the Potential Role of Human Cytomegalovirus (HCMV) Infections in Breast Cancer Carcinogenesis and Abnormal Immunity. *Cancers* **2019**, *11*, 1842. [CrossRef]
19. Manandhar, T.; Hò, G.-G.T.; Pump, W.C.; Blasczyk, R.; Bade-Doeding, C. Battle between Host Immune Cellular Responses and HCMV Immune Evasion. *Int. J. Mol. Sci.* **2019**, *20*, 3626. [CrossRef]
20. Rossini, G.; Cerboni, C.; Santoni, A.; Landini, M.P.; Landolfo, S.; Gatti, D.; Gribaudo, G.; Varani, S. Interplay between Human Cytomegalovirus and Intrinsic/Innate Host Responses: A Complex Bidirectional Relationship. *Mediat. Inflamm.* **2012**, *2012*, 1–16. [CrossRef] [PubMed]
21. Wilkinson, G.W.; Tomasec, P.; Stanton, R.J.; Armstrong, M.; Prod'Homme, V.; Aicheler, R.; McSharry, B.P.; Rickards, C.R.; Cochrane, D.; Llewellyn-Lacey, S.; et al. Modulation of natural killer cells by human cytomegalovirus. *J. Clin. Virol.* **2008**, *41*, 206–212. [CrossRef]
22. Hanley, P.J.; Bollard, C.M. Controlling Cytomegalovirus: Helping the Immune System Take the Lead. *Viruses* **2014**, *6*, 2242–2258. [CrossRef]
23. Avdic, S.; McSharry, B.P.; Steain, M.; Poole, E.; Sinclair, J.; Abendroth, A.; Slobedman, B. Human Cytomegalovirus-Encoded Human Interleukin-10 (IL-10) Homolog Amplifies Its Immunomodulatory Potential by Upregulating Human IL-10 in Monocytes. *J. Virol.* **2016**, *90*, 3819–3827. [CrossRef]
24. Wagner, C.S.; Walther-Jallow, L.; Buentke, E.; Ljunggren, H.-G.; Achour, A.; Chambers, B.J. Human cytomegalovirus-derived protein UL18 alters the phenotype and function of monocyte-derived dendritic cells. *J. Leukoc. Biol.* **2007**, *83*, 56–63. [CrossRef] [PubMed]
25. Fulop, T.; Larbi, A.; Pawelec, G. Human T Cell Aging and the Impact of Persistent Viral Infections. *Front. Immunol.* **2013**, *4*, 271. [CrossRef]
26. Bennett, J.M.; Glaser, R.; Malarkey, W.B.; Beversdorf, D.Q.; Peng, J.; Kiecolt-Glaser, J.K. Inflammation and reactivation of latent herpesviruses in older adults. *Brain Behav. Immun.* **2012**, *26*, 739–746. [CrossRef]
27. Goodier, M.R.; White, M.J.; Darboe, A.; Nielsen, C.M.; Goncalves, A.; Bottomley, C.; Moore, S.E.; Riley, E.M. Rapid NK cell differentiation in a population with near-universal human cytomegalovirus infection is attenuated by NKG2C deletions. *Blood* **2014**, *124*, 2213–2222. [CrossRef] [PubMed]
28. Gumá, M.; Budt, M.; Sáez, A.; Brckalo, T.; Hengel, H.; Angulo, A.; López-Botet, M. Expansion of CD94/NKG2C+ NK cells in response to human cytomegalovirus-infected fibroblasts. *Blood* **2006**, *107*, 3624–3631. [CrossRef] [PubMed]
29. King, P.T.; Ngui, J.; Farmer, M.W.; Hutchinson, P.; Holmes, P.W.; Holdsworth, S.R. Cytotoxic T lymphocyte and natural killer cell responses to non-typeable Haemophilus influenzae. *Clin. Exp. Immunol.* **2008**, *152*, 542–551. [CrossRef] [PubMed]
30. Mandal, A.; Viswanathan, C. Natural killer cells: In health and disease. *Hematol. Stem Cell Ther.* **2015**, *8*, 47–55. [CrossRef] [PubMed]
31. Anikeeva, N.; Sykulev, Y. Mechanisms controlling granule-mediated cytolytic activity of cytotoxic T lymphocytes. *Immunol. Res.* **2011**, *51*, 183–194. [CrossRef]
32. Martínez-Lostao, L.; Anel, A.; Pardo, J. How Do Cytotoxic Lymphocytes Kill Cancer Cells? *Clin. Cancer Res.* **2015**, *21*, 5047–5056. [CrossRef]
33. Osińska, I.; Popko, K.; Demkow, U. Perforin: An important player in immune response. *Central Eur. J. Immunol.* **2014**, *1*, 109–115. [CrossRef] [PubMed]
34. Ben Safta, T.; Ziani, L.; Favre, L.; Lamendour, L.; Gros, G.; Mami-Chouaib, F.; Martinvalet, D.; Chouaib, S.; Thiery, J. Granzyme B–Activated p53 Interacts with Bcl-2 To Promote Cytotoxic Lymphocyte–Mediated Apoptosis. *J. Immunol.* **2014**, *194*, 418–428. [CrossRef]
35. Curiel, T.J.; Coukos, G.; Zou, L.; Alvarez, X.; Cheng, P.; Mottram, P.; Evdemon-Hogan, M.; Conejo-Garcia, J.R.; Zhang, L.; Burow, M.; et al. Specific recruitment of regulatory T cells in ovarian carcinoma fosters immune privilege and predicts reduced survival. *Nat. Med.* **2004**, *10*, 942–949. [CrossRef] [PubMed]

36. Yigit, R.; Figdor, C.G.; Zusterzeel, P.L.; Pots, J.M.; Torensma, R.; Massuger, L.F. Cytokine analysis as a tool to understand tumour–host interaction in ovarian cancer. *Eur. J. Cancer* **2011**, *47*, 1883–1889. [CrossRef] [PubMed]
37. Barnett, J.C.; Bean, S.M.; Whitaker, R.S.; Kondoh, E.; Baba, T.; Fujii, S.; Marks, J.R.; Dressman, H.K.; Murphy, S.K.; Berchuck, A. Ovarian cancer tumor infiltrating T-regulatory (Treg) cells are associated with a metastatic phenotype. *Gynecol. Oncol.* **2010**, *116*, 556–562. [CrossRef] [PubMed]
38. Preston, C.C.; Maurer, M.J.; Oberg, A.L.; Visscher, D.W.; Kalli, K.R.; Hartmann, L.C.; Goode, E.L.; Knutson, K.L. The Ratios of CD8+ T Cells to CD4+CD25+ FOXP3+ and FOXP3- T Cells Correlate with Poor Clinical Outcome in Human Serous Ovarian Cancer. *PLoS ONE* **2013**, *8*, e80063. [CrossRef] [PubMed]
39. Yu, J.; Freud, A.G.; Caligiuri, M.A. Location and cellular stages of natural killer cell development. *Trends Immunol.* **2013**, *34*, 573–582. [CrossRef] [PubMed]
40. Korbel, D.S.; Finney, O.C.; Riley, E.M. Natural killer cells and innate immunity to protozoan pathogens. *Int. J. Parasitol.* **2004**, *34*, 1517–1528. [CrossRef] [PubMed]
41. Pegram, H.J.; Andrews, D.M.; Smyth, M.J.; Darcy, P.K.; Kershaw, M.H. Activating and inhibitory receptors of natural killer cells. *Immunol. Cell Biol.* **2010**, *89*, 216–224. [CrossRef] [PubMed]
42. Vivier, E.; Tomasello, E.; Baratin, M.; Walzer, T.; Ugolini, S. Functions of natural killer cells. *Nat. Immunol.* **2008**, *9*, 503–510. [CrossRef]
43. Webb, J.R.; Milne, K.; Watson, P.; DeLeeuw, R.J.; Nelson, B.H. Tumor-Infiltrating Lymphocytes Expressing the Tissue Resident Memory Marker CD103 Are Associated with Increased Survival in High-Grade Serous Ovarian Cancer. *Clin. Cancer Res.* **2014**, *20*, 434–444. [CrossRef] [PubMed]
44. Moody, R.; Wilson, K.; Jaworowski, A.; Plebanski, M. Natural Compounds with Potential to Modulate Cancer Therapies and Self-Reactive Immune Cells. *Cancers* **2020**, *12*, 673. [CrossRef]
45. Linhares, A.D.S.; Leitner, J.; Grabmeier-Pfistershammer, K.; Steinberger, P. Not All Immune Checkpoints Are Created Equal. *Front. Immunol.* **2018**, *9*, 1909. [CrossRef]
46. Dong, Y.; Sun, Q.; Zhang, X. PD-1 and its ligands are important immune checkpoints in cancer. *Oncotarget* **2017**, *8*, 2171–2186. [CrossRef]
47. Francisco, L.M.; Sage, P.T.; Sharpe, A.H. The PD-1 pathway in tolerance and autoimmunity. *Immunol. Rev.* **2010**, *236*, 219–242. [CrossRef]
48. Fife, B.T.; Bluestone, J.A. Control of peripheral T-cell tolerance and autoimmunity via the CTLA-4 and PD-1 pathways. *Immunol. Rev.* **2008**, *224*, 166–182. [CrossRef]
49. Francisco, L.M.; Salinas, V.H.; Brown, K.E.; Vanguri, V.K.; Freeman, G.J.; Kuchroo, V.K.; Sharpe, A.H. PD-L1 regulates the development, maintenance, and function of induced regulatory T cells. *J. Exp. Med.* **2009**, *206*, 3015–3029. [CrossRef]
50. E Latchman, Y.; Wood, C.R.; Chernova, T.; Chaudhary, D.; Borde, M.; Chernova, I.; Iwai, Y.; Long, A.J.; A Brown, J.; Nunes, R.; et al. PD-L2 is a second ligand for PD-1 and inhibits T cell activation. *Nat. Immunol.* **2001**, *2*, 261–268. [CrossRef] [PubMed]
51. Pardoll, D.M. The blockade of immune checkpoints in cancer immunotherapy. *Nat. Rev. Cancer* **2012**, *12*, 252–264. [CrossRef]
52. Dyck, L.; Mills, K.H. Immune checkpoints and their inhibition in cancer and infectious diseases. *Eur. J. Immunol.* **2017**, *47*, 765–779. [CrossRef] [PubMed]
53. Naran, K.; Nundalall, T.; Chetty, S.; Barth, S. Principles of Immunotherapy: Implications for Treatment Strategies in Cancer and Infectious Diseases. *Front. Microbiol.* **2018**, *9*, 3158. [CrossRef]
54. Shanmughapriya, S.; Senthilkumar, G.; Vinodhini, K.; Das, B.C.; Vasanthi, N.; Natarajaseenivasan, K. Viral and bacterial aetiologies of epithelial ovarian cancer. *Eur. J. Clin. Microbiol. Infect. Dis.* **2012**, *31*, 2311–2317. [CrossRef]
55. Ugel, S.; De Sanctis, F.; Mandruzzato, S.; Bronte, V. Tumor-induced myeloid deviation: When myeloid-derived suppressor cells meet tumor-associated macrophages. *J. Clin. Investig.* **2015**, *125*, 3365–3376. [CrossRef] [PubMed]
56. Sato, E.; Olson, S.H.; Ahn, J.; Bundy, B.; Nishikawa, H.; Qian, F.; Jungbluth, A.A.; Frosina, D.; Gnjatic, S.; Ambrosone, C.; et al. Intraepithelial CD8+ tumor-infiltrating lymphocytes and a high CD8+/regulatory T cell ratio are associated with favorable prognosis in ovarian cancer. *Proc. Natl. Acad. Sci. USA* **2005**, *102*, 18538–18543. [CrossRef]
57. Kumar, A.; Tripathy, M.K.; Pasquereau, S.; Al Moussawi, F.; Abbas, W.; Coquard, L.; Khan, K.A.; Russo, L.; Algros, M.-P.; Valmary-Degano, S.; et al. The Human Cytomegalovirus Strain DB Activates Oncogenic Pathways in Mammary Epithelial Cells. *EBioMedicine* **2018**, *30*, 167–183. [CrossRef] [PubMed]
58. Dziurzynski, K.; Wei, J.; Qiao, W.; Hatiboglu, M.A.; Kong, L.-Y.; Wu, A.; Wang, Y.; Cahill, D.; Levine, N.; Prabhu, S.; et al. Glioma-Associated Cytomegalovirus Mediates Subversion of the Monocyte Lineage to a Tumor Propagating Phenotype. *Clin. Cancer Res.* **2011**, *17*, 4642–4649. [CrossRef] [PubMed]
59. Bishop, R.K.; Oseguera, C.A.V.; Spencer, J.V. Human Cytomegalovirus interleukin-10 promotes proliferation and migration of MCF-7 breast cancer cells. *Cancer Cell Microenviron.* **2015**, *2*. [CrossRef]
60. Golubovskaya, V.; Wu, L. Different Subsets of T Cells, Memory, Effector Functions, and CAR-T Immunotherapy. *Cancers* **2016**, *8*, 36. [CrossRef]
61. Zhang, S.; Wu, M.; Wang, F. Immune regulation by CD8+ Treg cells: Novel possibilities for anticancer immunotherapy. *Cell. Mol. Immunol.* **2018**, *15*, 805–807. [CrossRef]
62. Zhang, S.; Ke, X.; Zeng, S.; Wu, M.; Lou, J.; Wu, L.; Huang, P.; Huang, L.; Wang, F.; Pan, S. Analysis of CD8+ Treg cells in patients with ovarian cancer: A possible mechanism for immune impairment. *Cell. Mol. Immunol.* **2015**, *12*, 580–591. [CrossRef]

63. Yang, Z.; Bjorkman, P.J. Structure of UL18, a peptide-binding viral MHC mimic, bound to a host inhibitory receptor. *Proc. Natl. Acad. Sci. USA* **2008**, *105*, 10095–10100. [CrossRef]
64. Smith, W.; Tomasec, P.; Aicheler, R.; Loewendorf, A.; Nemčovičová, I.; Wang, E.C.; Stanton, R.J.; Macauley, M.; Norris, P.; Willen, L.; et al. Human Cytomegalovirus Glycoprotein UL141 Targets the TRAIL Death Receptors to Thwart Host Innate Antiviral Defenses. *Cell Host Microbe* **2013**, *13*, 324–335. [CrossRef]
65. Prod'Homme, V.; Sugrue, D.M.; Stanton, R.J.; Nomoto, A.; Davies, J.; Rickards, C.R.; Cochrane, D.; Moore, M.; Wilkinson, G.W.G.; Tomasec, P. Human cytomegalovirus UL141 promotes efficient downregulation of the natural killer cell activating ligand CD112. *J. Gen. Virol.* **2010**, *91*, 2034–2039. [CrossRef]
66. Aiello, A.; Accardi, G.; Candore, G.; Caruso, C.; Colomba, C.; Di Bona, D.; Duro, G.; Gambino, C.M.; Ligotti, M.E.; Pandey, J.P. Role of Immunogenetics in the Outcome of HCMV Infection: Implications for Ageing. *Int. J. Mol. Sci.* **2019**, *20*, 685. [CrossRef]
67. Di Bona, D.; Accardi, G.; Aiello, A.; Bilancia, M.; Candore, G.; Colomba, C.; Caruso, C.; Duro, G.; Gambino, C.M.; Macchia, L.; et al. Association between γ marker, human leucocyte antigens and killer immunoglobulin-like receptors and the natural course of human cytomegalovirus infection: A pilot study performed in a Sicilian population. *Immunology* **2017**, *153*, 523–531. [CrossRef] [PubMed]
68. Pandey, J.P.; Kistner-Griffin, E.; Radwan, F.F.; Kaur, N.; Namboodiri, A.M.; Black, L.; Butler, M.A.; Carreón, T.; Ruder, A.M. Immunoglobulin genes influence the magnitude of humoral immunity to cytomegalovirus glycoprotein B. *J. Infect. Dis.* **2014**, *210*, 1823–1826. [CrossRef]
69. Di Bona, D.; Scafidi, V.; Plaia, A.; Colomba, C.; Nuzzo, D.; Occhino, C.; Tuttolomondo, A.; Giammanco, G.; De Grazia, S.; Montalto, G.; et al. HLA and Killer Cell Immunoglobulin-like Receptors Influence the Natural Course of CMV Infection. *J. Infect. Dis.* **2014**, *210*, 1083–1089. [CrossRef] [PubMed]
70. Hirano, F.; Kaneko, K.; Tamura, H.; Dong, H.; Wang, S.; Ichikawa, M.; Rietz, C.; Flies, D.B.; Lau, J.S.; Zhu, G.; et al. Blockade of B7-H1 and PD-1 by monoclonal antibodies potentiates cancer therapeutic immunity. *Cancer Res.* **2005**, *65*, 1089–1096. [PubMed]
71. Currie, A.J.; Prosser, A.; McDonnell, A.; Cleaver, A.L.; Robinson, B.W.S.; Freeman, G.J.; Van Der Most, R.G. Dual Control of Antitumor CD8 T Cells through the Programmed Death-1/Programmed Death-Ligand 1 Pathway and Immunosuppressive CD4 T Cells: Regulation and Counterregulation. *J. Immunol.* **2009**, *183*, 7898–7908. [CrossRef]
72. Wu, X.; Gu, Z.; Chen, Y.; Chen, B.; Chen, W.; Weng, L.; Liu, X. Application of PD-1 Blockade in Cancer Immunotherapy. *Comput. Struct. Biotechnol. J.* **2019**, *17*, 661–674. [CrossRef] [PubMed]
73. Zhu, X.; Lang, J. Programmed death-1 pathway blockade produces a synergistic antitumor effect: Combined application in ovarian cancer. *J. Gynecol. Oncol.* **2017**, *28*, e64. [CrossRef] [PubMed]
74. Zimmer, A.S.; Nichols, E.; Cimino-Mathews, A.; Peer, C.; Cao, L.; Lee, M.-J.; Kohn, E.C.; Annunziata, C.M.; Lipkowitz, S.; Trepel, J.B.; et al. A phase I study of the PD-L1 inhibitor, durvalumab, in combination with a PARP inhibitor, olaparib, and a VEGFR1–3 inhibitor, cediranib, in recurrent women's cancers with biomarker analyses. *J. Immunother. Cancer* **2019**, *7*, 197. [CrossRef] [PubMed]
75. Gallez-Hawkins, G.M.; Thao, L.; Palmer, J.; Dagis, A.; Li, X.; Franck, A.E.; Tegtmeier, B.; Lacey, S.F.; Diamond, D.J.; Forman, S.J.; et al. Increased Programmed Death-1 Molecule Expression in Cytomegalovirus Disease and Acute Graft-versus-Host Disease after Allogeneic Hematopoietic Cell Transplantation. *Biol. Blood Marrow Transplant.* **2009**, *15*, 872–880. [CrossRef]
76. Sester, U.; Presser, D.; Dirks, J.; Gärtner, B.C.; Köhler, H.; Sester, M. PD-1 Expression and IL-2 Loss of Cytomegalovirus- Specific T Cells Correlates with Viremia and Reversible Functional Anergy. *Arab. Archaeol. Epigr.* **2008**, *8*, 1486–1497. [CrossRef]
77. A Gutman, J.; Schmidt, C.; Freed, B.; Palmer, B. PD-1 Expression On Total and CMV-Specific T Cells In Early Post Transplant Is Associated With Donor Source, T Cell Maturation Profile, and Effectiveness Of CMV Control. *Blood* **2013**, *122*, 2062. [CrossRef]
78. Kato, T.; Nishida, T.; Murase, M.; Murata, M.; Naoe, T. Exhaustion of CMV Specific T Cells with Enhanced PD-1 Expression In Persistent Cytomegalovirus Infection After Allogeneic Stem Cell Transplantation. *Blood* **2010**, *116*, 3912. [CrossRef]
79. Pesce, S.; Greppi, M.; Tabellini, G.; Rampinelli, F.; Parolini, S.; Olive, D.; Moretta, L.; Moretta, A.; Marcenaro, E. Identification of a subset of human natural killer cells expressing high levels of programmed death 1: A phenotypic and functional characterization. *J. Allergy Clin. Immunol.* **2017**, *139*, 335–346.e3. [CrossRef]
80. Nduom, E.K.; Wei, J.; Yaghi, N.K.; Huang, N.; Kong, L.-Y.; Gabrusiewicz, K.; Ling, X.; Zhou, S.; Ivan, C.; Chen, J.Q.; et al. PD-L1 expression and prognostic impact in glioblastoma. *Neuro-Oncology* **2016**, *18*, 195–205. [CrossRef]
81. Qin, Z.; Zhang, L.; Xu, Y.; Zhang, X.; Fang, X.; Qian, D.; Liu, X.; Liu, T.; Li, L.; Yu, H.; et al. TLR3 regulates PD-L1 expression in human cytomegalovirus infected glioblastoma. *Int. J. Clin. Exp. Pathol.* **2018**, *11*, 5318–5326.
82. Herbein, G. The Human Cytomegalovirus, from Oncomodulation to Oncogenesis. *Viruses* **2018**, *10*, 408. [CrossRef] [PubMed]
83. Chan, G.; Bivins-Smith, E.R.; Smith, M.S.; Yurochko, A.D. NF-κB and phosphatidylinositol 3-kinase activity mediates the HCMV-induced atypical M1/M2 polarization of monocytes. *Virus Res.* **2009**, *144*, 329–333. [CrossRef] [PubMed]
84. Compton, T.; Kurt-Jones, E.A.; Boehme, K.W.; Belko, J.; Latz, E.; Golenbock, D.T.; Finberg, R.W. Human Cytomegalovirus Activates Inflammatory Cytokine Responses via CD14 and Toll-Like Receptor 2. *J. Virol.* **2003**, *77*, 4588–4596. [CrossRef] [PubMed]
85. Varani, S.; Landini, M.P. Cytomegalovirus-induced immunopathology and its clinical consequences. *Herpesviridae* **2011**, *2*, 6. [CrossRef] [PubMed]
86. Voigt, V.; Andoniou, C.E.; Schuster, I.S.; Oszmiana, A.; Ong, M.L.; Fleming, P.; Forrester, J.V.; Degli-Esposti, M.A. Cytomegalovirus establishes a latent reservoir and triggers long-lasting inflammation in the eye. *PLOS Pathog.* **2018**, *14*, e1007040. [CrossRef]

87. Van De Berg, P.J.; Heutinck, K.M.; Raabe, R.; Minnee, R.C.; La Young, S.; Pant, K.A.V.D.-V.D.; Bemelman, F.J.; Van Lier, R.A.; Berge, I.J.T. Human Cytomegalovirus Induces Systemic Immune Activation Characterized by a Type 1 Cytokine Signature. *J. Infect. Dis.* **2010**, *202*, 690–699. [CrossRef] [PubMed]
88. Forte, E.; Zhang, Z.; Thorp, E.B.; Hummel, M. Cytomegalovirus Latency and Reactivation: An Intricate Interplay With the Host Immune Response. *Front. Cell. Infect. Microbiol.* **2020**, *10*, 130. [CrossRef] [PubMed]
89. Grivennikov, S.I.; Greten, F.R.; Karin, M. Immunity, Inflammation, and Cancer. *Cell* **2010**, *140*, 883–899. [CrossRef]
90. Quinn, K.M.; Kartikasari, A.E.R.; Cooke, R.E.; Koldej, R.M.; Ritchie, D.S.; Plebanski, M. Impact of age-, cancer-, and treatment-driven inflammation on T cell function and immunotherapy. *J. Leukoc. Biol.* **2020**, *108*, 953–965. [CrossRef]
91. Rasmussen, C.B.; Kjaer, S.K.; Albieri, V.; Bandera, E.V.; Doherty, J.A.; Høgdall, E.; Webb, P.M.; Jordan, S.J.; Rossing, M.A.; Wicklund, K.G.; et al. Pelvic Inflammatory Disease and the Risk of Ovarian Cancer and Borderline Ovarian Tumors: A Pooled Analysis of 13 Case-Control Studies. *Am. J. Epidemiol.* **2016**, *185*, 8–20. [CrossRef]
92. Risch, H.A.; Howe, G.R. Pelvic inflammatory disease and the risk of epithelial ovarian cancer. *Cancer Epidemiol. Biomark. Prev.* **1995**, *4*, 447.
93. Shu, X.O.; Brinton, L.A.; Gao, Y.T.; Yuan, J.M. Population-based case-control study of ovarian cancer in Shanghai. *Cancer Res.* **1989**, *49*, 3670.
94. Ahmed, N.; Stenvers, K.L. Getting to Know Ovarian Cancer Ascites: Opportunities for Targeted Therapy-Based Translational Research. *Front. Oncol.* **2013**, *3*, 256. [CrossRef]
95. Kipps, E.; Tan, D.S.P.; Kaye, S.B. Meeting the challenge of ascites in ovarian cancer: New avenues for therapy and research. *Nat. Rev. Cancer* **2013**, *13*, 273–282. [CrossRef] [PubMed]
96. Kim, S.; Kim, B.; Song, Y.S. Ascites modulates cancer cell behavior, contributing to tumor heterogeneity in ovarian cancer. *Cancer Sci.* **2016**, *107*, 1173–1178. [CrossRef]
97. Kampan, N.C.; Madondo, M.T.; McNally, O.M.; Stephens, A.N.; Quinn, M.A.; Plebanski, M. Interleukin 6 Present in Inflammatory Ascites from Advanced Epithelial Ovarian Cancer Patients Promotes Tumor Necrosis Factor Receptor 2-Expressing Regulatory T Cells. *Front. Immunol.* **2017**, *8*, 1482. [CrossRef]
98. Govindaraj, C.; Scalzo-Inguanti, K.; Madondo, M.; Hallo, J.; Flanagan, K.; Quinn, M.; Plebanski, M. Impaired Th1 immunity in ovarian cancer patients is mediated by TNFR2+ Tregs within the tumor microenvironment. *Clin. Immunol.* **2013**, *149*, 97–110. [CrossRef] [PubMed]

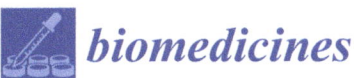

Review

Circulating Exosomal miRNAs as Biomarkers in Epithelial Ovarian Cancer

Meng-Shin Shiao [1], Jia-Ming Chang [2], Arb-Aroon Lertkhachonsuk [3], Naparat Rermluk [4] and Natini Jinawath [5,6,7,*]

1. Research Center, Faculty of Medicine Ramathibodi Hospital, Mahidol University, Bangkok 10400, Thailand; msshiao@gmail.com
2. Department of Computer Science, National Chengchi University, Taipei 11605, Taiwan; chang.jiaming@gmail.com
3. Division of Gynecologic Oncology, Department of Obstetrics and Gynecology, Faculty of Medicine Ramathibodi Hospital, Mahidol University, Bangkok 10400, Thailand; arbaroon.let@mahidol.ac.th
4. Department of Pathology, Faculty of Medicine Ramathibodi Hospital, Mahidol University, Bangkok 10400, Thailand; naparat.rer@mahidol.ac.th
5. Ramathibodi Comprehensive Cancer Center, Faculty of Medicine Ramathibodi Hospital, Mahidol University, Bangkok 10400, Thailand
6. Integrative Computational Bioscience Center (ICBS), Mahidol University, Nakhon Pathom 73170, Thailand
7. Program in Translational Medicine, Faculty of Medicine Ramathibodi Hospital, Mahidol University, Bangkok 10400, Thailand
* Correspondence: jnatini@hotmail.com or natini.jin@mahidol.ac.th

Abstract: Failure to detect early-stage epithelial ovarian cancer (EOC) is a major contributing factor to its low survival rate. Increasing evidence suggests that different subtypes of EOC may behave as distinct diseases due to their different cells of origins, histology and treatment responses. Therefore, the identification of EOC subtype-specific biomarkers that can early detect the disease should be clinically beneficial. Exosomes are extracellular vesicles secreted by different types of cells and carry biological molecules, which play important roles in cell-cell communication and regulation of various biological processes. Multiple studies have proposed that exosomal miRNAs present in the circulation are good biomarkers for non-invasive early detection of cancer. In this review, the potential use of exosomal miRNAs as early detection biomarkers for EOCs and their accuracy are discussed. We also review the differential expression of circulating exosomal miRNAs and cell-free miRNAs between different biofluid sources, i.e., plasma and serum, and touch on the issue of endogenous reference miRNA selection. Additionally, the current clinical trials using miRNAs for detecting EOCs are summarized. In conclusion, circulating exosomal miRNAs as the non-invasive biomarkers have a high potential for early detection of EOC and its subtypes, and are likely to be clinically important in the future.

Keywords: exosome; miRNA; biomarkers; epithelial ovarian cancer; liquid biopsy

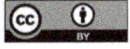

1. Introduction

Ovarian cancer (OC) is the eight most common cancer in women worldwide and remains the leading cause of mortality among gynecological malignancies in developed countries [1,2]. The estimated numbers of new OC cases and death in 2020 in the United States are 21,750 and 13,940, while globally the numbers are 313,959 and 207,252, respectively [1,2]. OC is mostly asymptomatic in its early stages; thus, the patients usually present with advanced-stage cancer, which is commonly associated with high mortality rate. Therefore, the development of a non-invasive diagnostic approach to accurately detect the disease early is one of the holy grails of combating OC and would lead to the increased overall survival.

Around 90% of the OC tumors are of epithelial origin (epithelial ovarian cancer; EOC), which can be further subdivided into different histopathological subtypes. Several EOC subtype classification systems have been proposed. The most widely applied system in the clinical practice was proposed by the World Health Organization (the WHO classification system) [3]. According to the recent WHO classification of tumors of the ovary, there are seven major subtypes of EOC: serous carcinoma, mucinous carcinoma, endometrioid carcinoma, clear-cell carcinoma, seromucinous carcinoma, malignant Brenner tumor and undifferentiated carcinoma. These tumors are mainly classified based on their histomorphological features; i.e., serous carcinoma has columnar cells resemble those of tubal-type epithelium; mucinous carcinoma has gastrointestinal-type mucin producing cells; clear-cell carcinoma has cells with clear cytoplasm with characteristic "hobnail" appearance; endometrioid carcinoma has cells resemble to the endometrial glands; Brenner tumors have cells similar to transitional/urothelial epithelium; seromucinous carcinoma has cells with both serous and endocervical-type mucin producing cells; and undifferentiated carcinoma have monotonous non-cohesive cells with lack of defining cell types. Furthermore, the serous carcinoma is classified into high-grade and low-grade serous carcinoma, which is based on the different degree of cytologic atypia and mitotic rate. High-grade serous carcinoma is featured with clear cytoplasm and pleomorphic/bizarre nucleus. Nuclei atypia with more than 12 mitoses per 10 high power fields in the worst area of tumors, multinucleated tumor giant cells and tumor architecture resemble epithelial cells of fallopian tube origin are also often seen in high-grade serous carcinoma [4–6]. Another system, dualistic classification of primary EOCs, is also widely applied in many research practices [7–9]. This system divides EOCs into two main types, type I and type II, by integrating the histopathologic classification with the molecular genetics findings. Currently, type I tumors, which have a relatively better clinical outcome, are subdivided into three groups: (i) endometriosis-related tumors that include endometrioid, clear cell and seromucinous carcinomas; (ii) low-grade serous carcinomas; and (iii) mucinous carcinomas and malignant Brenner tumors, while type II tumors are composed of the more aggressive high-grade serous carcinoma, carcinosarcoma and undifferentiated carcinoma [10].

Accurate diagnosis of the stage and subtype of EOC is very important because standard treatment options affect each subtype differently. The combination of paclitaxel and carboplatin chemotherapy usually produces good initial response rates in high-grade serous carcinoma (60–80%), but eventually most patients become platinum resistant and succumb to subsequent relapses. However, the majority of clear cell, mucinous and low-grade serous carcinoma are resistant to platinum chemotherapy, resulting in reduced usage of platinum for these subtypes. It has now become a standard practice to identify serous vs. non-serous EOC subtypes so that the suitable treatment can be selected for EOC patients [11].

2. Current Epithelial Ovarian Cancer (EOC) Biomarkers

In combination with histomorphology, immunohistochemistry (IHC) can help distinguish difficult-to-diagnose EOC subtypes [12–14]. p53 IHC is routinely used to distinguish low-grade from high-grade serous carcinoma; the pattern of p53 IHC staining in high-grade serous carcinoma is all or none (overexpression or complete absence), which reflects the underlying TP53 mutation. The combination of WT1 and p53 can be used to distinguish serous carcinoma from endometrioid carcinoma, while the combination of WT1, Napsin A and ER are used to distinguish clear-cell carcinoma from serous carcinoma. ER alone is used to distinguish endometrioid carcinoma from mucinous carcinoma. Recent studies from Kobel et al. proposed the use of the eight IHC biomarkers, namely WT1, p53, p16, Napsin A, PGR, TFF3, ARID1A and VIM, to classify subtypes of a large cohort of EOCs based on nominal logistic regression model [13,14]. After comparing the original diagnosis with the predicted histotypes, the IHC panel could correctly reclassify ~93% of the cases [13,14]. The most common misclassification involved reclassification from high-grade endometrioid to high-grade serous carcinoma, which are the two subtypes known to be difficult to distinguish by histomorphology. Additionally, supported evidence such as molecular alterations and clinical behaviors can help increase the accuracy of the subtype diagnosis.

In terms of molecular alterations, high-grade serous carcinoma is usually associated with *BRCA1* or *BRCA2* germline mutations and *TP53* somatic mutations, which are identified in 96% of the tumor samples [15]. Other than the three genes, mutations in *CSMD3*, *NF1*, *CDK12* and *RB1* are also commonly found [15]. Low-grade serous carcinoma has distinct underlying molecular mechanism than that of high-grade serous carcinoma. It is associated with *KRAS* and *BRAF* mutations but not *TP53* mutations [16,17]. Although it is believed that clear-cell and endometrioid carcinomas share similar molecular genetic profiles as they are both proposed to originate from endometriosis [18], the morphology and clinical behavior of the two subtypes are different. Genetic alterations in *ARID1A*, *PIK3CA* and *PTEN* occur in both subtypes, while microsatellite instability and *CTNNB1* mutations are more commonly observed in endometrioid carcinoma [10,19–21]. A recent study by Cochrane et al. proposed that clear-cell and endometrioid carcinomas may originate from different cell types of endometria as clear-cell tumors express much higher level of markers of the ciliated cells (cystathionine gamma-lyase (CTH), etc.), while endometrioid tumors express markers of the secretory cells of the endometrium (methylenetetrahydrofolate dehydrogenase 1 (MTHFD1) and ER) [22]. The authors further posited that clear-cell carcinoma may originate from the progenitor of ciliated cells. For mucinous carcinoma, *KRAS* alterations are found in more than 50% of the tumors [23–27].

Clinical screening of EOC includes imaging and serum biomarkers. Imaging tests include transabdominal and transvaginal ultrasound screening (TVS), computed tomography (CT) scan, magnetic resonance imaging (MRI) and positron emission tomography (PET) scan. Biomarker tests in the blood include the commonly used serum tumor markers; CA-125, cancer antigen 19-9 (CA19-9) and carcinoembryonic antigen (CEA). Most of the currently available tests give relatively low sensitivity and specificity, making them unable to detect early-stage EOCs and thus resulting in no significant changes of overall survival of EOC patients in the past 20 years [28]. The recently published study showed that neither the annual screening using serum CA-125 nor TSV can help reduce the mortality rate of ovarian cancer. This large randomized controlled trial in the UK, which recruited 202,562 postmenopausal women who were 50–74 years of age and conducted more than 16 years of follow-up, provides definitive new evidence that the existing general population screening approaches did not reduce ovarian cancer deaths [29]. Currently, OVA1 and its second-generation multivariate index assay (MIA), OVERA, are among the commonly used US Food and Drug Administration (FDA)-cleared assays that assess malignancy risk in adnexal masses planned for surgery. OVA1 has five serum protein biomarkers including CA-125, Transthyretin, Apolipoprotein A1, Transferrin and B2-microglobulin. OVERA substitutes B2-microglobulin and Transthyretin used in OVA1 with Human Epididymis secretory protein 4 (HE4) and Follicle-Stimulating Hormone (FSH). Both assays are used in combination with clinical assessment in women who have a pelvic mass to assess ovarian cancer risk prior to surgical treatment planning and are not a screening test. In addition, although OVA1 and OVERA have high sensitivities (92%, 91%), the specificities are quite low (42%, 69%) [30,31]. Therefore, it is critical to establish new strategies to efficiently screen the disease in its early stage, which is key to improving survival rate.

Taken together, novel biomarkers for early detection of EOCs, which are more effective and able to distinguish the subtypes to facilitate a timely clinical decision are urgently needed. Lately, exosomes have been extensively studied with an increasing number of reports showing their potential as a rich source of biomarkers. Exosomes are a type of extracellular membrane vesicles (EVs) with a diameter of 40–100 nm that are secreted by all cell type. Exosomes carry various biological molecules such as protein, lipid, mRNA and non-coding RNA including microRNA (miRNA) and long non-coding RNA (lncRNA) and transport them to a distant location via the circulatory system. They can be detected in various kinds of body fluids such as blood, urine and saliva. Several pathways have been proposed for biogenesis of exosomes [32]. One of the most well-studied pathways involves the generation of intracellular multivesicular bodies (MVBs) in two steps. First, the invagination of the plasma membrane and the formation of MVBs, which contains intraluminal vesicles (ILVs). Following the formation of MVBs, ILVs will be secreted to the extracellular compartment through the fusion of MVB to the plasma membrane and exocytosis, and they are now called exosomes. Exosomes are continuously being generated by and taken up by cells. Exosomes that are taken up are subsequently degraded by lysosomes or fused with preexisting early-sorting endosomes before disintegrating and releasing their contents into the endoplasmic reticulum and/or cytoplasm. Due to their lipid bilayer encapsulation, enzyme-sensitive molecular cargos are well preserved in exosomes [33].

Recent studies showed that exosomes play important roles in cell-cell communication and are particularly enriched in tumor microenvironment [34–36]. Among the biomolecules carried by exosomes, miRNAs are the most abundant, and have been shown to facilitate motility and invasiveness of ovarian cancer cells [37,38]. In addition, exosomes secreted by stromal cells may promote drug resistance of cancer cells [34,39,40]. One of the advantages of using miRNAs as liquid biopsy-based biomarker is that they are relatively stable in biofluids, which is particularly important because most of the specimens may not be processed immediately after collection in the clinic. Exosomal miRNAs are better protected from RNase degradation and are therefore more frequently studied as potential biomarkers than the non-exosomal circulating miRNA counterparts [41]. In this review, we focus on all the published exosomal studies so far that showed sensitivity and specificity of exosomal miRNAs in diagnosing and/or predicting the progression of EOC and its subtypes. Moreover, to address which biofluid source is suitable for circulating miRNA biomarker discovery, we summarize the reports showing differential profiles of circulating exosomal and cell-free miRNAs in different blood components (i.e., serum, plasma, platelet). As miRNAs in exosomes are only a small fraction of the entire transcriptomes, the optimal endogenous controls for expression profile normalization are still under debate, and thus we also discuss this topic in detail here. This comprehensive review of the exosomal miRNA biomarkers should provide more information for the future development of early detection biomarkers for EOCs.

3. Exosomal miRNAs as Diagnostic and Prognostic Biomarkers for EOCs

The first study that proposed the use of circulating exosomal miRNAs as diagnostic biomarkers for EOCs was published in 2008 by Taylor and Gercel-Taylor [42]. The authors identified eight exosomal miRNAs specifically up-regulated in the serum of patients with serous papillary adenocarcinoma, which is now referred to as high-grade serous carcinoma (Table 1). These eight miRNAs included the miR-200 family members (miR-200a, -200b, -200c, -141), miR-21, miR-203, miR-205 and miR-214. MiR-200c and miR-214 also showed higher expression in the patients with stage II and III disease comparing to those with stage I. The authors further concluded that since the expression of these miRNAs were similar between the ovarian tumor tissues and the circulating exosomes, miRNA profiling of the circulating exosomes could potentially be used as surrogate diagnostic markers for EOC instead of using a tissue biopsy.

Table 1. Circulating exosomal miRNAs identified as potential diagnostic biomarkers in EOCs. N/A: not available, HGSC: high-grade serous carcinoma.

References	Exosomal miRNAs	Bioliquid	Subtypes	Expression Pattern	Normalization Controls	Detection Methods
Taylor and Gercel-Taylor 2008 [42]	miR-21, miR-200a/b/c, miR-141, miR-203, miR-205, miR-214	Serum	HGSC	Up-regulated in HGSC	N/A	miRNA array
Meng et al., 2016 [43]	miR-200a/b/c miR-373	Serum	EOCs	Up-regulated in EOCs	miR-484 cel-miR-39	Taqman assay
Pan et al., 2018 [44]	miR-21 miR-100 miR-200b miR-320	Plasma	EOCs	Up-regulated in EOCs	RNU6, miR-484, cel-miR-39	Taqman assay
	miR-16 miR-93 miR-126 miR-223	Plasma	EOCs	Down-regulated in EOCs		
Kobayashi et al., 2018 [45]	miR-1290*	Serum	HGSC	Up-regulated in HGSC Down-regulated in non-HGSC	cel-miR-39	Taqman assay
Yoshimura et al., 2018 [46]	miR-99a-5p*	Serum	EOCs	Up-regulated in EOCs	N/A	Taqman assay
Kim et at., 2019 [47]	miR-145	Serum	EOCs	Up-regulated in EOCs	RNU48	Taqman assay
	miR-200c	Serum	HGSC	Up-regulated in HGSC		
	miR-21 and miR-93	Serum	non-HGSC	Up-regulated in non-HGSC		

* These exosomal miRNAs were first identified in HGSC cell lines. Circulating cell-free miRNAs were then quantified in the patient sera.

Meng et al. (2016) examined the possibility of using four circulating exosomal miRNAs in the serum to detect EOCs [43] (Table 1). The four exosomal miRNAs, miR-373 and miR-200 family members (miRNA-200a, 200b and 200c), were selected for studying as they were proposed to be associated with EOCs and breast cancers in the literature [48,49]. The authors observed significant up-regulation of the four exosomal miRNAs in EOCs as compared with benign tumors and healthy controls. However, no differential expression of the 4 miRNAs was observed in different EOC subtypes. Diagnostic performance was further tested by using each miRNA alone or by using a combination of all three miRNAs from the miR-200 family. The AUC values ranged from 0.655 to 0.914 using each miRNA and increased to 0.925 when using a model with all three miR-200 family members (Table 2). In addition, the authors found that the increased expression levels of miR-200b and miR-200c were associated with advanced stages, lymph node metastasis, high CA-125 values and a shorter overall survival, which indicates the potential of using these two miRNAs as prognostic biomarkers for disease progression. Of note, the authors also observed very low expression of the other two members of miR-200 family, i.e., miR-141 and miR-429, in EOC, which contradicts the findings in the study by Taylor and Gercel-Taylor [42].

Table 2. Sensitivity, specificity and area under the receiver operating characteristic (ROC) curve (AUC) of the circulating exosomal miRNAs used to detect epithelial ovarian cancers (EOCs) in the literature. HGSC: high-grade serous carcinoma, CCC: clear-cell carcinoma, ENC: endometroid carcinoma, MUC: mucinous carcinoma.

References	Exosomal miRNAs	Detected Subtype *	Sensitivity	Specificity	AUC	No. of Subjects
Meng et al., 2016 [43]	miR-200a	EOCs	0.839	0.900	0.914	HGSC n = 120; non-HGSC n = 15; unknown subtype n = 28; benign tumor n = 20; healthy n = 32
	miR-200b	EOCs	0.528	1.000	0.815	
	miR-200c	EOCs	0.311	1.000	0.655	
	miR-200a + b + c	EOCs	0.882	0.900	0.925	
Pan et al., 2018 [44]	miR-21	EOCs	0.610	0.820	0.740	HGSC n = 90; non-HGSC n = 13; unknown subtype n = 3; ovarian cystadenoma n = 8; healthy n = 29
	miR-100	EOCs	0.620	0.730	0.710	
	miR-200b	EOCs	0.640	0.860	0.868	
	miR-320	EOCs	0.560	0.690	0.658	
Kobayashi et al., 2018 ** [45]	miR-1290	EOCs	0.510	0.570	0.480	HGSC (n = 30); CCC (n = 18); ENC (n = 12); MUC (n = 10)
	miR-1290 + CA-125 [a]	EOCs	-	-	0.920	
	miR-1290	HGSC	0.630	0.850	0.710	
	miR-1290 + CA-125	HGSC	-	-	0.970	
	miR-1290	CCC	0.580	0.890	0.690	
	miR-1290 + CA-125	CCC	-	-	0.940	
	miR-1290	ENC	0.500	0.830	0.620	
	miR-1290 + CA-125	ENC	-	-	0.910	
	miR-1290	MUC	0.580	0.900	0.720	
	miR-1290 + CA-125	MUC	-	-	0.830	
	miR-1290	HGSC vs. non-HGSC	0.470	0.850	0.760	
	miR-1290 + CA-125 [b]	HGSC vs. non-HGSC	-	-	0.790	
Yoshimura et al., 2018 ** [46]	miR-99a-5p	EOCs	0.850	0.750	0.880	HGSC n = 32; CCC n = 15; ENC n = 9; MUC n = 6; Early stage (stage I-II) EOCs n = 31; benign tumor n = 26; healthy n = 20
	miR-99a-5p + CA-125 [c]	EOCs	-	-	0.950	
	miR-99a-5p	Early stage EOCs	0.900	0.750	0.850	
	miR-99a-5p + CA-125 [d]	Early stage EOCs	-	-	0.910	
	miR-99a-5p	EOCs vs. benign tumor	0.870	0.540	0.700	
	miR-99a-5p + CA-125 [e]	EOCs vs. benign tumor	-	-	0.810	
Kim et al., 2019 [47]	miR-21	EOCs	-	-	0.585	HGSC n = 39; non-HGSC n = 9, borderline tumor n = 10; benign ovarian cyst n = 10
	miR-93	EOCs	-	-	0.755	
	miR-145	EOCs	0.917	0.750	0.910	
	miR-145 + CA-125 [f]	EOCs	0.979	0.600	-	
	miR-200c	EOCs	0.729	0.900	0.802	
	miR-200c + CA-125 [f]	EOCs	0.938	0.700	-	
	miR-145 + miR-200c	EOCs	0.938	0.650	-	
	miR-145 + miR-200c + CA-125 [f]	EOCs	1.000	0.550	-	

* The detected group as compared with healthy controls (unless stated otherwise). ** These two studies first identified exosomal miRNAs in cell lines and then investigated the circulating cell-free miRNAs in the patient sera. [a] CA-125 alone had an AUC of 0.900; [b] CA-125 alone had an AUC of 0.690; [c] CA-125 alone had an AUC of 0.910; [d] CA-125 alone had an AUC of 0.840; [e] CA-125 alone had an AUC of 0.790; [f] CA-125 alone had an AUC of 0.801.

The same team later examined a collective list of 44 miRNAs with oncogenic or tumor suppressive function in EOC from the literature and further tested their quantities in the circulating plasma exosomes [44]. A total of 106 EOC patients, who mostly had high-grade serous carcinoma, and 29 healthy participants were compared. Among the 44 miRNAs, four (miR-21, -100, -200b and -320) were up-regulated, and four (miR-16, -93, -126 and -223) were down-regulated in the EOC cases (Table 1). The diagnostic performance using each of the four up-regulated miRNAs showed miR-200b as having the highest AUC (0.868) (Table 2). The author also pointed out some contradictory findings; although increased miR-200b expression in the circulating exosomes of EOC patients is associated with poorer prognosis [43], its overexpression in ovarian cancer cell lines resulted in reduced proliferation and increased apoptosis [50]. MiR-200b seems to have a dual role in EOC as it has been reported as having both oncogenic and tumor suppressive functions [51]. In addition, miR-200c, previously reported as having a significantly higher expression in the serum of EOC patients than in the healthy subjects [42,43], showed no significant differences between the two groups in this study.

Kobayashi et al. (2018) observed significant up-regulation of exosomal miR-1290 secreted by high-grade serous carcinoma cell lines in comparison to an immortalized normal ovarian epithelial cell line, and thus further examined the circulating cell-free miR-1290 in the serum of EOC patients [45]. A significant up-regulation of miR-1290 was observed in patients with high-grade serous carcinoma comparing to healthy controls (Table 1). The sensitivity and specificity of EOC detection were estimated in different subtypes by using miR-1290 expression level alone or in combination with CA-125. For all EOC cases and for each subtype, the AUC values ranged from 0.48 to 0.72 when using miR-1290 alone, and from 0.83 to 0.97 when using miR-1290 together with CA-125 (Table 2). Particularly, the highest AUC (0.97) obtained using the combination of miR-1290 and CA-125 belonged to the high-grade serous carcinoma subtype. Furthermore, a significantly higher expression of this miRNA in patients with high-grade serous than those with other non-high-grade serous subtypes was also observed. An AUC value of 0.79 was obtained when using a combination of miR-1290 and CA-125 to differentiate high-grade serous from other non-high-grade serous subtypes (Table 2). The authors concluded that miR-1290 can be used as a potential diagnostic biomarker for high-grade serous carcinoma.

The same group also examined the possibility of using exosomal miR-99a-5p, identified using the same method, to predict EOCs [46]. The authors further showed significant up-regulation of circulating cell-free miR-99a-5p in the serum of EOC patients as compared with patients with benign tumor or healthy subjects (Table 1). However, differences in the expression between subtypes were not observed for this miRNA. MiR-99a-5p showed sensitivity of 0.85 and specificity of 0.75 with an AUC of 0.88 for the detection of EOCs. In combination with CA-125, the AUC increased to 0.95. Even though the combination markers failed to distinguish different subtypes, it showed high accuracy in detecting EOC in the early stages (stage I-II) with an AUC of 0.91 (Table 2).

A recent study by Kim et al. hypothesized that the dysregulation of miRNAs in the EOC tissues should also be observed in the circulating exosomes [47]. The authors, thus, selected seven candidate miRNAs, namely miRNA-21, -93, -141, -145, -200a, -200b and -200c, which are either up-regulated of down-regulated in the EOC tissues (mostly high-grade serous subtypes) from the literature [52–55]. Using real-time quantitative PCR, they observed significant up-regulation of exosomal miR-21, -93, -145 and -200c in the serum of EOC patients comparing to subjects with benign or borderline tumor (Table 1). Furthermore, up-regulation of miR-21 and -93 was specific in non-high-grade serous subtypes, while high miR-200c expression was specific in high-grade serous carcinoma. Among the four exosomal miRNAs, two demonstrated good EOC-detecting accuracy with miR-145 showing 91.7% sensitivity, 75% specificity and an AUC of 0.910, and miR-200c showing 72.9% sensitivity, 90% specificity and an AUC of 0.802. (Table 2). Different combinations of the two miRNAs with or without CA-125 improved sensitivity but showed lower specificity to detect EOCs (Table 2). Therefore, the author proposed that using exosomal miR-145 alone might be the most promising diagnostic biomarker for EOCs.

In addition, they also found that up-regulation of miR-145 and -21 were significantly associated with distant metastasis in high-grade serous carcinoma patients.

Multiple studies suggested that miR-200c maybe a promising biomarker for detecting EOC, and it is also the most dysregulated miRNA in the circulatory system [56,57]. However, it showed high specificity to high-grade serous carcinoma, but lacked the power to distinguish between different subtypes of EOCs. The other members of miR-200 family including miR-200a and miR-200b, showed incongruent results in different studies. The two miRNAs were observed to be up-regulated in high-grade serous carcinoma in two studies [42,44], but were found to be lowly expressed in all subtypes in another study [47]. The inconsistency may result from different ethnic populations (Caucasians and Asians), or from different sources of exosomes (serum vs. plasma). This raises important concerns for identifying biomarkers used in liquid biopsy; different ethnic populations and different sources of biofluid for biomarker identification should always be taken into consideration when comparing the studies and analyzing the results.

The candidate exosomal miRNAs reviewed in this article were selected either based on the miRNA profiles in tumors [43,44,47] or by exosomes secreted by cancer cell lines [45,46]. They were not identified by large-scale screening of exosomal miRNAs in patient subjects. It is known that the expression of miRNAs in tumor tissues may not be consistent with the expression of circulating exosomal miRNAs [58,59]. For example, miR-145 has been reported to be significantly down-regulated in EOC tissues, particularly in high-grade serous carcinoma [52–55]. However, it is significantly up-regulated in the serum exosomes of EOC patients [47]. This indicates that there may be undiscovered selecting and sorting mechanisms, which control the encapsulation of specific miRNAs into exosomes before they are released to the tumor microenvironment for cell-cell communication [59–61]. Taken together, the optimal biofluid source, the availability of large case-control cohorts and the independent validation cohorts preferably with a substantial mixture of different ethnic population are required for the successful clinical translation of circulating exosomal miRNA biomarkers. Moreover, the high-throughput exosome isolation technology that can accurately capture circulating exosomes in a faster timeframe would greatly expedite the development of translational applications of exosome.

4. Circulating Exosomal miRNA and Cell-Free miRNA Expression Profiles in Different Blood-Based Sources

Plasma and serum are major biofluid sources in biobank repositories worldwide, which provide the most important resources for biomarker identification. As we mentioned in the previous section, the incongruence of reported exosomal miRNA expression may result from the use of different exosome sources (serum vs. plasma). In addition, the differences in the expression profiles of exosomal miRNAs and circulating cell-free miRNAs (cf-miRNA) between different sources have not yet been extensively reviewed. In this section, we focus on the literature that compared the expression patterns of exosomal miRNA and cf-miRNA between serum and plasma. We also discuss two studies that analyze miRNA profiles in the platelets, as there is increasing evidence that platelets are important sources of biomarkers, particularly for the diseases related to platelet dysfunctions, such as cancers [62–64].

Plasma and serum possess fundamental differences due to their distinct collection processes. Blood tubes for plasma collection contain EDTA to prevent coagulation. In addition, most biobanks collect plasma by centrifugation at high speed for a long period of time, i.e., at 1000–2000× g for 10–15 min, to separate cells and biofluid. As a result, the platelets are mixed with buffy coat layer (white blood cell layer) due to the high-speed centrifugation, and we are left with platelet-poor-plasma. For serum collection, blood tubes contain clot-activator, which result in the activation of platelets and the releasing of biological molecules, such as protein, DNA, RNA and microparticles (also known as extracellular vesicles), during the coagulation process [65]. Thus, the slightly different yet important fraction of exosomes related to platelet function may be found in serum, but not in plasma. This fact emphasizes the importance of exosome source selection for biomarker identification.

Hemolysis is one of the important confounding factors in cell-free miRNA biomarker discovery and may also affect the clinical interpretation if the hemolysis-susceptible miRNAs are used as a diagnostic/prognostic marker [66]. Several miRNAs have been used as potential indicators to evaluate hemolysis as they are relatively stable across all sources (e.g., miR-23a), or enriched in red blood cells (RBC) (e.g., miR-144, -16, -451, -486 and -92a) and in white blood cells (WBC) or platelets (e.g., let-7a, miR-150, -197, -199a, -223 and -574) [67–69]. Particularly, miR-223 is proposed to be abundantly released by activated platelets [70]. Juzenas et al. (2017) comprehensively analyzed the miRNA expression profiles from seven types of peripheral blood cells, serum, serum exosomes and whole blood [68]. They compared miRNAs in RBC, exosomal miRNAs and cf-miRNAs in serum, and suggested that the miRNAs commonly used as RBC-specific markers can also be found in exosomes or serum. For example, miR-16-5p and -451a apparently could be found across RBC, exosomes and serum, and thus their roles as hemolysis indicator may need to be reconsidered. Other markers such as miR-144-3p were found in RBC and exosomes but was absent in serum, while miR-144-5p could only be found in RBC but not in exosomes and serum. Based on the results of this study, several miRNAs were RBC-specific, including miR-142-3p, -454-3p, -19a-3p, -15b-3p and -421. In addition to using RBC-specific miRNAs to evaluate hemolysis effect, one study has suggested that the ratio between miR-23a and miR-451 can be an indicator of possible RBC lysis, which results in much higher concentration of miR-451 in the plasma and serum [67]. However, it is relatively difficult to define an optimal cutoff value for interpreting the extent of hemolysis.

One of the first studies published in 2008 by Hunter et al. first examined the expression of miRNAs in exosomes isolated in plasma and matched peripheral blood mononuclear cells (PBMC) from 51 healthy subjects [71]. The expression profiles of a total of 420 miRNAs were examined by reverse transcription quantitative real-time PCR (RT-qPCR). Among those, the authors identified miR-223 to be the most abundant miRNAs in both exosome and PBMC. The results showed that a quantity of miR-223 are more than 10 times higher than the second most abundant miRNA, miR-484, in both sources. The authors further compared the miRNA profiles in platelets isolated from 6 donors and in plasma-derived exosomes. Interestingly, miR-223 is also the most abundant miRNA in platelets, while one of the most abundant miRNAs, miR-484, was not detected in the platelets (Table 3).

Wang et al. (2012) published a comprehensive study not only compared the amount of cf-miRNAs in different blood-based sources, but also compared them using different probe-based RT-qPCR technologies, i.e., Taqman and LNA (locked nucleic acid) [72]. Even though the study did not analyze miRNA profiles in exosomes, the results are informative and can be a reference for comparing source-specific cf-miRNA and exosomal miRNA profiles. A total of 6 healthy donors were recruited and the cf-miRNA profiles in their plasma, serum, platelets and blood cells (RBC and WBC) were analyzed by either both or only one technique. Overall, the study showed that although the serum and plasma shared cf-miRNA contents, the profiles are different between the two sources (Table 3). Furthermore, the results between the two qPCR platforms showed low consistency (Table 3), probably because of the different pre-amplification steps. In line with other studies, miR-223 is the most abundant cf-miRNAs across various blood-based sources. The authors observed higher RNA concentration in serum than plasma and suggested that RNA/miRNAs may be released from blood cells and platelets into serum during coagulation process. Therefore, plasma may be the sample of choice when studying circulating cf-miRNAs, as RNA released during the coagulation process may change the true cf-miRNA repertoire.

Table 3. Exosomal miRNAs and circulating cell-free miRNAs showing differential expression between various bioliquid sources. N/A: not available.

Reference	Analytes	miRNA Sources	miRNAs	Detection Techniques	Normalization Controls	Contamination Indicators
Hunter et al., 2008 [71]	Exosomal miRNAs	Plasma	Higher in exosomes: miR-486, 328, 183, 32, 574, 27b, 222, 197, 151, 199a, 133b, 320, 96, 103, 17-5p	RT-qPCR panel (420 miRNAs)	RNU38B, RNU43, U6, 5S and 18S rRNA	N/A
		PBMC	Higher in PBMC: miR-150, 29a, 142-3p, 146b, 155, 532, 19a, 140, 21, 374, 181d, 345, let-7g, 15a, 19b, 142-5p, 106b, 26b, 195			
		Platelets	Most abundant miRNA: miR-223 (Note: miR-484 is not detected)			
Wang et al., 2012 [72]	Circulating cell-free miRNAs	Plasma	Most abundant in plasma: Taqman: miR-126, 146a, 150, 19b, 222, 223, 451, 617, 92a Exiqon: miR-15a, 16, 19b, 1974, 21, 223, 451, 486-5p, 92a	RT-qPCR (Taqman and Exiqon)	U6, RNU44 and RNU48	miR-150 as WBC lysis indicator; miR-16 as RBC lysis indicator; miR-126 as platelet activation indicator
		Serum	Most abundant in serum: Taqman: miR-17, 146a, 19b, 223, 24, 451, 519c, 92a Exiqon: miR-16, 126, 142-3p, 19b, 1974, 223, 451, 92a, 486-5p, 720			
		Platelets	Most abundant in platelet: Exiqon: miR-126, 16, 142-3p, 19b, 21, 223, 451			
		Plasma and serum	Most abundant in both plasma and serum: miR-126-3p, 16-5p, 191-5p, 223-3p, 451a, 484, 486-5p			
Cheng et al., 2014 [73]	Exosomal miRNAs	Plasma	Specific in plasma [a]: miR-664a-5p, 654-5p, 3620-3p, 4446-3p, 877-5p	Next-generation sequencing (NGS)	Reads per million mapped reads (RPM)	N/A
		Serum	Specific in serum [a]: miR-196b-5p, 502-3p, 16-2-3p, 550a-5p, 1180, -7-5p, 4732-5p, 532-3p, 204-5p, 942, 183-5p, 629-5p, 214-3p, 1292-5p, 550a-3p, 550b-2-5p, 500a-3p			

Table 3. Cont.

Reference	Analytes	miRNA Sources	miRNAs	Detection Techniques	Normalization Controls	Contamination Indicators
Blondal et al., 2013 [67]	Circulating cell-free miRNAs	Plasma and serum	119 miRNAs are found in both plasma and serum. Please see Appendix A in Blondal et al., 2013.	RT-qPCR (Exiqon)	Exiqon RNA spike-in kit	miR-23a-3p: stability indicator; miR-451: RBC lysis indicator
Ammerlaan and Betsou 2016 [74]	Circulating cell-free miRNAs	Plasma	Stably expressed in plasma: Let-7e*, miR-100, 105*, 106b*, 1228*, 1288, 1469, 150*, 1538, 183, 19b-1*, 3193, 320c, 342-3p, 342-5p, 3652, 3918, 3937, 4325, 503, 664, 92b*, 939, 99a	SmartChip Human miRNA Panel V3.0 (WaferGen)	Spike-in kit (WaferGen)	N/A
		Serum	Stably expressed in serum: Let-7d*, miR-106b*, 1231, 1237, 1273c, 1285, 1294, 1306, 142-5p, 155, 222, 29b, 302d*, 31, 3180-3p, 3192, 3652, 370, 371-5p, 423-3p, 4252, 4278, 4286, 4297, 503, 543, 611, 675, 873, 99a			
Foye et al., 2017 [75]	Circulating cell-free miRNAs	Plasma and serum	Most abundant in both serum and plasma: miR-128-1-5p, 19b-3p, 26a-5p, 302a-5p, 543, 544, 548g-3p, 585-3p, 6721-5p
Most dysregulated between serum and plasma: Let-7b-5p, miR-126-3p, 144-3p, 16-5p, 191-5p, 223-3p, 25-3p, 451a, 4454 + 7975, 873-3p	NanoString Human miRNA panel	Background subtraction and total mean normalization	miR-24-5p as WBC lysis indicator; miR-16-5p and miR-15b-3p as RBC lysis indicator [b]
Max et al., 2018 [76]	Circulating cell-free miRNAs	Plasma	Top 10 up-regulated in plasma: miR-144, 16-2 *, 18b, 3158, 3200, 451, 4685, 486, 517a, 550-1-3p	NGS	DESeq2 normalization	RBC-enriched miR-144, 451 and 486 are higher in plasma, and the platelet and PBMC-enriched miR-223 and 199a-5p are higher in serum.
		Serum	Top 10 up-regulated in serum: miR-223, 2355-5p, 411, 432, 487b, 493-5p, 495, 543, 582, 889			

* Indicates the opposite arm of the predominant miRNAs. [a] Results from further analysis by the authors of this review article. [b] Foye et al. identified higher WBC contamination in plasma.

Cheng et al. (2014) aimed to compare the profiles of intracellular miRNAs from peripheral blood cells, and cf-miRNAs and exosomal miRNAs in serum and plasma [73]. Exosomes were further isolated using differential ultracentrifugation (UC) or by commercial exosomal miRNA isolation kits (Norgen Biotek), and miRNAs were analyzed by next generation sequencing (NGS). For plasma, the UC protocol was superior to the commercial exosome isolation column as it did not pellet non-exosomal RNA or cellular RNA contaminants. The commercial kit performed better with serum samples and showed the same RNA profile as those observed in UC-isolated serum exosomes. This finding underscores the importance of standardizing sample collection, centrifugation of blood and handling for exosomal miRNA research. Overall, the results showed that miR-451a and miR-223-3p are the most abundant miRNAs across all samples for both cf-miRNAs and exosomal miRNAs isolated by different methods in plasma and serum. The other abundant miRNAs included miR-191-5p, -486-5p, 484, -16-5p, -126-3p. The authors also compared intracellular miRNAs profiles with those of the cell-free blood and exosomes to identify the unique miRNAs in each group for serum or plasma samples. Interestingly, not only exosomal miRNAs were resistant to RNaseA treatment, but there were also more miRNAs stably present in exosomes compared with cell-free fractions. Hence, the authors concluded that exosomes provide a good protection to miRNAs and therefore appear to be a better source for biomarker identification. Of note, as the authors did not perform exosomal miRNA profile comparison between serum and plasma, we, thus, carried out this analysis based on their results using the same inclusion criteria (miRNAs with mean reads per million (RPM) larger or equals to five). There are 5 and 17 exosomal miRNAs specifically found in plasma and serum, respectively (Table 3).

Other studies also identified miRNAs commonly seen in serum and plasma by using different platforms [67,74–76] including using Nanostring system, which performs quantification by digital counting of RNA molecules without PCR amplifications [75] (Table 3). Unfortunately, these studies only compared cf-miRNAs but not exosomal miRNAs. Of note, one of the studies identified that the abundant RBC-enriched miR-144, 451 and 486 were prevalent in plasma, while the platelet and PBMC-enriched miR-223 and 199a-5p were prevalent in serum [76]. Since biological diversity between patients may contribute to low reproducibility of miRNA profile, this study also investigated the effect of gender, fasting state and menstrual cycle on cf-miRNA levels in serum and plasma and concluded that these factors do not significantly affect cf-miRNA profiles and need not be controlled for [76].

In sum, the advantage of using exosomal miRNAs as biomarkers are that they are more stable in archival blood-based biospecimens (i.e., serum and plasma in biobanks) and resistant to ribonuclease degradation. No consensus has yet emerged on which specimen source is best for exosome work. On the contrary, in order to avoid miRNA contamination from blood cells, the specimen of choice for circulating cf-miRNA biomarker discovery is platelet-depleted plasma generated immediately after blood collection.

5. Concerns Regarding Endogenous Controls for Exosomal and Cell-Free miRNA Biomarkers

Reference genes/miRNAs have two main purposes: for evaluating techniques of miRNAs isolation as they are usually in a very small amount especially in cell-free blood or in the exosomes (spike-in or exogenous controls), and for normalization of expression levels across samples (endogenous controls). The most commonly used spike-in control is a miRNA from *Caenorhabditis elegans*, cel-mir-39, and it is added into the specimen lysate. The quantity of cel-mir-39 can help identify whether the isolation procedures is successful and consistent between samples. The most commonly used endogenous controls for circulating cf-miRNA are small nuclear and nucleolar RNA, such as U6, RNU44, RNU43 and RNU48 [77].

It is worth noting that the literature reviewed above used different reference genes for normalizing expression levels of exosomal and cf-miRNAs, implying that the selection of appropriate reference genes has not yet been standardized (Tables 1 and 3). It is particularly challenging to identify suitable reference genes for exosomes in different blood-based sources. Several studies identified most stable miRNAs for either cell-free or exosomal miRNAs, which may serve as reference genes in different specimen sources, using various platforms [67,75,78]. However, to use one or a set of miRNAs as universal reference genes for either cell-free and exosomal miRNAs are still under debate. One study using RT-qPCR platform proposed the use of cf-miR-23a as reference as it was relatively stable in plasma and serum and was not affected by hemolysis [67], while the other study using NanoString platform found that cf-miR-30e-5p is the most stable miRNA in both serum and plasma [75]. Gouin et al. applied two different platforms, namely NGS and NanoString miRNA panels, to identify the most stable exosomal miRNAs secreted by cardiosphere-derived cells from healthy donors [78]. Using a combination of four different algorithms (NormFinder, GeNorm, BestKeeper and delta Ct), the authors identified that exosomal miR-23a-3p was present and stably expressed across all samples. They further suggested that a combination of multiple exosomal miRNAs, including miR-23a-3p, miR-101-3p and miR-26a-5p, may yield stronger reference for normalization. Even though multiple studies showed the stability of miR-23a expression in both cf-miRNA and exosomal miRNA fractions, its stability may vary based on different types of tissue or cells that secrete exosomes. In a more recent study, Dai et al. combined RNA sequencing (RNA-Seq) data of exosomes in serum from three different cancer types (pancreatic adenocarcinoma, colorectal carcinoma and hepatocellular carcinoma) and from healthy donors to identify the most stable exosomal miRNAs across samples [79]. The candidate exosomal miRNAs were further verified in serum exosomes of EOC patients. Six exosomal miRNAs were observed to be stably expressed in the discovery cohort (pooled cancers and healthy donors) and validation cohort (EOCs). They are miR-125-5p, miR-192-3p, miR-4468, miR-4469, miR-6731-5p and miR-6835-3p. Among the six exosomal miRNAs, the combination of miR-4468 and miR-6835-3p gave the highest expression stability in both cohorts. It is worth mentioning that two exosomal miRNAs studies in EOC patients chose to use miR-484 over U6 as endogenous controls [43,44] (Table 1). Our preliminary unpublished data also showed that serum exosomal miR-484 has the smallest variation across healthy subjects, patients with benign tumors and patients with EOC. Furthermore, exosomal miR-484 has been used as endogenous control in the serum of breast cancer patients as well [48].

Taken together, we conclude that circulating exosomal and cf-miRNA profiles can be affected by many factors. These factors include individual genetic variations, specimen sources, various preanalytical factors including the extent of hemolysis, miRNA isolation protocols, different detection platforms (e.g., RT-qPCR, NanoString or NGS) or different qPCR techniques (e.g., Taqman and LNA assays), and the selection of reference genes. In order to be able to implement exosomal or cf-miRNA biomarkers in clinical setting, these factors will need to be carefully considered and standardized. Thorough evaluations of contamination of miRNAs from disrupted blood cells is suggested before using the data for biomarker identification. Finding a suitable set of standard reference genes for each specific setting remain one of the most challenging tasks for now.

6. Summary of Current Clinical Trials Using miRNAs as Biomarkers in Epithelial Ovarian Cancer

We explore clinical trials registered during years 2016–2021 in ClinicalTrials.gov by using key words "miRNA" or "microRNA" and set the disease to "ovarian cancer". A total of 12 projects were identified by the keyword search. Among these, only six trials are related to EOC. Two studies led by the same team in China, NCT03738319 and NCT03742856, are recruiting EOC patients for studying circulating exosomal miRNAs and long noncoding RNAs (lncRNA), and multi-omics analysis, respectively (Table 4). For NCT03738319, which focuses on identifying differential expression of exosomal miRNAs and lncRNAs in EOC patients, the team only recruit patients with high-grade serous carcinoma. The first stage aims to recruit 20 patients with high-grade serous carcinoma and 20 participants with benign gynecologic disease for prediction model construction. The second stage aims to recruit 120 participants with suspected high-grade serous carcinoma for validation. For multi-omics study (EOC subtype not specified), the trial plans to conduct whole-exome sequencing, transcriptome sequencing as well as obtaining data from proteomics and metabolomics studies. Of note, the status of these two trials is currently listed as "unknown".

Table 4. Summary of current clinical trials related to epithelial ovarian cancer that use miRNAs in the circulatory system or tissues as biomarkers. FIGO: Federation of Gynecology and Obstetrics.

NCT Number *	Study Title	EOC Subtype	Specimen	Expected Outcome **
NCT02758652	Molecular Mechanisms Leading to Chemoresistance in Epithelial Ovarian Cancer (CHEMOVA)	Not specified	Plasma	miRNA expression profiles of ovarian cancer patients in 5 years of trial period
NCT03776630	Exploring the Potential of Novel Biomarkers Based on Plasma microRNAs for a Better Management of Pelvic Gynecologic Tumors (GYNO-MIR)	Not specified	Plasma	To validate the previous finding on the prognostic value of the pre-/post-treatment variation of miR-200b concentrations in plasma with regards to progression-free survival (PFS)
NCT01391351	Search for predictors of therapeutic response in ovarian carcinoma	Not specified	Serum	Identify predictors of response to chemotherapy in ovarian carcinoma patients using the miRNA profile in serum before chemotherapy treatment
NCT03738319	Non-coding RNA in the exosomes of epithelial ovarian cancer	High-grade serous	Blood	Identify miRNA and lncRNA in exosomes of high-grade serous carcinoma as detection and prognostic biomarkers
NCT03742856	A Multi-omics Study of Epithelial Ovarian Cancer	Not specified	Blood and cancer tissue	The alteration of RNA expression, including mRNA, miRNA and lncRNA, will be compared between patients of different FIGO stages and different pathological subtypes
NCT03877796	Clinical Pre-screening Protocol for Ovarian Cancer	Not specified	FFPE tissue block	Identification of ovarian cancer patients with high likelihood of being sensitive to investigational cancer drug based on FFPE ovarian cancer tissue (Drug Response Predictor® (DRP))

* Registered data between 2016–2021 was last extracted from https://clinicaltrials.gov/, accessed on 3 July 2021. ** Only outcomes related to the use of miRNA expression as biomarkers are listed.

The other three clinical trials focus on the drug resistance and treatment response (Table 4). NCT02758652 aims to collect plasma, urine and tumor tissues from EOC patients to elucidate the expression profiles of miRNA. The results will be correlated with treatment responses, progression-free survival (PFS) and overall survival (OS) rate. NCT01391351 aims to search for predictors of therapeutic response, particularly for the combination of Taxol and Carboplatin or the combination of Taxol, carboplatin and avastin. MiRNA expression levels of the enrolled patients will be measured in serum on day 1 of receiving each course of treatment or before surgery. The ovarian cancer arm of NCT03776630 focuses on validating the prognostic value of plasma miR200b with regards to PFS after up-front or post-chemotherapy debulking and adjuvant chemotherapy. The last active clinical trial, NCT03877796, aims to verify a current commercial artificial intelligence (AI) algorithm, Drug Response Predictor (DRP), in EOC by using miRNAs from the formalin-fixed, paraffin-embedded (FFPE) tissue samples of patients to predict their response to investigational cancer drugs (Table 4).

7. Conclusions and Future Perspectives

In this review, we focus on the literature that observed significant dysregulation of exosomal miRNAs in EOC and showed the estimation of their sensitivities, specificities and AUC values in detecting EOC or the specific subtypes. We then discuss in detail about the factors that may influence the reproducibility of circulating exosomal and cf-miRNA biomarkers including the selection of biofluid source and normalization reference genes. However, we have noticed that the majority of published articles selected candidate exosomal miRNAs from the literature. The candidate exosomal miRNAs were not identified using a comprehensive screening of large number of miRNAs, which may require high-throughput deep sequencing technology, to acquire the complete catalogue of circulating exosomal miRNAs in EOC patients. A study by Elias et al. [80] is the first to combine NGS analysis of serum circulating cf-miRNA with machine learning techniques, namely a neural network model, to develop a diagnostic algorithm for EOC. This model, which had the AUC value of 0.90, significantly outperformed CA-125 and functioned well regardless of patient age, histology or stage; thus, ushering in the new era of machine-learning-driven biomarker discovery. Multiple studies have used machine learning algorithms to increase the prediction robustness of their miRNA prognostic biomarkers for EOC since then [81–83]. So far, the published candidate exosomal miRNA markers are mainly tested in the general EOC patients or only in high-grade serous carcinoma subtype, likely because it has the highest incidence. The other subtypes are gaining more attention lately because some of them show particularly higher prevalence in certain populations, i.e., clear-cell carcinoma has higher incidence in Asians than in Caucasians. Clear-cell carcinoma is also more resistant to chemotherapy, resulting in a higher mortality rate in general. Therefore, a set of exosomal miRNA biomarkers showing high sensitivity and specificity for every subtype would be highly beneficial.

Future work to accelerate the clinical application of exosomal miRNAs markers for early detection of EOCs may include: (1) using a larger cohort with adequate numbers of subjects for each subtype to provide a more powerful prediction accuracy; (2) recruiting subjects from different ethnic groups as EOC subtypes show various incidences in different populations; (3) the development of consensus protocols for biofluid (serum and plasma) collection, processing and long-term storage; (4) using the standardized high-throughput exosomal miRNA isolation, characterization and profiling platforms to better understand the biology underlying exosomal miRNAs; and (5) using multiple machine learning algorithms to identify candidates in different subtypes. With these solutions, we hope a prediction model for circulating exosomal miRNAs that can accurately diagnose EOC at an early stage can be realized in the near future.

Author Contributions: M.-S.S., J.-M.C., A.-A.L., N.R. and N.J. reviewed the literature and wrote the manuscript. All authors have read and agreed to the published version of the manuscript.

Funding: M.-S.S. is supported by New Researcher Grant Mahidol University (Fiscal Year 2561), Ministry of Science and Technology, Taiwan (108-2621-B-110-003-MY3). J.-M.C. is supported by Ministry of Science and Technology, Taiwan (108-2628-E-004-001-MY3). N.J. is supported by the government research grants managed by the Health Systems Research Institute (HSRI) (#HSRI 63-136 & 63-140), and the mid-career research grant joint-funded by the National Research Council of Thailand (NRCT) and Mahidol University (N41A640161).

Institutional Review Board Statement: Not applicable.

Informed Consent Statement: Not applicable.

Data Availability Statement: All the articles cited in this review can be found in Pubmed (https://pubmed.ncbi.nlm.nih.gov/ accessed on 3 July 2021).

Acknowledgments: We thank Artit Jinawath for his valuable input. We also thank the members of the Ramathibodi Tumor Biobank for their technical support.

Conflicts of Interest: The authors declare no conflict of interest.

References

1. Sung, H.; Ferlay, J.; Siegel, R.L.; Laversanne, M.; Soerjomataram, I.; Jemal, A.; Bray, F. Global Cancer Statistics 2020: GLOBOCAN Estimates of Incidence and Mortality Worldwide for 36 Cancers in 185 Countries. *CA Cancer J. Clin.* **2021**, *71*, 209–249. [CrossRef]
2. Siegel, R.L.; Mph, K.D.M.; Jemal, A. Cancer statistics. *CA Cancer J. Clin.* **2020**, *70*, 7–30. [CrossRef]
3. Kurman, R.J.; Carcangiu, M.L.; Herrington, C.S.; Young, R.H. (Eds.) *WHO Classification of Tumors of the Female Reproductive Organs*; World Health Organization: Washington, DC, USA, 2014.
4. Herrington, C.S.; McCluggage, W.G. The emerging role of the distal Fallopian tube and p53 in pelvic serous carcinogenesis. *J. Pathol.* **2009**, *220*, 5–6. [CrossRef]
5. Kindelberger, D.W.; Lee, Y.; Miron, A.; Hirsch, M.S.; Feltmate, C.; Medeiros, F.; Callahan, M.J.; Garner, E.O.; Gordon, R.W.; Birch, C.; et al. Intraepithelial Carcinoma of the Fimbria and Pelvic Serous Carcinoma: Evidence for a Causal Relationship. *Am. J. Surg. Pathol.* **2007**, *31*, 161–169. [CrossRef]
6. Lee, Y.; Medeiros, F.; Kindelberger, D.; Callahan, M.J.; Muto, M.G.; Crum, C.P. Advances in the Recognition of Tubal Intraepithelial Carcinoma. *Adv. Anat. Pathol.* **2006**, *13*, 1–7. [CrossRef]
7. Koshiyama, M.; Matsumura, N.; Konishi, I. Recent Concepts of Ovarian Carcinogenesis: Type I and Type II. *BioMed Res. Int.* **2014**, *2014*, 1–11. [CrossRef]
8. Koshiyama, M.; Matsumura, N.; Konishi, I. Subtypes of Ovarian Cancer and Ovarian Cancer Screening. *Diagnostics* **2017**, *7*, 12. [CrossRef]
9. Shih, I.-M.; Kurman, R.J. Ovarian Tumorigenesis: A proposed model based on morphological and molecular genetic analysis. *Am. J. Pathol.* **2004**, *164*, 1511–1518. [CrossRef]
10. Kurman, R.J.; Shih, I.-M. The Dualistic Model of Ovarian Carcinogenesis: Revisited, Revised, and Expanded. *Am. J. Pathol.* **2016**, *186*, 733–747. [CrossRef]
11. Van Zyl, B.; Tang, D.; Bowden, N.A. Biomarkers of platinum resistance in ovarian cancer: What can we use to improve treatment. *Endocr.-Relat. Cancer* **2018**, *25*, R303–R318. [CrossRef]
12. Köbel, M.; Kalloger, S.E.; Boyd, N.; McKinney, S.; Mehl, E.; Palmer, C.; Leung, S.; Bowen, N.; Ionescu, D.N.; Rajput, A.; et al. Ovarian Carcinoma Subtypes Are Different Diseases: Implications for Biomarker Studies. *PLoS Med.* **2008**, *5*, e232. [CrossRef] [PubMed]
13. Köbel, M.; Luo, L.; Grevers, X.; Lee, S.; Brooks-Wilson, A.; Gilks, C.B.; Le, N.D.; Cook, L.S. Ovarian Carcinoma Histotype: Strengths and Limitations of Integrating Morphology with Immunohistochemical Predictions. *Int. J. Gynecol. Pathol.* **2019**, *38*, 353–362. [CrossRef] [PubMed]
14. Köbel, M.; Rahimi, K.; Rambau, P.F.; Naugler, C.; Le Page, C.; Meunier, L.; De Ladurantaye, M.; Lee, S.; Leung, S.; Goode, E.L.; et al. An Immunohistochemical Algorithm for Ovarian Carcinoma Typing. *Int. J. Gynecol. Pathol.* **2016**, *35*, 430–441. [CrossRef]
15. The Cancer Genome Atlas Research Network Integrated genomic analyses of ovarian carcinoma. *Nature* **2011**, *474*, 609–615. [CrossRef]
16. Tsang, Y.T.; Deavers, M.T.; Sun, C.C.; Kwan, S.-Y.; Kuo, E.; Malpica, A.; Mok, S.C.; Gershenson, D.M.; Wong, K.-K. KRAS (but not BRAF) mutations in ovarian serous borderline tumour are associated with recurrent low-grade serous carcinoma. *J. Pathol.* **2013**, *231*, 449–456. [CrossRef]
17. McCluggage, W.G. Morphological subtypes of ovarian carcinoma: A review with emphasis on new developments and pathogenesis. *Pathology* **2011**, *43*, 420–432. [CrossRef]
18. Nezhat, F.; Datta, M.S.; Hanson, V.; Pejovic, T.; Nezhat, C.; Nezhat, C. The relationship of endometriosis and ovarian malignancy: A review. *Fertil. Steril.* **2008**, *90*, 1559–1570. [CrossRef]

19. McConechy, M.K.; Ding, J.; Senz, J.; Yang, W.; Melnyk, N.; Tone, A.A.; Prentice, L.M.; Wiegand, K.C.; McAlpine, J.N.; Shah, S.P.; et al. Ovarian and endometrial endometrioid carcinomas have distinct CTNNB1 and PTEN mutation profiles. *Mod. Pathol.* **2013**, *27*, 128–134. [CrossRef]
20. Samartzis, E.P.; Noske, A.; Dedes, K.J.; Fink, D.; Imesch, P. ARID1A Mutations and PI3K/AKT Pathway Alterations in Endometriosis and Endometriosis-Associated Ovarian Carcinomas. *Int. J. Mol. Sci.* **2013**, *14*, 18824–18849. [CrossRef]
21. Wiegand, K.C.; Shah, S.P.; Al-Agha, O.M.; Zhao, Y.; Tse, K.; Zeng, T.; Senz, J.; McConechy, M.K.; Anglesio, M.S.; Kalloger, S.E.; et al. ARID1AMutations in Endometriosis-Associated Ovarian Carcinomas. *New Engl. J. Med.* **2010**, *363*, 1532–1543. [CrossRef]
22. Cochrane, D.R.; Tessier-Cloutier, B.; Lawrence, K.M.; Nazeran, T.; Karnezis, A.N.; Salamanca, C.; Cheng, A.S.; McAlpine, J.N.; Hoang, L.N.; Gilks, C.B.; et al. Clear cell and endometrioid carcinomas: Are their differences attributable to distinct cells of origin? *J. Pathol.* **2017**, *243*, 26–36. [CrossRef] [PubMed]
23. Gemignani, M.L.; Schlaerth, A.C.; Bogomolniy, F.; Barakat, R.R.; Lin, O.; Soslow, R.; Venkatraman, E.; Boyd, J. Role of KRAS and BRAF gene mutations in mucinous ovarian carcinoma. *Gynecol. Oncol.* **2003**, *90*, 378–381. [CrossRef]
24. Mackenzie, R.; Kommoss, S.; Winterhoff, B.J.; Kipp, B.R.; Garcia, J.J.; Voss, J.; Halling, K.; Karnezis, A.; Senz, J.; Yang, W.; et al. Targeted deep sequencing of mucinous ovarian tumors reveals multiple overlapping RAS-pathway activating mutations in borderline and cancerous neoplasms. *BMC Cancer* **2015**, *15*, 1–10. [CrossRef]
25. Rechsteiner, M.; Zimmermann, A.-K.; Wild, P.J.; Caduff, R.; von Teichman, A.; Fink, D.; Moch, H.; Noske, A. TP53 mutations are common in all subtypes of epithelial ovarian cancer and occur concomitantly with KRAS mutations in the mucinous type. *Exp. Mol. Pathol.* **2013**, *95*, 235–241. [CrossRef]
26. Teer, J.K.; Yoder, S.; Gjyshi, A.; Nicosia, S.V.; Zhang, C.; Monteiro, A.N.A. Mutational heterogeneity in non-serous ovarian cancers. *Sci. Rep.* **2017**, *7*, 9728. [CrossRef]
27. Vereczkey, I.; Serester, O.; Dobos, J.; Gallai, M.; Szakacs, O.; Szentirmay, Z.; Toth, E. Molecular Characterization of 103 Ovarian Serous and Mucinous Tumors. *Pathol. Oncol. Res.* **2010**, *17*, 551–559. [CrossRef] [PubMed]
28. Poveda, A.; Romero, I. Advanced ovarian cancer: 20 years of ovarian cancer treatment. *Ann. Oncol.* **2016**, *27*, i72–i73. [CrossRef]
29. Menon, U.; Gentry-Maharaj, A.; Burnell, M.; Singh, N.; Ryan, A.; Karpinskyj, C.; Carlino, G.; Taylor, J.; Massingham, S.K.; Raikou, M.; et al. Ovarian cancer population screening and mortality after long-term follow-up in the UK Collaborative Trial of Ovarian Cancer Screening (UKCTOCS): A randomised controlled trial. *Lancet* **2021**, *397*, 2182–2193. [CrossRef]
30. Bristow, R.E.; Smith, A.; Zhang, Z.; Chan, D.W.; Crutcher, G.; Fung, E.T.; Munroe, D.G. Ovarian malignancy risk stratification of the adnexal mass using a multivariate index assay. *Gynecol. Oncol.* **2013**, *128*, 252–259. [CrossRef]
31. Coleman, R.L.; Herzog, T.J.; Chan, D.W.; Munroe, D.G.; Pappas, T.C.; Smith, A.; Zhang, Z.; Wolf, J. Validation of a second-generation multivariate index assay for malignancy risk of adnexal masses. *Am. J. Obstet. Gynecol.* **2016**, *215*, 82.e1. [CrossRef] [PubMed]
32. Pegtel, D.M.; Gould, S.J. Exosomes. *Annu. Rev. Biochem.* **2019**, *88*, 487–514. [CrossRef]
33. Kalluri, R.; LeBleu, V.S. The biology, function, and biomedical applications of exosomes. *Science* **2020**, *367*, eaau6977. [CrossRef]
34. Wendler, F.; Favicchio, R.; Simon, T.; Alifrangis, C.; Stebbing, J.; Giamas, G. Extracellular vesicles swarm the cancer microenvironment: From tumor–stroma communication to drug intervention. *Oncogene* **2016**, *36*, 877–884. [CrossRef] [PubMed]
35. Melo, S.; Luecke, L.B.; Kahlert, C.; Fernandez, A.; Gammon, S.; Kaye, J.; LeBleu, V.S.; Mittendorf, E.A.; Weitz, J.; Rahbari, N.; et al. Glypican-1 identifies cancer exosomes and detects early pancreatic cancer. *Nature* **2015**, *523*, 177–182. [CrossRef] [PubMed]
36. Hendriks, R.J.; Dijkstra, S.; Jannink, S.A.; Steffens, M.G.; Van Oort, I.M.; Mulders, P.F.; Schalken, J.A. Comparative analysis of prostate cancer specific biomarkers PCA3 and ERG in whole urine, urinary sediments and exosomes. *Clin. Chem. Lab. Med.* **2016**, *54*, 483–492. [CrossRef]
37. Nakamura, K.; Sawada, K.; Kinose, Y.; Yoshimura, A.; Toda, A.; Nakatsuka, E.; Hashimoto, K.; Mabuchi, S.; Morishige, K.-I.; Kurachi, H.; et al. Exosomes Promote Ovarian Cancer Cell Invasion through Transfer of CD44 to Peritoneal Mesothelial Cells. *Mol. Cancer Res.* **2016**, *15*, 78–92. [CrossRef]
38. Nakamura, K.; Sawada, K.; Yoshimura, A.; Kinose, Y.; Nakatsuka, E.; Kimura, T. Clinical relevance of circulating cell-free microRNAs in ovarian cancer. *Mol. Cancer* **2016**, *15*, 1–10. [CrossRef] [PubMed]
39. Colombo, M.; Raposo, G.; Théry, C. Biogenesis, Secretion, and Intercellular Interactions of Exosomes and Other Extracellular Vesicles. *Annu. Rev. Cell Dev. Biol.* **2014**, *30*, 255–289. [CrossRef] [PubMed]
40. Yeung, C.L.A.; Co, N.-N.; Tsuruga, T.; Yeung, T.-L.; Kwan, S.Y.; Leung, C.S.; Li, Y.; Lu, E.S.; Kwan, K.; Wong, K.-K.; et al. Exosomal transfer of stroma-derived miR21 confers paclitaxel resistance in ovarian cancer cells through targeting APAF1. *Nat. Commun.* **2016**, *7*, 11150. [CrossRef]
41. Nik Mohamed Kamal, N.N.S.B.; Shahidan, W.N.S. Non-Exosomal and Exosomal Circulatory MicroRNAs: Which Are More Valid as Biomarkers? *Front. Pharmacol.* **2020**, *10*, 1500. [CrossRef]
42. Taylor, D.D.; Gercel-Taylor, C. MicroRNA signatures of tumor-derived exosomes as diagnostic biomarkers of ovarian cancer. *Gynecol. Oncol.* **2008**, *110*, 13–21. [CrossRef] [PubMed]
43. Meng, X.; Müller, V.; Milde-Langosch, K.; Trillsch, F.; Pantel, K.; Schwarzenbach, H. Diagnostic and prognostic relevance of circulating exosomal miR-373, miR-200a, miR-200b and miR-200c in patients with epithelial ovarian cancer. *Oncotarget* **2016**, *7*, 16923–16935. [CrossRef] [PubMed]
44. Pan, C.; Stevic, I.; Müller, V.; Ni, Q.; Oliveira-Ferrer, L.; Pantel, K.; Schwarzenbach, H. Exosomal micro RNA s as tumor markers in epithelial ovarian cancer. *Mol. Oncol.* **2018**, *12*, 1935–1948. [CrossRef]

45. Kobayashi, M.; Sawada, K.; Nakamura, K.; Yoshimura, A.; Miyamoto, M.; Shimizu, A.; Ishida, K.; Nakatsuka, E.; Kodama, M.; Hashimoto, K.; et al. Exosomal miR-1290 is a potential biomarker of high-grade serous ovarian carcinoma and can discriminate patients from those with malignancies of other histological types. *J. Ovarian Res.* **2018**, *11*, 81. [CrossRef]
46. Yoshimura, A.; Sawada, K.; Nakamura, K.; Kinose, Y.; Nakatsuka, E.; Kobayashi, M.; Miyamoto, M.; Ishida, K.; Matsumoto, Y.; Kodama, M.; et al. Exosomal miR-99a-5p is elevated in sera of ovarian cancer patients and promotes cancer cell invasion by increasing fibronectin and vitronectin expression in neighboring peritoneal mesothelial cells. *BMC Cancer* **2018**, *18*, 1–13. [CrossRef]
47. Kim, S.; Choi, M.C.; Jeong, J.-Y.; Hwang, S.; Jung, S.G.; Joo, W.D.; Park, H.; Song, S.H.; Lee, C.; Kim, T.H.; et al. Serum exosomal miRNA-145 and miRNA-200c as promising biomarkers for preoperative diagnosis of ovarian carcinomas. *J. Cancer* **2019**, *10*, 1958–1967. [CrossRef] [PubMed]
48. Eichelser, C.; Stückrath, I.; Müller, V.; Milde-Langosch, K.; Wikman, H.; Pantel, K.; Schwarzenbach, H. Increased serum levels of circulating exosomal microRNA-373 in receptor-negative breast cancer patients. *Oncotarget* **2014**, *5*, 9650–9663. [CrossRef] [PubMed]
49. Humphries, B.; Yang, C. The microRNA-200 family: Small molecules with novel roles in cancer development, progression and therapy. *Oncotarget* **2015**, *6*, 6472–6498. [CrossRef]
50. Zuberi, M.; Mir, A.R.; Das, J.; Ahmad, I.; Javid, J.; Yadav, P.; Masroor, M.; Ahmad, S.; Ray, P.C.; Saxena, A. Expression of serum miR-200a, miR-200b, and miR-200c as candidate biomarkers in epithelial ovarian cancer and their association with clinicopathological features. *Clin. Transl. Oncol.* **2015**, *17*, 779–787. [CrossRef]
51. Muralidhar, G.G.; Barbolina, M.V. The miR-200 Family: Versatile Players in Epithelial Ovarian Cancer. *Int. J. Mol. Sci.* **2015**, *16*, 16833–16847. [CrossRef]
52. Nam, E.J.; Yoon, H.; Kim, S.W.; Kim, H.; Kim, Y.T.; Kim, J.H.; Kim, S. MicroRNA Expression Profiles in Serous Ovarian Carcinoma. *Clin. Cancer Res.* **2008**, *14*, 2690–2695. [CrossRef] [PubMed]
53. Li, Y.; Yao, L.; Liu, F.; Hong, J.; Chen, L.; Zhang, B.; Zhang, W. Characterization of microRNA expression in serous ovarian carcinoma. *Int. J. Mol. Med.* **2014**, *34*, 491–498. [CrossRef] [PubMed]
54. Elgaaen, B.V.; Olstad, O.K.; Haug, K.B.F.; Brusletto, B.; Sandvik, L.; Staff, A.C.; Gautvik, K.M.; Davidson, B. Global miRNA expression analysis of serous and clear cell ovarian carcinomas identifies differentially expressed miRNAs including miR-200c-3p as a prognostic marker. *BMC Cancer* **2014**, *14*, 80. [CrossRef]
55. Ibrahim, F.F.; Jamal, R.; Syafruddin, S.E.; Ab Mutalib, N.S.; Saidin, S.; MdZin, R.R.; Mollah, M.M.H.; Mokhtar, N.M. MicroRNA-200c and microRNA-31 regulate proliferation, colony formation, migration and invasion in serous ovarian cancer. *J. Ovarian Res.* **2015**, *8*, 56. [CrossRef]
56. Sulaiman, S.A.; Ab Mutalib, N.-S.; Jamal, R. miR-200c Regulation of Metastases in Ovarian Cancer: Potential Role in Epithelial and Mesenchymal Transition. *Front. Pharmacol.* **2016**, *7*. [CrossRef]
57. Moga, M.A.; Bălan, A.; Dimienescu, O.G.; Burtea, V.; Dragomir, R.M.; Anastasiu, C.V. Circulating miRNAs as Biomarkers for Endometriosis and Endometriosis-Related Ovarian Cancer—An Overview. *J. Clin. Med.* **2019**, *8*, 735. [CrossRef]
58. Chan, M.; Liaw, C.S.; Ji, S.M.; Tan, H.H.; Wong, C.Y.; Thike, A.A.; Tan, P.H.; Ho, G.H.; Lee, A.S.-G. Identification of Circulating MicroRNA Signatures for Breast Cancer Detection. *Clin. Cancer Res.* **2013**, *19*, 4477–4487. [CrossRef]
59. Pigati, L.; Yaddanapudi, S.C.S.; Iyengar, R.; Kim, D.-J.; Hearn, S.A.; Danforth, D.; Hastings, M.; Duelli, D.M. Selective Release of MicroRNA Species from Normal and Malignant Mammary Epithelial Cells. *PLoS ONE* **2010**, *5*, e13515. [CrossRef]
60. Kobayashi, M.; Salomon, C.; Tapia, J.; Illanes, S.E.; Mitchell, M.D.; Rice, G.E. Ovarian cancer cell invasiveness is associated with discordant exosomal sequestration of Let-7 miRNA and miR-200. *J. Transl. Med.* **2014**, *12*, 4. [CrossRef]
61. Villarroya-Beltri, C.; Gutierrez-Vazquez, C.; Sanchez-Cabo, F.; Pérez-Hernández, D.; Vázquez, J.; Martin-Cofreces, N.; Martinez-Herrera, D.J.; Pascual-Montano, A.; Mittelbrunn, M.; Sánchez-Madrid, F. Sumoylated hnRNPA2B1 controls the sorting of miRNAs into exosomes through binding to specific motifs. *Nat. Commun.* **2013**, *4*, 2980. [CrossRef] [PubMed]
62. Lomnytska, M.; Pinto, R.; Becker, S.; Engström, U.; Gustafsson, S.; Bjorklund, C.; Templin, M.; Bergstrand, J.; Xu, L.; Widengren, J.; et al. Platelet protein biomarker panel for ovarian cancer diagnosis. *Biomark. Res.* **2018**, *6*, 2. [CrossRef]
63. Michael, J.V.; Wurtzel, J.G.T.; Mao, G.F.; Rao, A.K.; Kolpakov, M.A.; Sabri, A.; Hoffman, N.E.; Rajan, S.; Tomar, D.; Madesh, M.; et al. Platelet microparticles infiltrating solid tumors transfer miRNAs that suppress tumor growth. *Blood* **2017**, *130*, 567–580. [CrossRef]
64. Yun, S.-H.; Sim, E.-H.; Goh, R.-Y.; Park, J.-I.; Han, J.-Y. Platelet Activation: The Mechanisms and Potential Biomarkers. *BioMed Res. Int.* **2016**, *2016*, 1–5. [CrossRef]
65. Heijnen, H.F.; Schiel, A.E.; Fijnheer, R.; Geuze, H.J.; Sixma, J.J. Activated platelets release two types of membrane vesicles: Microvesicles by surface shedding and exosomes derived from exocytosis of multivesicular bodies and alpha-granules. *Blood* **1999**, *94*, 3791–3799. [CrossRef]
66. Kirschner, M.B.; Edelman, J.B.; Kao, S.C.-H.; Vallely, M.P.; Van Zandwijk, N.; Reid, G. The Impact of Hemolysis on Cell-Free microRNA Biomarkers. *Front. Genet.* **2013**, *4*, 94. [CrossRef]
67. Blondal, T.; Nielsen, S.J.; Baker, A.; Andreasen, D.; Mouritzen, P.; Teilum, M.W.; Dahlsveen, I.K. Assessing sample and miRNA profile quality in serum and plasma or other biofluids. *Methods* **2012**, *59*, S1–S6. [CrossRef] [PubMed]

68. Juzenas, S.; Venkatesh, G.; Hübenthal, M.; Hoeppner, M.P.; Du, Z.G.; Paulsen, M.; Rosenstiel, P.; Senger, P.; Hofmann-Apitius, M.; Keller, A.; et al. A comprehensive, cell specific microRNA catalogue of human peripheral blood. *Nucleic Acids Res.* **2017**, *45*, 9290–9301. [CrossRef] [PubMed]
69. Pritchard, C.C.; Kroh, E.; Wood, B.; Arroyo, J.; Dougherty, K.J.; Miyaji, M.M.; Tait, J.F.; Tewari, M. Blood Cell Origin of Circulating MicroRNAs: A Cautionary Note for Cancer Biomarker Studies. *Cancer Prev. Res.* **2011**, *5*, 492–497. [CrossRef]
70. Laffont, B.; Corduan, A.; Plé, H.; Duchez, A.-C.; Cloutier, N.; Boilard, E.; Provost, P. Activated platelets can deliver mRNA regulatory Ago2 microRNA complexes to endothelial cells via microparticles. *Blood* **2013**, *122*, 253–261. [CrossRef]
71. Hunter, M.P.; Ismail, N.; Zhang, X.; Aguda, B.D.; Lee, E.J.; Yu, L.; Xiao, T.; Schafer, J.; Lee, M.-L.T.; Schmittgen, T.D.; et al. Detection of microRNA Expression in Human Peripheral Blood Microvesicles. *PLoS ONE* **2008**, *3*, e3694. [CrossRef]
72. Wang, K.; Yuan, Y.; Cho, J.-H.; McClarty, S.; Baxter, D.; Galas, D.J. Comparing the MicroRNA Spectrum between Serum and Plasma. *PLoS ONE* **2012**, *7*, e41561. [CrossRef]
73. Cheng, L.; Sharples, R.A.; Scicluna, B.J.; Hill, A.F. Exosomes provide a protective and enriched source of miRNA for biomarker profiling compared to intracellular and cell-free blood. *J. Extracell. Vesicles* **2014**, *3*. [CrossRef] [PubMed]
74. Ammerlaan, W.; Betsou, F. Intraindividual Temporal miRNA Variability in Serum, Plasma, and White Blood Cell Subpopulations. *Biopreserv. Biobank.* **2016**, *14*, 390–397. [CrossRef] [PubMed]
75. Foye, C.; Yan, I.K.; David, W.; Shukla, N.; Habboush, Y.; Chase, L.; Ryland, K.; Kesari, V.; Patel, T. Comparison of miRNA quantitation by Nanostring in serum and plasma samples. *PLoS ONE* **2017**, *12*, e0189265. [CrossRef] [PubMed]
76. Max, K.E.A.; Bertram, K.; Akat, K.M.; Bogardus, K.A.; Li, J.; Morozov, P.; Ben-Dov, I.Z.; Li, X.; Weiss, Z.; Azizian, A.; et al. Human plasma and serum extracellular small RNA reference profiles and their clinical utility. *Proc. Natl. Acad. Sci. USA* **2018**, *115*, E5334–E5343. [CrossRef]
77. Gee, H.; Buffa, F.; Camps, C.; Ramachandran, A.; Leek, R.; Taylor, M.; Patil, M.; Sheldon, H.; Betts, G.; Homer, J.; et al. The small-nucleolar RNAs commonly used for microRNA normalisation correlate with tumour pathology and prognosis. *Br. J. Cancer* **2011**, *104*, 1168–1177. [CrossRef]
78. Gouin, K.; Peck, K.; Antes, T.; Johnson, J.L.; Li, C.; Vaturi, S.D.; Middleton, R.; de Couto, G.; Walravens, A.; Rodriguez-Borlado, L.; et al. A comprehensive method for identification of suitable reference genes in extracellular vesicles. *J. Extracell. Vesicles* **2017**, *6*, 1347019. [CrossRef]
79. Dai, Y.; Cao, Y.; Köhler, J.; Lu, A.; Xu, S.; Wang, H. Unbiased RNA-Seq-driven identification and validation of reference genes for quantitative RT-PCR analyses of pooled cancer exosomes. *BMC Genom.* **2021**, *22*, 1–13. [CrossRef]
80. Elias, K.M.; Fendler, W.; Stawiski, K.; Fiascone, S.J.; Vitonis, A.F.; Berkowitz, R.S.; Frendl, G.; Konstantinopoulos, P.; Crum, C.P.; Kedzierska, M.; et al. Diagnostic potential for a serum miRNA neural network for detection of ovarian cancer. *eLife* **2017**, *6*, e28932. [CrossRef]
81. Dong, J.; Xu, M. A 19-miRNA Support Vector Machine classifier and a 6-miRNA risk score system designed for ovarian cancer patients. *Oncol. Rep.* **2019**, *41*, 3233–3243. [CrossRef]
82. Johnson, S.C.; Chakraborty, S.; Drosou, A.; Cunnea, P.; Tzovaras, D.; Nixon, K.; Zawieja, D.C.; Muthuchamy, M.; Fotopoulou, C.; Moore, J.E., Jr. Inflammatory state of lymphatic vessels and miRNA profiles associated with relapse in ovarian cancer patients. *PLoS ONE* **2020**, *15*, e0230092. [CrossRef] [PubMed]
83. Ray, M.; Ruffalo, M.M.; Bar-Joseph, Z. Construction of integrated microRNA and mRNA immune cell signatures to predict survival of patients with breast and ovarian cancer. *Genes Chromosom. Cancer* **2018**, *58*, 34–42. [CrossRef] [PubMed]

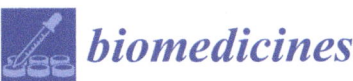

Review

Current Treatments and New Possible Complementary Therapies for Epithelial Ovarian Cancer

Maritza P. Garrido [1,2,*], Allison N. Fredes [1], Lorena Lobos-González [3], Manuel Valenzuela-Valderrama [4], Daniela B. Vera [1] and Carmen Romero [1,2,*]

[1] Laboratorio de Endocrinología y Biología de la Reproducción, Hospital Clínico Universidad de Chile, Santiago 8380456, Chile; allison.fredes@ug.uchile.cl (A.N.F.); daniela.vera@gmail.com (D.B.V.)
[2] Departamento de Obstetricia y Ginecología, Facultad de Medicina, Universidad de Chile, Santiago 8380453, Chile
[3] Centro de Medicina Regenerativa, Facultad de Medicina, Clínica Alemana-Universidad del Desarrollo, Santiago 7710162, Chile; llobos@udd.cl
[4] Laboratorio de Microbiología Celular, Instituto de Investigación y Postgrado, Facultad de Ciencias de la Salud, Universidad Central de Chile, Santiago 8320000, Chile; manuel.valenzuela@ucentral.cl
* Correspondence: mgarrido@hcuch.cl (M.P.G.); cromero@hcuch.cl (C.R.)

Abstract: Epithelial ovarian cancer (EOC) is one of the deadliest gynaecological malignancies. The late diagnosis is frequent due to the absence of specific symptomatology and the molecular complexity of the disease, which includes a high angiogenesis potential. The first-line treatment is based on optimal debulking surgery following chemotherapy with platinum/gemcitabine and taxane compounds. During the last years, anti-angiogenic therapy and poly adenosine diphosphate-ribose polymerases (PARP)-inhibitors were introduced in therapeutic schemes. Several studies have shown that these drugs increase the progression-free survival and overall survival of patients with ovarian cancer, but the identification of patients who have the greatest benefits is still under investigation. In the present review, we discuss about the molecular characteristics of the disease, the recent evidence of approved treatments and the new possible complementary approaches, focusing on drug repurposing, non-coding RNAs, and nanomedicine as a new method for drug delivery.

Keywords: epithelial ovarian cancer; drug repurposing; non-coding RNAs; nanocarriers; anti-angiogenic therapy

1. Introduction

Anti-tumoral therapies are constantly evolving, mainly because of growing evidence about the physiopathological mechanisms involved in tumoral progression and drug resistance [1]. The approved treatments for ovarian cancer, one of the deadliest gynaecological malignancies, are limited and have had few changes in the last decades compared to the observed progress in therapies against other cancers [2]. The introduction of anti-angiogenic therapy [3] and poly adenosine diphosphate-ribose polymerases (PARP)-inhibitors [4] have been the most recent changes on therapeutic schemes, increasing the progression-free survival of EOC patients but with some important drawbacks. At present, there are many proposals for complementary therapies to the existent, including other anti-angiogenic compounds, immune checkpoint inhibitors, tropomyosin receptor kinases (TRK)-inhibitors, biological compounds as non-coding RNAs, and drug repositioning, which will be reviewed in the following sections. In addition, advances in drug delivery encourage the use of previously discarded drugs due to their toxicity or hydrophobic properties. The current work aims to provide an overview of current and potential new therapeutic options that are being tested in ovarian cancer, considering both preclinical and clinical evidence.

2. Epithelial Ovarian Cancer

Ovarian cancer is the most lethal gynaecological cancer worldwide. According to the American Cancer Society, in the United States, more than 21,400 women will receive a new diagnosis of ovarian cancer, and more than 13,700 women will die from ovarian cancer each year [5]. Unfortunately, there is no reliable test to screen for ovarian cancer, and symptoms are often confused with other diseases, which delays the diagnoses and treatments and results in poor survival rates [6].

Ovarian cancer staging is used to predict clinical behaviour and to select the appropriate therapeutic approach for patients. There are two main criteria: (1) the tumour-node-metastasis (TNM) system, based on tumour size, local growth (T), the extent of lymph node metastases (N) and occurrence of distant metastases (M) [7], and (2) the International Federation of Gynecology and Obstetrics (FIGO) classification. This system considers the fallopian tube and peritoneal origins of ovarian tumours collectively. The classification is based on the location, compromise of lymph nodes, peritoneal dissemination, ascites and metastasis to extra-abdominal organs, ranging from stage I through stage IV [8,9].

Around 85 to 90% of ovarian cancers have an epithelial origin (EOC) [10,11]. Half of them correspond to serous carcinomas, 10% to endometrioid subtype, and about 6% to clear cell and mucinous carcinoma [10]. EOC has heterogeneous nature and can be classified depending on its morphologic and molecular features. Based on that, the dualistic model confirms two major histologic types of EOC, type I and type II [12,13]. Type I tumours develop in a stepwise progression from well-established precursor lesions, such as borderline tumours and endometriosis lesions that in turn originate from cystadenomas and adenofibromas (low-grade serous carcinomas, low-grade endometrioid, clear cell, malignant Brenner tumour and mucinous carcinomas) [12,14]. These neoplasms are present as large masses, confined to one ovary with better prognosis but, importantly, seem not to respond well to adjutant chemotherapy, being the optimal debulking surgery the best option [15–17].

On the other hand, type II carcinomas evolve rapidly, are highly aggressive with rapid growth, and tend to spread sooner [12]. These tumours are relatively sensitive to platinum and taxane-based chemotherapy [18]. Some examples of type II carcinomas are high-grade serous (HGS) EOC, high-grade endometrioid carcinoma, carcinosarcomas and undifferentiated carcinomas [12,14].

It is commonly proposed that serous tumours, the more frequent histological type of EOC, derive from two origins, cortical inclusion cysts from ovarian surface epithelium or malignant precursors from fimbrial epithelium [19–21]. Fimbrial cells could be implanted on the disrupted ovarian surface forming inclusion cysts, and later, a malignant lesion [22]. Recent evidence suggests that the dominant origin of HGS-EOC is the fimbrial epithelium, unlike low-grade serous, endometrioid, mucinous, or clear-cell ovarian cancer that arise from ovarian surface epithelium [20–22].

The stage and histological subtype of EOC are essential considerations to optimize the patients' treatment because therapeutical success is poor when the cancer is detected in advanced stages. For instance, the 5-year relative survival rate in patients with invasive EOC is only 31%, while in localized EOC, it is 93% [23]. Moreover, studies have showed that survival rates of patients with EOC depend on the histological type. For example, patients with type II EOC had a significantly higher incidence of advanced disease (FIGO stages III/IV) than type I patients (79.8% vs. 38% respectively) being the overall survival and progression-free survival significantly higher in patients with type I tumours [24]. In addition, some studies have found a markedly higher mortality in patients with advanced mucinous and clear cell carcinoma, compared to higher survival rates of patients with HGS-EOC and endometrioid subtypes [25,26].

Current knowledge indicates that molecular characteristics of each patient with EOC should be considered to choose the best existing treatment, and personalized medicine should be considered in patients with EOC in the next future.

3. Molecular Characteristics of Epithelial Ovarian Cancer

The ovary is a complex organ, which involves cyclic changes in endocrine, inflammatory, and nervous components. These characteristics influence not only the pathogenesis of EOC, but also its molecular heterogenicity and, potentially, the therapeutic response of these patients.

3.1. SOMATIC and Germinal Mutations

Type I tumours are more genetically stable than type II tumours. Somatic mutations usually found in type I tumours include the genes of the RAF kinase family, Kirsten rat sarcoma virus protein (KRAS), beta-catenin, phosphatase and tensin homolog (PTEN), transforming growth factor-beta receptor II (TGF-β RII), phosphatidylinositol-4,5-bisphosphate 3-kinase subunit alpha (PIK3CA), and AT-rich interactive domain-containing protein 1A (ARID1A) [12,27].

In contrast, type II tumours rarely display the mutations found in type I tumours. They are chromosomally unstable and TP53 mutations are frequent (96% of HGS-EOC) [28]. Other recurrent mutations in type II tumours affect retinoblastoma protein (RB) and Notch signalling pathway [28]. Less frequent but not less important are genetic alterations in breast cancer type 1 susceptibility proteins (BRCA), because mutation or inactivation of BRCA genes and its downstream genes (via promoter methylation) occurs in up to 40–50% of HGS-EOC [19]. It is important to note that characteristic mutations of type I tumours could be found in type II tumours; however, these molecular changes are rarely important drivers in type II tumours [28] (Figure 1).

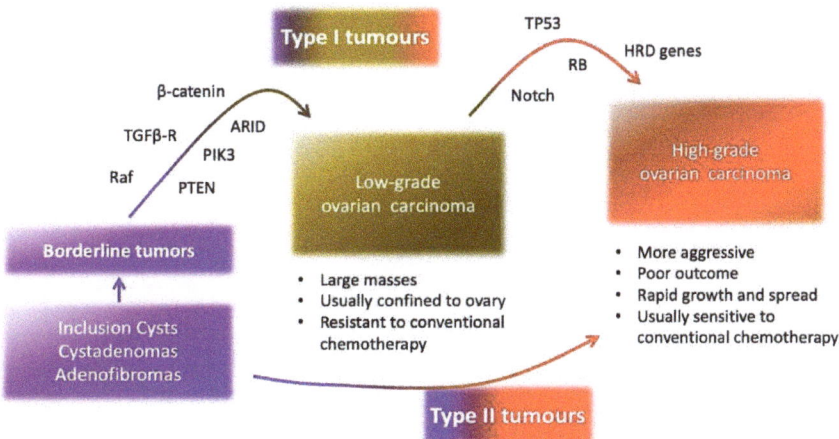

Figure 1. Main characteristics of type I and type II ovarian tumours. Type I tumours are characterized by sequential and low growth from the cyst and borderline tumours. In contrast, the evolution of type II tumours from pre-neoplastic lesions is quicker, resulting in an aggressive phenotype. Tumour evolution involves the acquisition of mutations in onco-suppressor genes as RAF kinase, beta-catenin, phosphatase and tensin homolog (PTEN), transforming growth factor-beta receptor (TGF-βR), phosphatidylinositol-4,5-bisphosphate 3-kinase (PIK3), AT-rich interactive domain-containing protein (ARID), TP53, retinoblastoma protein (RB), homologous recombinant deficiency (HRD) genes, and Notch pathway.

Recent advances in EOC therapy have been modest, with few therapeutic options that significantly improve patients´ survival. A better knowledge of molecular characteristics of EOC requires further development of molecular-targeted therapies, which are just being explored in this neoplasm.

3.2. Angiogenesis in Ovarian Cancer

Angiogenesis, or the generation of new blood vessels from other pre-existing, displays a considerable role in EOC [29,30]. In cancer cells, angiogenesis is enhanced to ensure the oxygen and nutrients supply, allowing tumoral growth and its dissemination. Many humoral factors are secreted by EOC cells to reach endothelial cells during tumour angiogenesis, promoting its proliferation, migration, and differentiation [30]. One of the most studied angiogenic factors is vascular endothelial growth factor (VEGF), which is largely produced and secreted by EOC cells [31–33]. This knowledge was used to develop the drug bevacizumab (Avastin), a monoclonal antibody against VEGF, which is currently used to treat EOC in advanced stages [3], a topic that will be discussed in detail later.

Besides VEGF, other important pro-angiogenic molecules produced by EOC cells are neurotrophins. They display important functions in the nervous system and are involved in the correct ovarian performance [34,35]. Nerve growth factor (NGF) and brain-derived neurotrophic factor (BDNF) act as direct and indirect angiogenic factors, and their importance in EOC angiogenesis has been studied by several researchers [36–38]. Additionally, EOC produces a broad range of other angiogenic molecules, including placental growth factor (PlGF) [39,40], fibroblast growth factors (FGF) [41–44], platelet-derived growth factor (PDGF) [42,45] and angiopoietins [46].

Current studies have shown that the effects of angiogenic factors are not limited to endothelial cells, but they also produce autocrine stimulation in EOC cells [45–47]. The expression pattern of angiogenic factors could differ among histological types and significantly influences the progression-free survival and therapy response of patients with EOC [48], which should be considered for cancer treatment.

4. Current Therapies for Epithelial Ovarian Cancer
4.1. First-Line Chemotherapy

The current treatment for EOC is debulking surgery. In advanced stages, the primary cytoreductive surgery followed by adjuvant chemotherapy remains the standard treatment for EOC [49,50]. Since the 80´s, the first-line chemotherapy has been based on platinum compounds, and during the 90's taxanes were introduced, so depending on local guidelines, the standard chemotherapy is based only on platinum compounds or its combination especially in platinum-refractory or platinum-resistant patients [51,52]. In women with optimally debulked EOC (who did not receive the neoadjuvant treatment), adjuvant chemotherapy is not considered a reasonable option [51]. Intraperitoneal chemotherapy was introduced in the last decade, and some clinical trials have shown an advantage over intravenous administration, improving patients' survival and tolerability [53–55].

Although complete remission is generally reached, most tumours will recur within two years, and rapid emergence of resistance to chemotherapy is observed [56]. The mechanisms responsible for chemoresistance to cisplatin and paclitaxel are diverse and include altered expression of membrane transporters, drug inactivation/detoxification, and resistance to cell death, among others [57,58]. However, beyond this acquired resistance, a plausible explanation for this phenomenon is the multiplication of a population of ovarian cancer tumour-initiating cells or stem-like cells, possibly originating from the ovary's hilum region, that is proposed to initiate primary tumor growth, metastasis, and relapse of disease, but also for the development of chemoresistance [59,60].

To overcome platinum resistance, the United States food and drug administration (U.S. FDA) approved in 2006 the use of gemcitabine in combination with carboplatin to treat women with advanced ovarian cancer that relapsed at least six months after initial therapy [61,62]. Gemcitabine is a synthetic nucleoside inhibitor that increases the accumulation of cisplatin lesions producing cytotoxic synergy [63–65], enhancing the response to cisplatin treatment.

4.2. PARP Inhibitors

The poly adenosine diphosphate-ribose polymerases (PARP) are essential enzymes involved in most cellular processes, including cell stress response, chromatin remodelling, DNA repair, and apoptosis [66–68]. They work by stabilizing PARP enzymes, inhibiting their activity, which prevents DNA repair and leads to cell death [68,69]. The four most used PARP inhibitors are olaparib (Lynparza), niraparib (Zejula), rucaparib (Rubraca) and talazoparib (Talzenna) [68]. These drugs are targeted agents for EOC with somatic or germinal mutations of BRCA1/2 genes or other genes that produce homologous recombination deficiency (HRD). HGS-EOC, the most common histological type of EOC, is characterized by frequent genetic and epigenetic alterations that produce HRD, most commonly BRCA1 and BRCA2 genes [28]. HRD is present in around a third of HGS-EOC, producing an aggressive phenotype [70–72].

The PARP inhibitor olaparib is the most studied in the context of cancer and was approved by the U.S. FDA as maintenance therapy for patients with EOC who have a partial or complete response to chemotherapy and have BRCA1/2 mutations [73]. Similarly, the U.S. FDA approved rucaparib as a single agent for treating relapsed ovarian cancer with mutations in BRCA genes in patients who had received two or more lines of chemotherapy [74]. Unlike the other PARP inhibitors, veliparib has not shown anti-proliferative activity, but radio and chemo-sensitizing effects were reported in cancer cells [75].

Regarding PARP inhibitors' progress in EOC, Table 1 summarizes the most recent studies. It stands out an international clinical trial that evaluated carboplatin, paclitaxel, and veliparib induction therapy followed by veliparib maintenance therapy in patients with HGS-EOC, which showed a significantly longer progression-free survival than carboplatin plus paclitaxel induction therapy alone [76], suggesting that veliparib in association with chemotherapy or radiotherapy, could be used as chemosensitivity agent in HGS-EOC.

Additionally, PARP inhibitors have been studied as a single agent after chemotherapy or in combination with molecular-target agents. For instance, niraparib, which was approved in 2019 by U.S. FDA [77] has been tested in combination with pembrolizumab, an antibody against the programmed cell death receptor 1 (anti-PD1) in patients with platinum-resistant ovarian cancer. The use of niraparib plus the PD-1 inhibitor showed promising anti-tumoral activity in these patients, and importantly, responses of cancer patients without BRCA mutations (non-HRD) were higher than expected with either agent as monotherapy [78], which extend the groups of patients with the potential benefit of the use of PARP inhibitors.

Other interesting associations studied include PARP inhibitors combined with anti-angiogenic therapy, such as cediranib (VEGF receptor inhibitor) or bevacizumab [79–81] as described in Table 1.

Even though BRCA mutations are the best predictors of the efficacy of PARP inhibitors, these drugs have shown positive effects in patients without BRCA mutations or non-HRD, which suggests that the use of PARP inhibitors may be extended to HGS-EOC, independently of the presence of HRD.

Table 1. Summary of latest studies performed with PARP inhibitors in ovarian cancer patients.

Drugs	Study and Patients	Main Findings	Ref.
Chemotherapy in combination with veliparib (ABT-888) and as maintenance therapy	Phase III study. Advanced HGS-EOC [1]	Veliparib increased progression-free survival compared to chemotherapy therapy alone in the HRD [2] cohort	[76]
Niraparib (Zejula) and pembrolizumab	Phase II study. Recurrent, platinum-resistant ovarian cancer	Responses of patients non-HRD were higher than expected either agent as monotherapy	[78]
Cediranib and olaparib (Lynparza)	Phase II/III study. Recurrent platinum-sensitive HGS-EOC	Drugs improved progression-free survival in patients with BRCA1/2 mutations	[79,80]
Chemotherapy with bevacizumab and olaparib (Lynparza) as maintenance therapy	Phase III study. Advanced HGS and endometroid EOC	The addition of olaparib increased progression-free survival in patients with HRD-positive tumours	[81]
Niraparib (Zejula) as maintenance therapy	Phase III study. Platinum-sensitive, recurrent ovarian cancer	Increase of progression-free survival in patients with or without BRCA mutations.	[82]
Olaparib (Lynparza) as maintenance treatment	platinum-sensitive relapsed ovarian cancer	Increased median overall survival of patients with BRCA mutations	[83]

[1] HGS-EOC: high-grade serous epithelial ovarian cancer. [2] HRD: homologous recombination deficiency.

4.3. Anti-Angiogenic Therapy (Bevacizumab)

Since exacerbated angiogenesis is a crucial characteristic of EOC cells and VEGF-A is the most expressed angiogenic factor in ovarian tumours, a therapy based on a human monoclonal antibody against VEGF-A seems promissory for EOC treatment. In this context, the U.S. FDA approved in 2018 the use of bevacizumab (Avastin), a monoclonal antibody against VEGF-A as first-line treatment for epithelial ovarian, fallopian tube, or primary peritoneal cancer stage III or IV in combination with carboplatin and paclitaxel [3]. Similarly, the European Commission approves the use of bevacizumab in combination with standard chemotherapy as a treatment for women with the first recurrence of platinum-sensitive ovarian cancer and first-line chemotherapy following surgery in women with advanced ovarian cancer [84].

Bevacizumab has been studied in clinical trials that include patients with recurrent platinum-sensitive and platinum-resistant ovarian cancer. In the first case, OCEANS trial showed that the addition of bevacizumab to gemcitabine and carboplatin therapy improved the progression-free survival of patients [85]. Alike, AURELIA trial, that studied the combination of bevacizumab to chemotherapy in patients with platinum-resistant EOC, shows that the benefit of bevacizumab therapy in advanced EOC was modest, increasing in a few months the progression-free survival of patients and without significant changes in the overall survival of intervened patients [86]. Similar results were obtained in the trial GOG-0218, a phase III randomized trial of bevacizumab in women with newly diagnosed ovarian cancer, that showed no survival differences for patients who received bevacizumab compared with chemotherapy alone [87].

To a better understanding of the real benefit of using bevacizumab in ovarian cancer patients, a meta-analysis that included 7 studies with patients with advanced ovarian cancer was performed [88]. This study concluded that bevacizumab treatment increased progression-free survival in patients with both advanced and recurrent disease, but its use was associated with an increase of overall survival only in patients with recurrent disease [88]. Although bevacizumab therapy is extended to many countries and is considered one of the greatest advances in the treatment of ovarian cancer, some researchers consider that this therapy could be not cost-effective [89,90].

The inhibition of VEGF-mediated signalling leads to tumour vasculature normalization, improving chemotherapy delivery which results in increased tumour toxicity and a decreased formation of ascites fluid [91,92]. This knowledge suggests that selecting appropriate patients for bevacizumab treatment could contribute to improve therapeutic efficacy. Results from the trial GOG 0218 show that patients with ascites treated with bevacizumab had a significant improvement in progression-free and overall survival, which was not observed in patients without ascites, suggesting that ascites predicts treatment benefit of bevacizumab in patients with advanced EOC [93]. Similarly, a phase I study in patients with diverse cancers tested intraperitoneal bevacizumab for treating refractory malignant ascites. Preliminary results of this study showed that bevacizumab exhibited short-term anti-tumoral efficacy and palliated symptoms [94]. Given that over one-third of women with ovarian cancer will develop ascites [95], bevacizumab therapy should be considered in this subgroup of patients.

Further, it is believed that polymorphisms of several genes involved in angiogenic pathways could be associated with the efficacy of bevacizumab in cancer treatment [96], including genetic variants in the renin-angiotensin system [97]. In ovarian cancer patients, it was described that a specific polymorphism of interleukin 8 (IL-8) may predict the response to bevacizumab-based chemotherapy [98]. Another recent study suggests that patients with ovarian cancer that express low levels of the tumour-suppressor micro-RNA-25 (miR-25) will have significant benefit from bevacizumab treatment in terms of progression-free survival and overall survival [99].

Currently, other anti-angiogenic compounds are being tested to improve the response of EOC treatment (Figure 2). For instance, aflibercept is an antiangiogenic soluble fusion protein that acts as a "VEGF trap" and inhibits VEGF-A and VEGF-B, as well as PlGF signaling [100,101]. Two clinical trials show that aflibercept was effective in controlling malignant ascites with a safety profile [102,103], even though the drug shows a significant risk of fatal bowel perforation of patients with very advanced cancer, which suggests that the benefit-risk balance should be discussed with each patient.

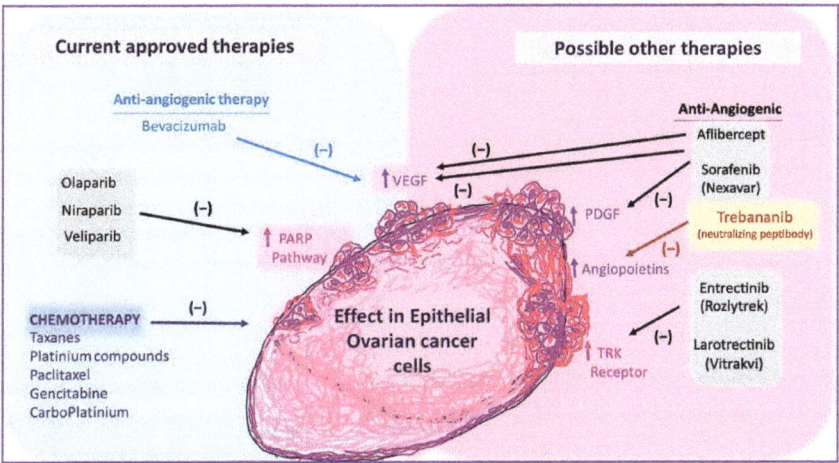

Figure 2. Summary of current and new possible therapies for ovarian cancer treatment. VEGF: vascular endothelial growth factor. PARP: poly adenosine diphosphate-ribose polymerases. TRK: tropomyosin receptor kinases. PDGF: platelet-derived growth factor.

Even though VEGF is the most studied angiogenic factor in ovarian cancer, other important pro-angiogenic molecules could be upregulated in response to anti-VEGF therapy. This theory could explain the failure or resistance to anti-angiogenic therapy in some patients.

5. Inhibitors of Other Angiogenic Factors That Are Being Tested in EOC

Apart from VEGF, EOC cells could yield and release several other angiogenic factors such as angiopoietins, neurotrophins, and PDGF, among others [30,38–40,46,104]. Based on this knowledge, specific inhibitors of these molecules (summarized in Table 2) have been developed. An example is trebananib (AMG-386), an angiopoietin 1 and 2 neutralizing chimeric protein (peptibody). It binds angiopoietins thereby preventing the interaction with their cell surface receptors, inhibiting angiogenesis and tumoral growth [105]. Trebananib has been tested in combination with carboplatin and paclitaxel as first-line treatment for advanced ovarian cancer in the clinical trial TRINOVA-1/3. Unfortunately, the trial shows that the addition of trebananib to standard therapy was minimally effective and did not improve the progression-free survival of patients [106,107].

Table 2. Summary of several new anti-angiogenic options under study in EOC.

Drugs	Mechanism	Study and Patients	Main Findings	Ref.
Trebananib (AMG 386)	Neutralizing peptibody that targets angiopoietin 1 and 2	Phase III study, tested with carboplatin and paclitaxel	Trebananib did not improve the progression-free survival of patients with advanced ovarian cancer	[106,107]
Sorafenib (Nexavar)	Protein kinase inhibitor of VEGF and PDGF receptors	Phase II study tested in combination with topotecan or bevacizumab	Clinical activity was observed in patients with ovarian cancer heavily-pretreated, bevacizumab-naive and platinum-resistant disease.	[108,109]
Entrectinib (Rozlytrek)	pan-TRK inhibitors (TRK receptors)	Phase I/II trials. At least one dose after standard treatments	Entrectinib was well tolerated and induced a durable response in patients with NTRK fusion-positive solid tumours.	[110]

Because anti-angiogenic therapy is a key point in EOC and most of the angiogenic and growth factors have in common the activation of tyrosine kinase (RK)-mediated signalling, selective or non-selective TK inhibitors have emerged as alternative drugs in the context of EOC therapy. For instance, sorafenib (Nexavar) is a multiple protein kinase inhibitor that decreases the signalling of VEGF and PDGF receptors [111,112] and is approved by the U.S. FDA for the treatment of patients with advanced renal cell carcinoma and unresectable hepatocellular carcinoma [113]. Unfortunately, a clinical trial shows that sorafenib had only modest anti-tumoral activity and substantial toxicity in patients with recurrent ovarian cancer [114], but this combination with other drugs shows better results. For instance, using sorafenib in combination with topotecan (topoisomerase inhibitor) as maintenance therapy improves the progression-free survival of patients with platinum-resistant ovarian cancer [108]. Similarly, a phase II study showed a clinical benefit of the combination of sorafenib and bevacizumab in bevacizumab-naïve EOC patients who were heavily pre-treated with platinum. However, the study highlights the importance of close monitoring and dose modifications in these patients due to toxicity of the drug combination [109], which puts into question the effectiveness and security of the use of tyrosine kinase inhibitors in EOC.

6. Anti-Neurotrophins Therapies as Possible New Approaches in EOC

Neurotrophins and their receptors are a group of molecules whose importance in the nervous system is widely known. In the last decades, their contribution to the homeostasis of other non-neuronal tissues has been described. For instance, neurotrophins dysregulation has been reported in some ovarian pathologies such as polycystic ovarian syndrome [115,116] and EOC [30,38].

Neurotrophins and their receptors display a crucial role in the progression of EOC, acting as autocrine growth factors and angiogenic factors [36–38,117]. The most studied neurotrophins, NGF and BDNF, bind their high-affinity tropomyosin receptor kinases (TRK) A and B, respectively [118]. In EOC, their upregulation has been associated with poor survival rates [37,119]. Therefore, neurotrophins and their receptors have been proposed as potential therapeutic targets in EOC.

TRK fusion is a phenomenon present in diverse kinds of cancer [120]. In EOC, the presence of TRK fusions in patients' biopsies is not documented, but it is assumed, because of the critical contribution of neurotrophins and their receptors to EOC progression. Based on this, two clinical trials are testing pan-TRK inhibitors in patients with neoplasms, including EOC (NCT02568267 and NCT03215511). These inhibitors are small molecules that bind to TRK receptors, prevent neurotrophins-TRK interaction and, therefore, TRK activation [121]. In 2018 and 2019, the U.S. FDA approved larotrectinib (Vitrakvi) and entrectinib (Rozlytrek) respectively for the treatment of adult and paediatric patients with solid tumours that have TRK gene fusions [122,123]. Another recently developed TRK inhibitor is loxo-195 (Selitrectinib), a second-generation drug that overcomes the acquired resistance to first-generation TRK-inhibitors [124].

A recent report on the use of TRK-inhibitors in EOC shows that entrectinib induced durable and clinically meaningful responses in patients with TRK fusion-positive solid tumours, being well tolerated with a manageable safety profile. However, only 2% of these participants had ovarian cancer [110], so the usefulness of TRK inhibitors as a complementary therapy in EOC needs further study.

7. Immune Checkpoint Inhibitors as an Alternative for Ovarian Cancer Treatment

Cells with tumour potential are constantly produced in the human body but the immune system oversees their elimination. Immune checkpoints are modulators of immune response which is crucial for self-tolerance, preventing autoimmunity and the shutdown of exacerbated responses. In this context, regulatory T cells (Treg) and inhibitory surface molecules, including cytotoxic T lymphocyte-associated protein 4 (CTLA4), programmed cell death receptor 1 (PD1) and its ligand (PD-L1), are induced during immune responses and represent immune checkpoints [125,126]. Cancer cells manipulate these mechanisms to avoid the immune response, preventing their elimination [127].

Different inhibitors of immune checkpoints have been developed to treat solid cancers and some of them have been tested in patients with EOC. In November 2021, there were more than 120 clinical trials using checkpoint inhibitors in ovarian cancer patients inscribed in clinicaltrials.gov (accessed on 7 December 2021), whose results are summarized in Table 3. These studies concluded that the expression of PD-L1 in EOC cells, the histotype, and previous treatment are associated with the success of immune therapies.

The phase Ib KEYNOTE-028 study tested pembrolizumab in 26 patients with PDL1-positive advanced ovarian cancer, showing modest but durable anti-tumor activity with an overall response rate (ORR) of 11.5% [130]. Phase II of this study (KEYNOTE-100 cohort) tested the same drug in 376 patients with recurrent ovarian cancer [131]. The study showed a higher ORR in HGS-EOC and clear cell ovarian cancer subgroups, a better response in patients with five or more lines of previous treatment, and an increased ORR in patients with a high presence of PDL1 (combined positive score > 10). In addition, the study showed that 8% of patients had a complete or partial response to pembrolizumab monotherapy, while progressive disease was reported in 57.2% of patients [131].

Among other current immunologic therapies, a clinical trial intends to test the drug ipilimumab (anti- CTLA-4 antibody) in ovarian cancer patients (NCT00060372). Although the preliminary reports are available only for patients with hematopoietic malignancies, they showed encouraging results [135]. On the other hand, given that ovarian cancers express high levels of mesothelin [136], a clinical trial is testing a monoclonal antibody anti-mesothelin (ABBV-428) as monotherapy in patients with several cancers, including ovarian cancer (NCT02955251). ABBV-428 targets mesothelin via a C-terminal single-chain variable fragment flanking Fc-modified human IgG1 and CD40 via an N-terminal single-chain variable fragment, which produces the activation of CD40 [137]. CD40 acts via ligation on antigen-presenting cells, stimulating T-cell activation and proliferation [138]. Unfortunately, the first results of this trial showed minimal clinical activity in a small cohort of patients with advanced ovarian cancer [137].

Table 3. Summary of clinical trials using inhibitors of immune checkpoints with published results in ovarian cancer patients.

Drug	Study and Patients	Main Findings	Ref.
Niraparib in combination with pembrolizumab (anti-PD-1 antibody)	Phase I/II study in recurrent platinum-resistant ovarian cancer	The results of the combination were better than for single agents (ORR [1] was 18%). Antitumor activity was independent of BRCA mutation or HRD status and irrespective of PD-L1 expression	[78]
Pembrolizumab with cisplatin and gemcitabine	Phase II study in platinum-resistant ovarian cancer	Pembrolizumab addition did not appear to provide benefit beyond chemotherapy alone in the 18 patients treated.	[128]
SC-003 (anti-dipeptidase 3 antibody) and budigalimab (anti-DP-1)	Phase Ia/Ib in platinum-resistant/refractory ovarian cancer	Low and not durable responses in the 3 patients with the combined treatment. Low safety profile of SC-003	[129]
Pembrolizumab as single agent	Phase II study in patients with advanced and recurrent ovarian cancer	ORR of 7.4% in patients with one to three prior lines of treatment and 9.9% in patients with four or more lines of treatments. ORR 10.0% in patients with CPS [2] $\geq$ 10	[130,131]
Varlilumab (anti-CD27 antibody) and nivolumab (anti-PD-1 antibody)	Phase I/II study in patients advanced and refractory ovarian cancer	Increase in PD-L1 expression and CD8+ T cells in ovarian biopsies, changes related with a better outcome. Possible benefit in a group of resistant to PD-1 inhibitor monotherapy	[132,133]
Nivolumab and ipilimumab (anti-CTLA-4 antibody)	Phase II in patients with recurrent or persistent ovarian cancer	The combined use of nivolumab and ipilimumab in EOC showed a longer progression-free disease compared to nivolumab alone	[134]

[1] ORR: overall response rate. [2] CPS: combined positive score.

Another interesting approach regarding immunotherapies is the development of cell-specific vaccines. For instance, DPX-Survivac (DepoVax) is a vaccine that generates a tumour-specific immune response, particularly by cells that express the protein survivin, using survivin HLA class I peptides [139]. Because ovarian cancer is one of the neoplasms that express higher amounts of this protein, a clinical trial tested the combination of DPX-Survivac, a low dose of cyclophosphamide and epacadostat, an inhibitor of indoleamine 2,3-dioxygenase-1 (IDO1) which may reverse tumour-associated immune suppression (NCT02785250). Preliminary results of this study showed encouraging results in 3 of 10 patients, 2 of them with a disease control for more than 12 months [140].

A current perspective using immune checkpoint inhibitors is the combination of these drugs with anti-angiogenic therapies [141] and with PARP inhibitors [142] which could decrease primary resistance, improving therapy results. This is because PARP inhibitors activate the generation of type I interferon response, which upregulates chemokines that leads to T-cell recruitment and to PD-L1 upregulation on cancer cells [143,144]. In addition, BRCA dysfunction increases T-cell recruitment to the tumour site and increases the expression of immune response genes as PD1 and PD-L1 [145,146]. The combined use of immune checkpoint inhibitors with PARP inhibitors promotes the sensibilization to the second ones in breast cancer cell lines [147] and greater anti-tumoral activity than either drug alone, suggesting that this combination could be a rational strategy. In ovarian cancer patients, the combination of olaparib and durvalumab was tested in heavily pretreated patients, showing clinical activity in patients without BRCA mutations [148]. Another phase I study tested olaparib and tremelimumab in women with heavily pre-treated and recurrent BRCA-associated ovarian cancer. Preliminary results of this study showed acceptable tolerability and therapeutic effect [149].

8. Drug Repurposing for Complementary Treatment for Ovarian Cancer

Drug repurposing is the process of identifying new therapeutic uses for existing or available drugs. It is an effective strategy in discovering molecules with new therapeutic implications [150,151]. Because existing drugs have studies of pharmacokinetics and safety in humans, the approval for further therapeutical use is shorter than the conventional development of a new drug, which could be especially beneficial in lower-income countries. The increased knowledge about the mechanisms involved in the progression of EOC has promoted several studies of repurposed drugs as possible complementary therapies (summarized in Table 4 and Figure 3), and most of them are addressed in the following sections.

Table 4. Summary of the main findings of studies using repurposing drugs for ovarian cancer treatment.

Drugs	Mechanism	Study and Patients	Main Findings	Ref.
Chloroquine	Autophagy inhibitor	Phase I/II study with advanced platinum-resistant epithelial ovarian cancer	Reverses cisplatin resistance in vitro. In patients, 30% expressed autophagy-related proteins but did not correlate with patient benefit	[152,153]
Ivermectin	Autophagy inhibitor	In vivo and in vitro studies	Synergistically suppresses tumour growth in combination with cisplatin or paclitaxel	[154,155]
Statins	HMG-CoA [1] reductase inhibitors	Observational studies	Statin use was inversely associated with ovarian cancer risk, particularly mucinous and endometrioid subtypes	[156]
Bisphosphonates	Inhibitors of mevalonic acid pathway	In vitro studies	Zoledronate displayed additive and synergistic anti-tumoral effects with pitavastatin on cell growth, tumour-promoting cytokines, and mediators	[157,158]
Disulfiram	Aldehyde dehydrogenase inhibitor	Observational and in vitro studies	ALDH1A1 [2] -positive cells are negatively correlated with progression-free survival in HGS-EOC patients. In vitro enhancement of cisplatin-induced apoptosis	[159,160]
Arsenic trioxide	Pro-oxidative compound	In vitro and in vivo studies	Increases sensibility of ovarian cancer cells to PARP inhibitors and synergically suppress tumour growth with cisplatin and paclitaxel treatment	[161,162]
Metformin	mTOR [3] inhibitor	Observational studies in type 2 diabetic patients. Phase II study in non-diabetic patients	Decreases in ovarian cancer incidence and mortality in type 2 diabetic patients. Tumours from metformin-treated patients presented a decrease of cancer stem cells markers and an increased sensitivity to cisplatin ex vivo.	[163–165]
NSAIDs [4]	COX [5] inhibitors	In vitro and in vivo studies	Anti-inflammatory effects. Increases paclitaxel sensitivity and restores cisplatin sensitivity	[166–168]

[1] HMG-CoA: β-Hydroxy β-methylglutaryl-coenzyme A. [2] ALDH1A1: aldehyde dehydrogenase 1 family member A1. [3] mTOR: mammalian target of rapamycin. [4] NSAIDs: non-steroidal anti-inflammatory drugs. [5] COX: cyclooxygenase.

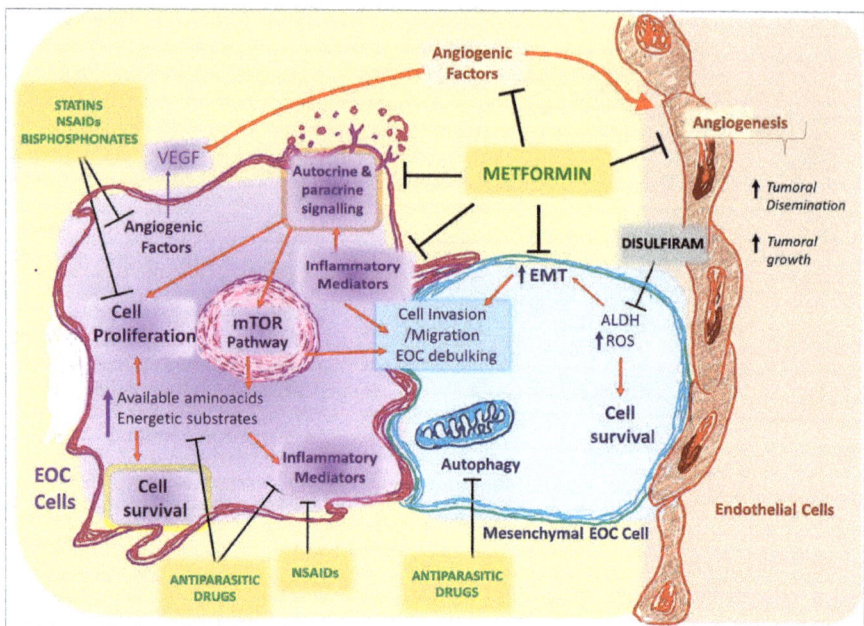

Figure 3. Repurposed drugs with anti-tumoral effects in epithelial ovarian cancer cells (in vitro and in vivo) and their molecular targets. EOC: epithelial ovarian cancer. VEGF: vascular endothelial growth factor. EMT: epithelial-mesenchymal transition. ALDH: aldehyde dehydrogenase. ROS: reactive oxygen species. NSAIDs: non-steroidal anti-inflammatories.

8.1. Autophagy Inhibitors (Antiparasitic Drugs)

Autophagy is an evolutionary form of self-digestion whose pathways are involved in protein and organelle degradation, and its imbalance is observed in several human diseases, such as EOC [169–171]. Autophagy increases during nutrient and growth factor deprivation, endoplasmic reticulum stress, development, or accumulation of protein aggregates [169].

The tumour microenvironment has exceptionally stressful conditions, including hypoxia and nutrient deprivation, and autophagy allows cancer cells to survive under these metabolic stress conditions [172]. In cancer cells, it is described that autophagy plays a dual role. On the one hand, it promotes cell death and cell cycle arrest, which usually prevents tumour development [173–175]. On the other hand, autophagy operates as a mechanism for tumour adaptation, reducing damaged cellular parts, recycling intracellular components to supply metabolic substrates, and maintaining cellular homeostasis, promoting tumour survival and growth in advanced cancers [176,177]. In addition, it is involved in the increase of resistance of anticancer drugs and other essential processes, including oxidative stress, inflammation and modulates tumour immunology [178–180]. In EOC cells, the increase of autophagy leads to cisplatin resistance, and their inhibition mediates cisplatin sensitivity [181,182]. Therefore, it is believed that autophagy inhibition can re-sensitize resistant cancer cells to chemotherapy and increase its cytotoxicity.

Chloroquine and its derivatives are common autophagy inhibitors. These compounds could be accumulated in intercellular acid vesicles as lysosomes, thereby inhibiting lysosome–autophagosome fusion [183]. In 2018, a case report showed that a 60-year-old woman with advanced and not resected intra-abdominal EOC achieved a complete response to chemotherapy after receiving hydroxychloroquine and quinacrine [184]. This finding fostered the interest of several researchers in the anti-tumoral effects of antimalarials in ovarian cancer.

In vitro experiments have shown that chloroquine reverses cisplatin resistance in EOC cells, producing autophagy inhibition and lethal DNA damage by inducing p21WAF1/CIP1 expression [152]. Besides, autophagy inhibitors have been tested in combination with other anti-tumoral compounds. In glioblastoma cells, hydroxychloroquine potentiates the anti-cancer effect of bevacizumab [185]. These findings encouraged a phase I/II trial that assesses hydroxychloroquine and itraconazole in women with advanced platinum-resistant EOC (HYDRA-01). The study shows that even if a high presence of autophagy markers was detected in 30% of patients, the drug combination did not show patient benefits [153]. It is important to highlight that this study included a heavily pre-treated platinum-resistant EOC population; therefore, the effect of autophagy inhibitors in EOC patients without previous treatment or in less advanced stages of the disease is still unknown.

Another broad-spectrum antiparasitic drug whose anti-tumoral effects are mediated by the increases of autophagy is ivermectin [186]. In ovarian cancer cells, ivermectin synergistically suppresses tumour growth in combination with cisplatin [155] or paclitaxel [154], and its anticancer mechanism involves the modulation of long non-coding RNAs with multiple targets [187]. However, these effects have not been tested in humans yet.

8.2. Lipid-Lowering Medications

Statins are a group of drugs widely used to reduce cholesterol biosynthesis inhibiting the enzyme HMG-CoA reductase [188]. A Danish study performed in 2012 showed that statin use in patients with cancer was associated with reducing cancer-related mortality [189]. In agreement with this, a meta-analysis conducted with different studies of statins and gynaecological cancers showed that the use of these drugs was inversely associated with ovarian cancer risk [190].

However, some studies showed no association between the use of statins and reduced risk of ovarian cancer [191,192]. Therefore, the evidence suggests a protective role of statins in ovarian cancer, but this is not conclusive. To elucidate this controversy, researchers have performed studies using EOC cells as well as more detailed analyses of published studies. In vitro experiments have shown that statins (lovastatin and atorvastatin) inhibit cell proliferation, suppress anchorage-independent growth, induce apoptosis, autophagy, cellular stress, and cell cycle arrest [193–195] in different EOC cell lines. Currently, there is a clinical trial recruiting patients with platinum-sensitive ovarian cancer to test the effect of simvastatin in the progression of the disease (NCT04457089).

The conflicting evidence about the positive effects of statin in ovarian cancer patients could be explained by a differential effect according to the histotype of ovarian carcinoma. A recent systematic review [156] that included 9 studies of statins in ovarian cancer showed a new perspective. The study concluded that the use of hydrophilic statins was associated with a decrease of risk of ovarian cancer (unlike hydrophobic, whose use increased the risk), particularly in mucinous and endometroid subtypes, a higher protective effect with long term use of statins (>5 years) and a most significant benefit with the combination of statins with other drugs, as salicylic acid.

8.3. Bisphosphonates

Bisphosphonates are pharmacological agents used against osteoclast-mediated bone loss [196]. Nitrogen-containing bisphosphonates (second generation of these drugs) inhibit the activity of farnesyl pyrophosphate synthase, a key regulatory enzyme in the mevalonic acid pathway. This substrate is critical to producing sterols and isoprenoid lipids whose deficiency produces osteoclast apoptosis [197,198].

In vitro studies have shown that pamidronate, incadronate, alendronate, risedronate and zoledronate had direct inhibitory effects on cell proliferation of several ovarian cancer cell lines [157,199]. However, these results are not consistent with a few studies performed with ovarian cancer patients. A systematic revision [157] studied the relationship between the use of bisphosphonate and the risk of endometrial and ovarian cancer. The study evidenced that the use of bisphosphonates for more than one year was associated with a reduced risk of endometrial cancer, but ovarian cancer risk remains unchanged. However, this meta-analysis included only four studies with ovarian cancer patients.

On the other hand, another study evaluated the effect of bisphosphonates and lipid-lowering medications in EOC cells. Results showed that the treatment with pitavastatin and zoledronate displayed additive and synergistic anti-proliferative effects on most ovarian cancer cell lines [157]. Another study in EOC cell lines showed that tumour-promoting cytokines and mediators, such as transforming growth factor (TGF)-β1, VEGF, interleukin (IL)-8, and IL-6, were suppressed up to 90% after the treatment with statins and zoledronate [158].

Because ovarian cancer affects women in the age of 65 years and older more frequently than younger [5,200] and osteoporosis is the most prevalent disease in menopausal women [201,202], the use of bisphosphonates in association with other known medications as statins could be an interesting field that should continue to be investigated.

8.4. Pro-Oxidative Drugs

In the context of repurposing drugs, some pro-oxidative agents have shown anti-tumoral activity in EOC cells. An evident example is disulfiram, one of three drugs approved by the U.S. FDA to treat alcohol dependence, whose mechanism involves the irreversible inhibition of aldehyde dehydrogenase (ALDH1A1) [203]. ALDH1A1 is not only a hepatic enzyme implicated in the major oxidative pathway of alcohol metabolism; it is also considered a stem cell marker that promotes epithelial-mesenchymal transition (EMT) progress in EOC cells [204,205]. The activity of ALDH1A1 is significantly higher in taxane- and platinum-resistant cell lines, and notably, the presence of ALDH1A1-positive cells is negatively correlated with progression-free survival in HGS-EOC patients [159]. Therefore, inhibitors of this enzyme could be helpful in the context of EOC.

In ovarian cancer cells, the treatment with disulfiram produces dose and time-dependent cytotoxic effects, enhancing cisplatin-induced apoptosis, and consequentially their association with the cofactor copper increases intracellular ROS levels, triggering apoptosis of ovarian cancer with stem cell phenotype [160]. In the same way, it was reported that disulfiram caused irreversible cell damage in EOC cells by redox-related proteotoxicity associated with induction of heat shock proteins HSP70, HSP40, and HSP32 [206].

Another pro-oxidative compound with anti-tumoral effects in EOC cells is arsenic trioxide (As_2O_3). The treatment with this compound is used as first-line and consolidation/maintenance treatments in haematological pathologies such as promyelocytic myeloid leukaemia [207]. Arsenic trioxide has been tested on ovarian cancer cell lines in both in vitro and animal models [208]. It can sensitize ovarian cancer cells to PARP inhibitors and cisplatin resistance [161], it has anti-angiogenic and antiproliferative activities by decreasing the expression of VEGFA and topoisomerase II, respectively [209,210], and produces cell growth inhibition and increase of apoptosis in adherent and suspension ovarian cancer cells, along with a synergism with cisplatin and paclitaxel treatment [162,211,212]. These findings encouraged two clinical trials registered in ClinicalTrials.gov (accessed on 7 December 2021) database testing the effect of arsenic trioxide in platinum resistance relapsed ovarian cancer (NCT04518501) and recurrent and metastatic ovarian cancer with P53 mutation (NCT04489706).

8.5. mTOR Inhibitors

One of the most studied signalling pathways in cancer is the mechanistic target of rapamycin (mTOR), two protein complexes that regulate cell growth, survival, metabolism, nutrient input, drug resistance, and immunity [213,214]. One example of mTOR inhibitor is itraconazole, a broad-spectrum antifungal agent, that had anti-proliferative effects in EOC and endothelial cells [215]. Currently, there are two clinical trials studying itraconazole in the context of EOC. The first aims to evaluate the effects of itraconazole and tamoxifen in platinum-refractory/resistant or recurrent ovarian cancer (NCT03458221). The second is the previously mentioned study HYDRA-01 that tested the combination of hydroxychloroquine and itraconazole in women with heavily pre-treated platinum-resistant EOC. This study is the only one with results, which unfortunately did not show a patient benefit [153].

Biguanides

Other widely studied mTOR inhibitors are biguanides, of which metformin, phenformin, and buformin are the main representatives. Due to reports of lactic acidosis (the more serious adverse effect), phenformin and buformin were withdrawn from clinical use in most countries during the 1970s [216]. Metformin, which has a much lower risk of lactic acidosis, is the most used biguanide for treating type 2 diabetes and metabolic disorders [216]. In the context of EOC, both metformin and phenformin have shown anti-proliferative effects in-vitro and in-vivo [217,218], but most studies have been conducted using metformin.

In humans, metformin intake has been associated with decreased cancer incidence and mortality in type 2 diabetic patients [219], including women with EOC [163,164]. Besides, in vitro studies have shown that metformin exerts multiple and pleiotropic anti-tumoral effects in EOC cells [218,220]. One of the most studied molecular targets of metformin is the adenosine monophosphate-activated protein kinase (AMPK), a key sensor of the energetic status of the cell [221]. AMPK activation inhibits mTOR complex 1 (mTORC1), impairing cancer cell survival, protein synthesis (which regulates cell proliferation and immune cell differentiation), and tumoral metabolism [222]. Although metformin is a known activator of AMPK, studies have reported that their anti-tumoral effects are dependent and independent of AMPK inhibition [223,224].

The treatment of HGS-EOC cells with metformin or phenformin decreases cell proliferation and produces changes in their cell metabolism, increasing glycolysis and inhibiting oxidative phosphorylation by alteration of mitochondrial shuttle metabolites [225,226]. In addition, studies have shown that metformin enhances cisplatin cytotoxicity in EOC cells [128] and produces chemo-sensitizing effects in cisplatin- and paclitaxel-resistant EOC cells [227].

Some targets of metformin in EOC cells include angiogenic factors that are overexpressed by tumoral cells such as VEGF or NGF; the proteins sterol regulatory elementbinding protein 1 (SREBP) and acetyl-CoA carboxylase (ACC) (critical proteins involved in fatty acid synthesis), c-MYC transcription factor, cyclins, cell cycle regulators and EMT proteins [218,228]. In addition, metformin elicits anticancer effects through the sequential modulation of the endoribonuclease Dicer [229], an important component of microRNAs biogenesis, which is dysregulated in EOC, which is further discussed later.

Tumour cells grow in environments with scarce nutrients and oxygen, known as the tumour microenvironment [230]. The resulting microenvironments contribute to the development of cellular subpopulations with different metabolic characteristics. These populations include stem-like cells, which adapt to reduced oxygen availability, switching between glycolysis and oxidative phosphorylation as energy sources and metabolites [230]. Epidemiologic and preclinical studies suggest a selective anti-tumoral effect of metformin on stem-like EOC cells [231–234], which plays an essential role in chemoresistance and ovarian cancer recurrence [60,235]. In this context, a phase II trial evaluated the impact of metformin on stem-like EOC cells and carcinoma-associated mesenchymal stem cells in nondiabetic patients with advanced EOC [165]. Results showed that tumours from metformin-treated patients decrease cancer stem cells markers and increase sensitivity to cisplatin ex vivo. Additionally, metformin altered the methylation signature in carcinomaassociated mesenchymal stem cells, which prevented the chemoresistance mediated by these cells in vitro [236].

Biguanides have been tested with other antitumoral agents, such as PARP inhibitors. Phenformin and metformin have shown a synergistic effect with olaparib, reducing cell survival, tumorigenesis, and decreasing mesenchymal markers of drug-resistant ovarian cancer cells [237], so the association of metformin with other new anti-tumoral drugs could be an important research matter.

Because metformin has additional beneficial effects against cancer, including anti-inflammatory, anti-aging, and antithrombotic properties [238], it was proposed as a plausible complementary therapy to first-line treatments for EOC patients. Most in vitro studies have corroborated the anti-tumoral potential of this drug; however, few clinical trials have tested metformin in non-diabetic patients with EOC. Although there is much in-vitro evidence indicating that metformin could be helpful as an anti-tumoral drug, many questions remain to be answered, such as its anti-tumoral mechanism, dose, timing, and the optimal therapeutic window (before cytoreduction? during chemotherapy cycles? both?). It is relevant to continue studying the anti-tumoral effects of metformin in patients with earlier stages and without previous treatment, along with establishing the best dose and optimal therapeutic window that could benefit to EOC patients, as well as the combination with other possible drugs.

8.6. Non-Steroidal Anti-Inflammatory Drugs (NSAIDs)

NSAIDs are widely used to relieve pain, reduce inflammation, and bring down a high temperature [239]. The primary mechanism of action of NSAIDs is the inhibition of the enzymes cyclooxygenases (COX) 1 and 2 and, therefore, prostaglandin (PG) synthesis [239]. Long-term use of NSAIDs has been associated with reduced incidence of several epithelial cancers [240–242]. A molecular explanation is that chronic inflammation promotes carcinogenesis by inducing proliferation, angiogenesis, metastasis, and chemotherapy resistance [243], so the use of NSAIDs could be an adequate possibility to improve cancer treatments targeting the inflammation.

In addition to the direct anti-tumoral effects of NSAIDs in cancer cells, their use could be beneficial as complementary use to chemotherapy. It is thought that the combination of cell death and PGE2 release due to cisplatin treatment results in a wound-like response and initiates a stem-like program, which favours cancer progression. In bladder cancer cells, the use of combined cisplatin and COX-2 inhibitor celecoxib prevents cisplatin resistance and restores cisplatin sensitivity in vivo and in vitro [166,167]. In neuroblastoma, diclofenac (a known NSAIDs drug) enhanced chemotherapy-induced apoptosis via upregulation of p53 [244]. Particularly in EOC, it is described that COX inhibitors increase paclitaxel sensitivity in taxane-resistant EOC cells [245].

Among NSAIDs, diclofenac is a relevant drug in cancer therapy. One significant footprint of human cancers is the metabolic switch which favours glycolytic pathways to obtain energy in the form of ATP (Warburg effect) [246]. Cancer cells increase glucose uptake, and as a result of an increased glycolysis rate, high concentrations of lactate are produced [247]. Lactate is considered an immunosuppressive metabolite [248], and under low glucose, tumour cells uptake and oxidize lactate, which means that lactate is used as an energetic source by cancer cells [247,249]. Research performed in a murine glioma model demonstrated that diclofenac (but not ibuprofen, another known NSAID), decreased lactate dehydrogenase A and lactate secretion. Additionally, it was described that diclofenac inhibited the uptake of lactate in colorectal cancer cells, being the most potent inhibitor among other NSAIDs [250].

This in vitro evidence suggests that NSAIDs could be helpful not only as anti-inflammatory agents, but also as inhibitors of cell metabolism, as the drug metformin.

9. Non-Coding RNA-Based Therapeutics for Ovarian Cancer

Non-coding RNAs are one of the latest emergent tools for targeting-cell therapy. Around 98% of the human genome corresponds to non-protein-coding sequences, and a substantial part of them are non-protein-coding RNA transcripts (ncRNAs) [251]. ncRNAs are RNA molecules that are not translated into proteins but have crucial cellular functions so that their dysregulation can lead to the development of different pathologies such as cancer [252]. The ncRNAs are classified according to their size into small non-coding RNAs and long non-coding RNAs (lncRNA), greater than 200 nucleotides [253].

Among the small ncRNAs, microRNAs (miRs) play a key role in the initiation and progression of ovarian cancer [254]. miRs are short sequences of nucleotides that bind messenger RNAs and interfere in protein translation [255], so they are post-transcriptional regulators. In cancer, there is a miR disbalance, with a predominance of oncomiRs (that inhibits the transcription of oncosupressor proteins) and a decrease of tumour-suppressor miRs, resulting in an increase of oncoproteins [255]. Because one miR regulates several messenger RNAs (and several different proteins) involved in critical tumoral processes such as proliferation, migration, invasion, and angiogenesis [254], the use of miR-based therapy has been attractive for most researchers. Among different miRs, dysregulation of Let-7, miR-200 family, miR-17-92, miR-21, miR-145, and miR-23b have been reported in ovarian cancer, being the first one of the most studied miR in the context of EOC [256]. miR-145 is an onco-suppressor miR that is downregulated in EOC biopsies and EOC cells. Studies have shown that overexpression of miR-145 decreases the cell proliferation, migration, invasion, and tumoral formation of EOC cells [257]. In addition, the role of this miR in tumoral metabolism has been documented. miR-145 negatively regulates the Warburg effect in bladder cancer cells [258] and inhibits the mitochondrial function of EOC cells [259], suggesting that its reinstatement could contribute to the energetic depletion of tumoral cells. Significantly, cisplatin mediates downregulation of miR-145 in cisplatin-resistant EOC cells [260] and upregulation of miR-145 sensitizes EOC cells to paclitaxel, suggesting a crucial role of miR-145 in chemotherapy resistance. Because miRs are "natural" molecules present in all bodies, with likely no adverse effects in other tissues [253], the re-establishment of levels of onco-suppressor miRs as miR-145 could be an interesting proposition as a future complementary treatment in EOC.

On the other hand, lncRNAs are also involved in miRs disbalance. They play an important role in gene expression and may even function as miRs sponges, which may cause a decrease in the effect of some miRs [261,262].

Metastasis-associated lung adenocarcinoma transcript 1 (MALAT1) is one of the best-described lncRNAs and its up-regulation has been associated with progression and chemoresistance in different types of cancers [263–265]. In ovarian cancer, MALAT is overexpressed in epithelial ovarian cancer tissues and cell lines, promoting proliferation and metastasis via the PI3K-AKT pathway [266,267]. Recent studies in prostatic cancer cells determined that MALAT1 promotes the proliferation, migration, and invasion of tumour cells by acting as a miR-145 sponge, suppressing its anti-tumoral activity, and the downregulation of MALAT1 increases miR-145 and decreases cell migration and invasion [268]. These observations led to the proposition of oncogenic sponge lncRNAs as possible therapeutic targets for cancer treatment, and their specific modulation could be an interesting approach in EOC.

10. New Methods of Drug Delivery (Nanomedicine)

For decades, the anti-tumoral drugs were chemically modified to increase their half-life and biodistribution. However, the tissue-specific drug delivery using nanotechnology (nanocarriers) is set to spread rapidly and gained much interest as a promising diagnostic and therapeutic strategy (Figure 4).

Research groups have explored new methods of drug delivery, such as nanoparticles, in different ovarian cancer models, with the purpose to improve the effectiveness of chemotherapy [269]. In this context, nanocarriers that address chemotherapeutic drugs or new anti-tumoral biological molecules, such as miRs or small interference RNAs (siRNAs) have been tested in vivo. They could be directly delivered into target cancer cells, resulting in enhanced therapeutic impact with less toxicity, biocompatibility, good biodegradability and increased therapeutic impact than free drugs, with fewer side-effects [269–271].

Targeted drug delivery has become a new paradigm in cancer therapy [271] using a range of nanomaterials based on organic, inorganic, lipid, or glycan compounds and synthetic polymers [272]. For instance, nanoparticles in base to hyaluronic acid encapsulating both paclitaxel and focal adhesion kinase (FAK) siRNA were developed as a selective delivery system against chemoresistant EOC cells. This nanoformulation strongly decreased the tumoral growth of EOC xenografts and patient-derivate xenografts [273]. Similarly, iron-oxide nanoparticles (Fe_2O_3) have emerged as one of the extensively utilized nanostructures in different models of EOC, because of their superparamagnetic features, which enables their accumulation in animal tumours, and appear as a candidate for properties such as antioxidant, antibiofilm, antimicrobial, and antitumoral activities [274–276]. A recent work showed that Fe_2O_3 nanoparticles display cytotoxic activity in metastatic ovarian teratocarcinoma cells by augmenting the level of reactive oxygen species (ROS), destabilizing mitochondrial membrane, and enhancing of programmed cell death [277]. Other nanocarrier examples include cationic liposomes with polyethylene glycol and glycolic acid-based nanoparticles, which may incorporate chemotherapeutics such as paclitaxel or doxorubicin and small interference RNAs (siRNA) producing synergistic antitumoral effects in in vitro and in vivo models of EOC cells [278–280].

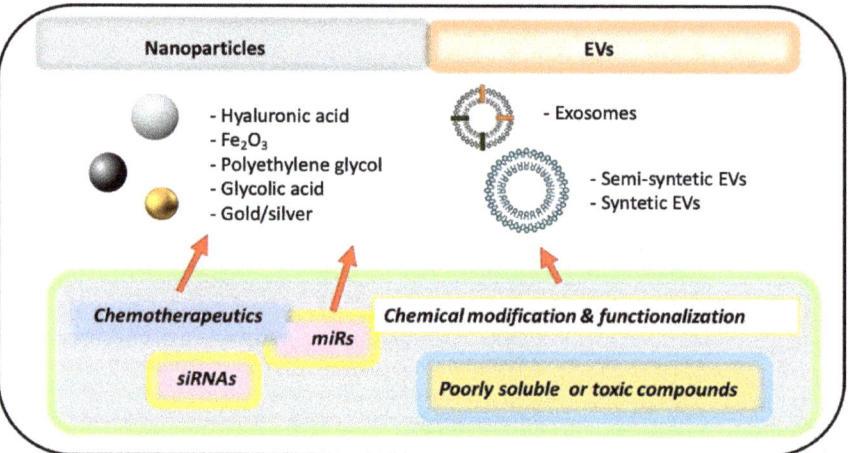

Figure 4. Some examples of advances in monotherapies and drug delivery for ovarian cancer. Most nanocarriers are under study in different models of ovarian cancer. It is expected that they could improve the delivery, half-life, and distribution of ovarian cancer therapies. Some examples of nanocarriers are nanoparticles, exosomes and modified extracellular vesicles (EVs). miRs: microRNAs. siRNAs: small interference RNAs.

Another recent approach of molecular agents that are tested in several ovarian cancer models is the use of extracellular vesicles (EVs). They are continuously produced and released by cells and contain proteins, messenger RNA, and miRs that can be transferred to another cell and become functional in the new location [281]. EVs play an important role in cancer diagnosis [282] or prognosis [283] and drug resistance [284] and it is proposed that they could be used as a delivery vehicle of chemotherapeutics [285]. Two main kinds of EVs are produced to carrier and deliver anti-tumoral therapies: EVs-based semisynthetic nanoparticles and EVs mimetic nanoparticles. The first is naturally isolated EVs with surface and membrane modifications; while EVs mimetic nanoparticles are artificial structures [286] that could efficiently encapsulate a different kind of anti-tumoral molecules. Among EVs, exosomes, a subtype of EVs with a diameter less than 150 nm, are fully considered as possible nanocarriers due to their size and the capacity to carry a wide variety of molecular cargos [281].

A recent work shows that stem cell-derived EVs can release the encapsulated miR-424, suppressing tumorigenesis and angiogenesis of ovarian tumours in vivo [287]. Not only biological compound could be delivered by EVs, but also hydrophobic or toxic chemotherapeutics. For instance, exosomes from tumour cells (modified with biomimetic porous silicon nanoparticles) were used as drug nanocarriers for targeting doxorubicin [288]. This nanoformulation enhanced tumour accumulation, extravasation from blood vessels, and penetration into deep tumour parenchyma of doxorubicin in a model of mouse hepatocellular carcinoma [288]. In ovarian cancer cells, researchers have studied the encapsulation of triptolide (a natural product isolated from the Chinese herbal) in exosomes from EOC cells, obtaining a high drug encapsulation efficiency and uptake by SKOV3 cells [289]. In vivo, this exosome formulation showed more potent inhibition of tumour growth and less toxic effects on the liver and spleen than free triptolide extract, concluding that exosome delivery could be helpful to address and decrease the side effects of antitumoral agents [289].

Inspired by the self-assembly that occurs in cells and exosomes, researchers designed a biomimetic lipid/dextran hybrid nanocarrier loaded with a siRNA for multidrug resistance protein 1 (MDR1) and the drug paclitaxel, which reversed the chemoresistance in both in vitro and in vivo models of EOC cells [168]. These synthetic structures based on exosomes could be a promising strategy for EOC treatment because they can overcome some difficulties inherent to the natural purification of exosomes, such as the problematic obtention and variable retrieval of extracts, which should be studied for the following years.

11. Main Conclusions

EOC is a neoplasm with high mortality and late diagnosis. Because of its molecular heterogenicity and different patient's therapeutically response, personalized medicine should be incorporated into current practice during the next years.

It is necessary to understand better the molecular characteristics of ovarian cancer tumours and the new possible drugs or biological agents that could be useful in each patient. Based on this, immune checkpoints inhibitors, PARP inhibitors, and anti-angiogenic therapies constitute great advances for EOC treatment, and the testing of its combinations appears to be a reasonable alternative. Besides, there are several new possible and complementary therapies, including neurotrophic receptors inhibitors, repurposing drugs, non-coding RNAs, and the development of different nanoformulations under study, mainly in preclinical stages and pretend to offer new therapeutic alternatives for EOC patients.

Author Contributions: Conceptualization, M.P.G. and C.R.; investigation, M.P.G., A.N.F., L.L.-G., M.V.-V., D.B.V. and C.R.; writing—original draft preparation, M.P.G., M.V-V. and C.R.; writing—review and editing, M.P.G. All authors have read and agreed to the published version of the manuscript.

Funding: This research received no external funding. The APC was funded by Universidad de Chile.

Institutional Review Board Statement: Not applicable.

Informed Consent Statement: Not applicable.

Data Availability Statement: Not applicable.

Conflicts of Interest: The authors declare no conflict of interest.

References

1. Falzone, L.; Salomone, S.; Libra, M. Evolution of Cancer Pharmacological Treatments at the Turn of the Third Millennium. *Front. Pharm.* **2018**, *9*, 1300. [CrossRef]
2. U.S. Food and Drug Administration (FDA). Drugs Approved for Ovarian, Fallopian Tube, or Primary Peritoneal Cancer. 2021. Available online: https://www.cancer.gov/about-cancer/treatment/drugs/ovarian (accessed on 7 December 2021).
3. U.S. Food and Drug Administration (FDA). FDA Approves Bevacizumab in Combination with Chemotherapy for Ovarian Cancer. 2018. Available online: https://www.fda.gov/drugs/resources-information-approved-drugs/fda-approves-bevacizumab-combination-chemotherapy-ovarian-cancer (accessed on 7 December 2021).
4. Valabrega, G.; Scotto, G.; Tuninetti, V.; Pani, A.; Scaglione, F. Differences in PARP Inhibitors for the Treatment of Ovarian Cancer: Mechanisms of Action, Pharmacology, Safety, and Efficacy. *Int. J. Mol. Sci.* **2021**, *22*, 4203. [CrossRef]
5. American Cancer Society. Key Statistics for Ovarian Cancer. 2021. Available online: https://www.cancer.org/cancer/ovarian-cancer/about/key-statistics.html (accessed on 7 December 2021).
6. Jayde, V.; White, K.; Blomfield, P. Symptoms and diagnostic delay in ovarian cancer: A summary of the literature. *Contemp. Nurse* **2009**, *34*, 55–65. [CrossRef]
7. Telloni, S.M. Tumor Staging and Grading: A Primer. *Methods Mol. Biol.* **2017**, *1606*, 1–17. [CrossRef]

8. Mutch, D.G.; Prat, J. 2014 FIGO staging for ovarian, fallopian tube and peritoneal cancer. *Gynecol. Oncol.* **2014**, *133*, 401–404. [CrossRef]
9. Javadi, S.; Ganeshan, D.M.; Qayyum, A.; Iyer, R.B.; Bhosale, P. Ovarian Cancer, the Revised FIGO Staging System, and the Role of Imaging. *AJR Am. J. Roentgenol.* **2016**, *206*, 1351–1360. [CrossRef] [PubMed]
10. American Cancer Society. About Ovarian Cancer. 2018. Available online: https://www.cancer.org/cancer/ovarian-cancer/about/what-is-ovarian-cancer.html (accessed on 7 December 2021).
11. Cancer Research UK. Epithelial Ovarian Cancer. 2021. Available online: https://www.cancerresearchuk.org/about-cancer/ovarian-cancer/types/epithelial-ovarian-cancers/epithelial (accessed on 7 December 2021).
12. Shih, I.M.; Kurman, R.J. Ovarian tumorigenesis: A proposed model based on morphological and molecular genetic analysis. *Am. J. Pathol.* **2004**, *164*, 1511–1518. [CrossRef]
13. Kurman, R.J.; Shih, I.M. The Dualistic Model of Ovarian Carcinogenesis: Revisited, Revised, and Expanded. *Am. J. Pathol.* **2016**, *186*, 733–747. [CrossRef] [PubMed]
14. Li, J.; Abushahin, N.; Pang, S.; Xiang, L.; Chambers, S.K.; Fadare, O.; Kong, B.; Zheng, W. Tubal origin of 'ovarian' low-grade serous carcinoma. *Mod. Pathol.* **2011**, *24*, 1488–1499. [CrossRef]
15. Trimbos, J.B.; Parmar, M.; Vergote, I.; Guthrie, D.; Bolis, G.; Colombo, N.; Vermorken, J.B.; Torri, V.; Mangioni, C.; Pecorelli, S.; et al. International Collaborative Ovarian Neoplasm trial 1 and Adjuvant ChemoTherapy in Ovarian Neoplasm trial: Two parallel randomized phase III trials of adjuvant chemotherapy in patients with early-stage ovarian carcinoma. *J. Natl. Cancer Inst.* **2003**, *95*, 105–112. [CrossRef]
16. Esin, E.; Bilgetekin, İ.; Başal, F.B.; Duran, A.O.; Demirci, U.; Öksüzoğlu, B. Controversies in the efficacy of adjuvant chemotherapy in different epithelial ovarian carcinoma histologies. *J. Oncol. Sci.* **2019**, *5*, 96–99. [CrossRef]
17. Lheureux, S.; Braunstein, M.; Oza, A.M. Epithelial ovarian cancer: Evolution of management in the era of precision medicine. *CA Cancer J. Clin.* **2019**, *69*, 280–304. [CrossRef] [PubMed]
18. Lengyel, E. Ovarian cancer development and metastasis. *Am. J. Pathol.* **2010**, *177*, 1053–1064. [CrossRef]
19. Kurman, R.J.; Shih, I.M. Molecular pathogenesis and extraovarian origin of epithelial ovarian cancer—Shifting the paradigm. *Hum. Pathol.* **2011**, *42*, 918–931. [CrossRef]
20. Zeppernick, F.; Meinhold-Heerlein, I.; Shih, I.M. Precursors of ovarian cancer in the fallopian tube: Serous tubal intraepithelial carcinoma—An update. *J. Obs. Gynaecol. Res.* **2015**, *41*, 6–11. [CrossRef]
21. Klotz, D.M.; Wimberger, P. Cells of origin of ovarian cancer: Ovarian surface epithelium or fallopian tube? *Arch. Gynecol. Obs.* **2017**, *296*, 1055–1062. [CrossRef]
22. Kurman, R.J.; Shih, I.M. The origin and pathogenesis of epithelial ovarian cancer: A proposed unifying theory. *Am. J. Surg. Pathol.* **2010**, *34*, 433–443. [CrossRef] [PubMed]
23. American Cancer Society. Survival Rates for Ovarian Cancer. 2021. Available online: https://www.cancer.org/cancer/ovarian-cancer/detection-diagnosis-staging/survival-rates.html (accessed on 23 November 2021).
24. Braicu, E.I.; Sehouli, J.; Richter, R.; Pietzner, K.; Denkert, C.; Fotopoulou, C. Role of histological type on surgical outcome and survival following radical primary tumour debulking of epithelial ovarian, fallopian tube and peritoneal cancers. *Br. J. Cancer* **2011**, *105*, 1818–1824. [CrossRef]
25. Zhou, J.; Wu, S.G.; Wang, J.; Sun, J.Y.; He, Z.Y.; Jin, X.; Zhang, W.W. The Effect of Histological Subtypes on Outcomes of Stage IV Epithelial Ovarian Cancer. *Front. Oncol.* **2018**, *8*, 577. [CrossRef]
26. Ebrahimi, V.; Khalafi-Nezhad, A.; Ahmadpour, F.; Jowkar, Z. Conditional disease-free survival rates and their associated determinants in patients with epithelial ovarian cancer: A 15-year retrospective cohort study. *Cancer Rep.* **2021**, e1416. [CrossRef]
27. Jones, S.; Wang, T.L.; Shih Ie, M.; Mao, T.L.; Nakayama, K.; Roden, R.; Glas, R.; Slamon, D.; Diaz, L.A., Jr.; Vogelstein, B.; et al. Frequent mutations of chromatin remodeling gene ARID1A in ovarian clear cell carcinoma. *Science* **2010**, *330*, 228–231. [CrossRef] [PubMed]
28. Cancer Genome Atlas Research Network. Integrated genomic analyses of ovarian carcinoma. *Nature* **2011**, *474*, 609–615. [CrossRef] [PubMed]
29. Bamberger, E.S.; Perrett, C.W. Angiogenesis in epithelian ovarian cancer. *Mol. Pathol.* **2002**, *55*, 348–359. [CrossRef]
30. Garrido, M.P.; Torres, I.; Vega, M.; Romero, C. Angiogenesis in Gynecological Cancers: Role of Neurotrophins. *Front. Oncol.* **2019**, *9*, 913. [CrossRef]
31. Campos, X.; Munoz, Y.; Selman, A.; Yazigi, R.; Moyano, L.; Weinstein-Oppenheimer, C.; Lara, H.E.; Romero, C. Nerve growth factor and its high-affinity receptor trkA participate in the control of vascular endothelial growth factor expression in epithelial ovarian cancer. *Gynecol. Oncol.* **2007**, *104*, 168–175. [CrossRef]
32. Sopo, M.; Anttila, M.; Hamalainen, K.; Kivela, A.; Yla-Herttuala, S.; Kosma, V.M.; Keski-Nisula, L.; Sallinen, H. Expression profiles of VEGF-A, VEGF-D and VEGFR1 are higher in distant metastases than in matched primary high grade epithelial ovarian cancer. *BMC Cancer* **2019**, *19*, 584. [CrossRef]
33. Fujimoto, J.; Sakaguchi, H.; Hirose, R.; Ichigo, S.; Tamaya, T. Biologic implications of the expression of vascular endothelial growth factor subtypes in ovarian carcinoma. *Cancer* **1998**, *83*, 2528–2533. [CrossRef]
34. Dissen, G.A.; Garcia-Rudaz, C.; Ojeda, S.R. Role of neurotrophic factors in early ovarian development. *Semin. Reprod. Med.* **2009**, *27*, 24–31. [CrossRef]

35. Streiter, S.; Fisch, B.; Sabbah, B.; Ao, A.; Abir, R. The importance of neuronal growth factors in the ovary. *Mol. Hum. Reprod.* **2016**, *22*, 3–17. [CrossRef] [PubMed]
36. Vera, C.; Tapia, V.; Vega, M.; Romero, C. Role of nerve growth factor and its TRKA receptor in normal ovarian and epithelial ovarian cancer angiogenesis. *J. Ovarian Res.* **2014**, *7*, 82. [CrossRef]
37. Au, C.W.; Siu, M.K.; Liao, X.; Wong, E.S.; Ngan, H.Y.; Tam, K.F.; Chan, D.C.; Chan, Q.K.; Cheung, A.N. Tyrosine kinase B receptor and BDNF expression in ovarian cancers—Effect on cell migration, angiogenesis and clinical outcome. *Cancer Lett.* **2009**, *281*, 151–161. [CrossRef]
38. Tapia, V.; Gabler, F.; Munoz, M.; Yazigi, R.; Paredes, A.; Selman, A.; Vega, M.; Romero, C. Tyrosine kinase A receptor (trkA): A potential marker in epithelial ovarian cancer. *Gynecol. Oncol.* **2011**, *121*, 13–23. [CrossRef] [PubMed]
39. Lassus, H.; Sihto, H.; Leminen, A.; Nordling, S.; Joensuu, H.; Nupponen, N.N.; Butzow, R. Genetic alterations and protein expression of KIT and PDGFRA in serous ovarian carcinoma. *Br. J. Cancer* **2004**, *91*, 2048–2055. [CrossRef] [PubMed]
40. Wang, Y.; Hu, C.; Dong, R.; Huang, X.; Qiu, H. Platelet-derived growth factor-D promotes ovarian cancer invasion by regulating matrix metalloproteinases 2 and 9. *Asian Pac. J. Cancer Prev.* **2011**, *12*, 3367–3370. [PubMed]
41. Sun, Y.; Fan, X.; Zhang, Q.; Shi, X.; Xu, G.; Zou, C. Cancer-associated fibroblasts secrete FGF-1 to promote ovarian proliferation, migration, and invasion through the activation of FGF-1/FGFR4 signaling. *Tumor Biol.* **2017**, *39*, 1010428317712592. [CrossRef] [PubMed]
42. Madsen, C.V.; Steffensen, K.D.; Olsen, D.A.; Waldstrom, M.; Sogaard, C.H.; Brandslund, I.; Jakobsen, A. Serum platelet-derived growth factor and fibroblast growth factor in patients with benign and malignant ovarian tumors. *Anticancer Res.* **2012**, *32*, 3817–3825.
43. Student, V.; Andrys, C.; Soucek, O.; Spacek, J.; Tosner, J.; Sedlakova, I. Importance of basal fibroblast growth factor levels in patients with ovarian tumor. *Ceska Gynekol.* **2018**, *83*, 169–176.
44. Meng, Q.H.; Xu, E.; Hildebrandt, M.A.; Liang, D.; Lu, K.; Ye, Y.; Wagar, E.A.; Wu, X. Genetic variants in the fibroblast growth factor pathway as potential markers of ovarian cancer risk, therapeutic response, and clinical outcome. *Clin. Chem.* **2014**, *60*, 222–232. [CrossRef] [PubMed]
45. Matei, D.; Emerson, R.E.; Lai, Y.C.; Baldridge, L.A.; Rao, J.; Yiannoutsos, C.; Donner, D.D. Autocrine activation of PDGFRalpha promotes the progression of ovarian cancer. *Oncogene* **2006**, *25*, 2060–2069. [CrossRef]
46. Brunckhorst, M.K.; Xu, Y.; Lu, R.; Yu, Q. Angiopoietins promote ovarian cancer progression by establishing a procancer microenvironment. *Am. J. Pathol.* **2014**, *184*, 2285–2296. [CrossRef] [PubMed]
47. Berchuck, A.; Olt, G.J.; Everitt, L.; Soisson, A.P.; Bast, R.C., Jr.; Boyer, C.M. The role of peptide growth factors in epithelial ovarian cancer. *Obstet. Gynecol.* **1990**, *75*, 255–262. [PubMed]
48. Smith, G.; Ng, M.T.; Shepherd, L.; Herrington, C.S.; Gourley, C.; Ferguson, M.J.; Wolf, C.R. Individuality in FGF1 expression significantly influences platinum resistance and progression-free survival in ovarian cancer. *Br. J. Cancer* **2012**, *107*, 1327–1336. [CrossRef] [PubMed]
49. American Cancer Society. Treatment of Invasive Epithelial Ovarian Cancers, by Stage. 2020. Available online: https://www.cancer.org/cancer/ovarian-cancer/treating/by-stage.html (accessed on 24 November 2021).
50. Kim, A.; Ueda, Y.; Naka, T.; Enomoto, T. Therapeutic strategies in epithelial ovarian cancer. *J. Exp. Clin. Cancer Res.* **2012**, *31*, 14. [CrossRef] [PubMed]
51. Eisenhauer, E.A. Real-world evidence in the treatment of ovarian cancer. *Ann. Oncol.* **2017**, *28*, viii61–viii65. [CrossRef]
52. Kampan, N.C.; Madondo, M.T.; McNally, O.M.; Quinn, M.; Plebanski, M. Paclitaxel and Its Evolving Role in the Management of Ovarian Cancer. *Biomed. Res. Int.* **2015**, *2015*, 413076. [CrossRef]
53. Markman, M.; Bundy, B.N.; Alberts, D.S.; Fowler, J.M.; Clark-Pearson, D.L.; Carson, L.F.; Wadler, S.; Sickel, J. Phase III trial of standard-dose intravenous cisplatin plus paclitaxel versus moderately high-dose carboplatin followed by intravenous paclitaxel and intraperitoneal cisplatin in small-volume stage III ovarian carcinoma: An intergroup study of the Gynecologic Oncology Group, Southwestern Oncology Group, and Eastern Cooperative Oncology Group. *J. Clin. Oncol.* **2001**, *19*, 1001–1007. [CrossRef]
54. Armstrong, D.K.; Bundy, B.; Wenzel, L.; Huang, H.Q.; Baergen, R.; Lele, S.; Copeland, L.J.; Walker, J.L.; Burger, R.A.; Gynecologic Oncology, G. Intraperitoneal cisplatin and paclitaxel in ovarian cancer. *N. Engl. J. Med.* **2006**, *354*, 34–43. [CrossRef]
55. Walker, J.L.; Brady, M.F.; Wenzel, L.; Fleming, G.F.; Huang, H.Q.; DiSilvestro, P.A.; Fujiwara, K.; Alberts, D.S.; Zheng, W.; Tewari, K.S.; et al. Randomized Trial of Intravenous Versus Intraperitoneal Chemotherapy Plus Bevacizumab in Advanced Ovarian Carcinoma: An NRG Oncology/Gynecologic Oncology Group Study. *J. Clin. Oncol.* **2019**, *37*, 1380–1390. [CrossRef]
56. Pogge von Strandmann, E.; Reinartz, S.; Wager, U.; Muller, R. Tumor-Host Cell Interactions in Ovarian Cancer: Pathways to Therapy Failure. *Trends Cancer* **2017**, *3*, 137–148. [CrossRef]
57. Galluzzi, L.; Senovilla, L.; Vitale, I.; Michels, J.; Martins, I.; Kepp, O.; Castedo, M.; Kroemer, G. Molecular mechanisms of cisplatin resistance. *Oncogene* **2012**, *31*, 1869–1883. [CrossRef]
58. Alqahtani, F.Y.; Aleanizy, F.S.; El Tahir, E.; Alkahtani, H.M.; AlQuadeib, B.T. Paclitaxel. *Profiles Drug Subst. Excip. Relat. Methodol.* **2019**, *44*, 205–238. [CrossRef]
59. Ottevanger, P.B. Ovarian cancer stem cells more questions than answers. *Semin. Cancer Biol.* **2017**, *44*, 67–71. [CrossRef]
60. Kenda Suster, N.; Virant-Klun, I. Presence and role of stem cells in ovarian cancer. *World J. Stem. Cells* **2019**, *11*, 383–397. [CrossRef]

61. Pfisterer, J.; Plante, M.; Vergote, I.; Bois, A.d.; Hirte, H.; Lacave, A.J.; Wagner, U.; Stähle, A.; Stuart, G.; Kimmig, R.; et al. Gemcitabine Plus Carboplatin Compared with Carboplatin in Patients With Platinum-Sensitive Recurrent Ovarian Cancer: An Intergroup Trial of the AGO-OVAR, the NCIC CTG, and the EORTC GCG. *J. Clin. Oncol.* **2006**, *24*, 4699–4707. [CrossRef] [PubMed]
62. U.S. Food and Drug Administration (FDA). GEMZAR (Gemcitabine) for Injection, for Intravenous Use. 1996. Available online: https://www.accessdata.fda.gov/drugsatfda_docs/label/2019/020509s082lbl.pdf (accessed on 24 November 2021).
63. Peters, G.J.; Van Moorsel, C.J.; Lakerveld, B.; Smid, K.; Noordhuis, P.; Comijn, E.C.; Weaver, D.; Willey, J.C.; Voorn, D.; Van der Vijgh, W.J.; et al. Effects of gemcitabine on cis-platinum-DNA adduct formation and repair in a panel of gemcitabine and cisplatin-sensitive or -resistant human ovarian cancer cell lines. *Int. J. Oncol.* **2006**, *28*, 237–244. [CrossRef] [PubMed]
64. Moufarij, M.A.; Phillips, D.R.; Cullinane, C. Gemcitabine potentiates cisplatin cytotoxicity and inhibits repair of cisplatin-DNA damage in ovarian cancer cell lines. *Mol. Pharm.* **2003**, *63*, 862–869. [CrossRef]
65. Lorusso, D.; Di Stefano, A.; Fanfani, F.; Scambia, G. Role of gemcitabine in ovarian cancer treatment. *Ann. Oncol.* **2006**, *17* (Suppl. S5), v188–v194. [CrossRef]
66. Benjamin, R.C.; Gill, D.M. ADP-ribosylation in mammalian cell ghosts. Dependence of poly(ADP-ribose) synthesis on strand breakage in DNA. *J. Biol. Chem.* **1980**, *255*, 10493–10501. [CrossRef]
67. Durkacz, B.W.; Omidiji, O.; Gray, D.A.; Shall, S. (ADP-ribose)n participates in DNA excision repair. *Nature* **1980**, *283*, 593–596. [CrossRef]
68. Rose, M.; Burgess, J.T.; O'Byrne, K.; Richard, D.J.; Bolderson, E. PARP Inhibitors: Clinical Relevance, Mechanisms of Action and Tumor Resistance. *Front. Cell Dev. Biol.* **2020**, *8*, 564601. [CrossRef] [PubMed]
69. Dale Rein, I.; Solberg Landsverk, K.; Micci, F.; Patzke, S.; Stokke, T. Replication-induced DNA damage after PARP inhibition causes G2 delay, and cell line-dependent apoptosis, necrosis and multinucleation. *Cell Cycle* **2015**, *14*, 3248–3260. [CrossRef]
70. How, J.A.; Jazaeri, A.A.; Fellman, B.; Daniels, M.S.; Penn, S.; Solimeno, C.; Yuan, Y.; Schmeler, K.; Lanchbury, J.S.; Timms, K.; et al. Modification of Homologous Recombination Deficiency Score Threshold and Association with Long-Term Survival in Epithelial Ovarian Cancer. *Cancers* **2021**, *13*, 946. [CrossRef]
71. Da Cunha Colombo Bonadio, R.R.; Fogace, R.N.; Miranda, V.C.; Diz, M. Homologous recombination deficiency in ovarian cancer: A review of its epidemiology and management. *Clinics* **2018**, *73*, e450s. [CrossRef] [PubMed]
72. Bowtell, D.D.; Bohm, S.; Ahmed, A.A.; Aspuria, P.J.; Bast, R.C., Jr.; Beral, V.; Berek, J.S.; Birrer, M.J.; Blagden, S.; Bookman, M.A.; et al. Rethinking ovarian cancer II: Reducing mortality from high-grade serous ovarian cancer. *Nat. Rev. Cancer* **2015**, *15*, 668–679. [CrossRef]
73. U.S. Food and Drug Administration (FDA). FDA Approved Olaparib (LYNPARZA, AstraZeneca Pharmaceuticals LP) for the Maintenance Treatment of Adult Patients with Deleterious or Suspected Deleterious Germline or Somatic BRCA-Mutated (gBRCAm or sBRCAm) Advanced Epithelial Ovarian, Fallopian Tube or Primary Peritoneal Cancer who are in Complete or Partial Response to First-Line Platinum-Based. 2018. Available online: https://www.fda.gov/drugs/fda-approved-olaparib-lynparza-astrazeneca-pharmaceuticals-lp-maintenance-treatment-adult-patients (accessed on 24 November 2021).
74. Balasubramaniam, S.; Beaver, J.A.; Horton, S.; Fernandes, L.L.; Tang, S.; Horne, H.N.; Liu, J.; Liu, C.; Schrieber, S.J.; Yu, J.; et al. FDA Approval Summary: Rucaparib for the Treatment of Patients with Deleterious BRCA Mutation-Associated Advanced Ovarian Cancer. *Clin. Cancer Res.* **2017**, *23*, 7165–7170. [CrossRef]
75. Buck, J.; Dyer, P.J.C.; Hii, H.; Carline, B.; Kuchibhotla, M.; Byrne, J.; Howlett, M.; Whitehouse, J.; Ebert, M.A.; McDonald, K.L.; et al. Veliparib Is an Effective Radiosensitizing Agent in a Preclinical Model of Medulloblastoma. *Front. Mol. Biosci.* **2021**, *8*, 633344. [CrossRef]
76. Coleman, R.L.; Fleming, G.F.; Brady, M.F.; Swisher, E.M.; Steffensen, K.D.; Friedlander, M.; Okamoto, A.; Moore, K.N.; Efrat Ben-Baruch, N.; Werner, T.L.; et al. Veliparib with First-Line Chemotherapy and as Maintenance Therapy in Ovarian Cancer. *N. Engl. J. Med.* **2019**, *381*, 2403–2415. [CrossRef] [PubMed]
77. U.S. Food and Drug Administration (FDA). FDA Approves Niraparib for HRD-Positive Advanced Ovarian Cancer. 2019. Available online: https://www.fda.gov/drugs/resources-information-approved-drugs/fda-approves-niraparib-hrd-positive-advanced-ovarian-cancer (accessed on 24 November 2021).
78. Konstantinopoulos, P.A.; Waggoner, S.; Vidal, G.A.; Mita, M.; Moroney, J.W.; Holloway, R.; Van Le, L.; Sachdev, J.C.; Chapman-Davis, E.; Colon-Otero, G.; et al. Single-Arm Phases 1 and 2 Trial of Niraparib in Combination With Pembrolizumab in Patients With Recurrent Platinum-Resistant Ovarian Carcinoma. *JAMA Oncol.* **2019**, *5*, 1141–1149. [CrossRef] [PubMed]
79. Liu, J.F.; Barry, W.T.; Birrer, M.; Lee, J.M.; Buckanovich, R.J.; Fleming, G.F.; Rimel, B.; Buss, M.K.; Nattam, S.; Hurteau, J.; et al. Combination cediranib and olaparib versus olaparib alone for women with recurrent platinum-sensitive ovarian cancer: A randomised phase 2 study. *Lancet Oncol.* **2014**, *15*, 1207–1214. [CrossRef]
80. Liu, J.F.; Brady, M.F.; Matulonis, U.A.; Miller, A.; Kohn, E.C.; Swisher, E.M.; Tew, W.P.; Cloven, N.G.; Muller, C.; Bender, D.; et al. A phase III study comparing single-agent olaparib or the combination of cediranib and olaparib to standard platinum-based chemotherapy in recurrent platinum-sensitive ovarian cancer. *J. Clin. Oncol.* **2020**, *38*, 6003. [CrossRef]
81. Ray-Coquard, I.; Pautier, P.; Pignata, S.; Perol, D.; Gonzalez-Martin, A.; Berger, R.; Fujiwara, K.; Vergote, I.; Colombo, N.; Maenpaa, J.; et al. Olaparib plus Bevacizumab as First-Line Maintenance in Ovarian Cancer. *N. Engl. J. Med.* **2019**, *381*, 2416–2428. [CrossRef]

82. Mirza, M.R.; Monk, B.J.; Herrstedt, J.; Oza, A.M.; Mahner, S.; Redondo, A.; Fabbro, M.; Ledermann, J.A.; Lorusso, D.; Vergote, I.; et al. Niraparib Maintenance Therapy in Platinum-Sensitive, Recurrent Ovarian Cancer. *N. Engl. J. Med.* **2016**, *375*, 2154–2164. [CrossRef] [PubMed]
83. Poveda, A.; Floquet, A.; Ledermann, J.A.; Asher, R.; Penson, R.T.; Oza, A.M.; Korach, J.; Huzarski, T.; Pignata, S.; Friedlander, M.; et al. Final overall survival (OS) results from SOLO2/ENGOT-ov21: A phase III trial assessing maintenance olaparib in patients (pts) with platinum-sensitive, relapsed ovarian cancer and a BRCA mutation. *J. Clin. Oncol.* **2020**, *38*, 6002. [CrossRef]
84. European Medicines Agency. EPAR Summary for the Public: Avastin. 2017. Available online: https://www.ema.europa.eu/en/documents/overview/avastin-epar-summary-public_en.pdf (accessed on 24 November 2021).
85. Aghajanian, C.; Blank, S.V.; Goff, B.A.; Judson, P.L.; Teneriello, M.G.; Husain, A.; Sovak, M.A.; Yi, J.; Nycum, L.R. OCEANS: A randomized, double-blind, placebo-controlled phase III trial of chemotherapy with or without bevacizumab in patients with platinum-sensitive recurrent epithelial ovarian, primary peritoneal, or fallopian tube cancer. *J. Clin. Oncol.* **2012**, *30*, 2039–2045. [CrossRef]
86. Pujade-Lauraine, E.; Hilpert, F.; Weber, B.; Reuss, A.; Poveda, A.; Kristensen, G.; Sorio, R.; Vergote, I.; Witteveen, P.; Bamias, A.; et al. Bevacizumab combined with chemotherapy for platinum-resistant recurrent ovarian cancer: The AURELIA open-label randomized phase III trial. *J. Clin. Oncol.* **2014**, *32*, 1302–1308. [CrossRef] [PubMed]
87. Tewari, K.S.; Burger, R.A.; Enserro, D.; Norquist, B.M.; Swisher, E.M.; Brady, M.F.; Bookman, M.A.; Fleming, G.F.; Huang, H.; Homesley, H.D.; et al. Final Overall Survival of a Randomized Trial of Bevacizumab for Primary Treatment of Ovarian Cancer. *J. Clin. Oncol.* **2019**, *37*, 2317–2328. [CrossRef]
88. Liu, S.; Kasherman, L.; Fazelzad, R.; Wang, L.; Bouchard-Fortier, G.; Lheureux, S.; Krzyzanowska, M.K. The use of bevacizumab in the modern era of targeted therapy for ovarian cancer: A systematic review and meta-analysis. *Gynecol. Oncol.* **2021**, *161*, 601–612. [CrossRef] [PubMed]
89. Cohn, D.E.; Kim, K.H.; Resnick, K.E.; O'Malley, D.M.; Straughn, J.M., Jr. At what cost does a potential survival advantage of bevacizumab make sense for the primary treatment of ovarian cancer? A cost-effectiveness analysis. *J. Clin. Oncol.* **2011**, *29*, 1247–1251. [CrossRef] [PubMed]
90. Lesnock, J.L.; Farris, C.; Krivak, T.C.; Smith, K.J.; Markman, M. Consolidation paclitaxel is more cost-effective than bevacizumab following upfront treatment of advanced epithelial ovarian cancer. *Gynecol. Oncol.* **2011**, *122*, 473–478. [CrossRef] [PubMed]
91. Nagy, J.A.; Chang, S.H.; Dvorak, A.M.; Dvorak, H.F. Why are tumour blood vessels abnormal and why is it important to know? *Br. J. Cancer* **2009**, *100*, 865–869. [CrossRef]
92. Jain, R.K. Normalization of tumor vasculature: An emerging concept in antiangiogenic therapy. *Science* **2005**, *307*, 58–62. [CrossRef]
93. Ferriss, J.S.; Java, J.J.; Bookman, M.A.; Fleming, G.F.; Monk, B.J.; Walker, J.L.; Homesley, H.D.; Fowler, J.; Greer, B.E.; Boente, M.P.; et al. Ascites predicts treatment benefit of bevacizumab in front-line therapy of advanced epithelial ovarian, fallopian tube and peritoneal cancers: An NRG Oncology/GOG study. *Gynecol. Oncol.* **2015**, *139*, 17–22. [CrossRef] [PubMed]
94. Kou, F.; Gong, J.; Li, Y.; Li, J.; Zhang, X.; Li, J.; Shen, L. Phase I study of intraperitoneal bevacizumab for treating refractory malignant ascites. *J. Int. Med. Res.* **2021**, *49*, 300060520986664. [CrossRef] [PubMed]
95. Ayantunde, A.A.; Parsons, S.L. Pattern and prognostic factors in patients with malignant ascites: A retrospective study. *Ann. Oncol.* **2007**, *18*, 945–949. [CrossRef] [PubMed]
96. Liang, X.; Li, H.; Coussy, F.; Callens, C.; Lerebours, F. An update on biomarkers of potential benefit with bevacizumab for breast cancer treatment: Do we make progress? *Chin. J. Cancer Res.* **2019**, *31*, 586–600. [CrossRef]
97. Moreno-Munoz, D.; de la Haba-Rodriguez, J.R.; Conde, F.; Lopez-Sanchez, L.M.; Valverde, A.; Hernandez, V.; Martinez, A.; Villar, C.; Gomez-Espana, A.; Porras, I.; et al. Genetic variants in the renin-angiotensin system predict response to bevacizumab in cancer patients. *Eur. J. Clin. Invest.* **2015**, *45*, 1325–1332. [CrossRef]
98. Schultheis, A.M.; Lurje, G.; Rhodes, K.E.; Zhang, W.; Yang, D.; Garcia, A.A.; Morgan, R.; Gandara, D.; Scudder, S.; Oza, A.; et al. Polymorphisms and clinical outcome in recurrent ovarian cancer treated with cyclophosphamide and bevacizumab. *Clin. Cancer Res.* **2008**, *14*, 7554–7563. [CrossRef] [PubMed]
99. Li, J.; Yue, H.; Li, W.; Zhu, G.; Zhu, T.; Chen, R.; Lu, X. Bevacizumab confers significant improvements in survival for ovarian cancer patients with low miR-25 expression and high miR-142 expression. *J. Ovarian. Res.* **2021**, *14*, 166. [CrossRef]
100. Papadopoulos, N.; Martin, J.; Ruan, Q.; Rafique, A.; Rosconi, M.P.; Shi, E.; Pyles, E.A.; Yancopoulos, G.D.; Stahl, N.; Wiegand, S.J. Binding and neutralization of vascular endothelial growth factor (VEGF) and related ligands by VEGF Trap, ranibizumab and bevacizumab. *Angiogenesis* **2012**, *15*, 171–185. [CrossRef]
101. Ciombor, K.K.; Berlin, J. Aflibercept–a decoy VEGF receptor. *Curr. Oncol. Rep.* **2014**, *16*, 368. [CrossRef]
102. Colombo, N.; Mangili, G.; Mammoliti, S.; Kalling, M.; Tholander, B.; Sternas, L.; Buzenet, G.; Chamberlain, D. A phase II study of aflibercept in patients with advanced epithelial ovarian cancer and symptomatic malignant ascites. *Gynecol. Oncol.* **2012**, *125*, 42–47. [CrossRef] [PubMed]
103. Gotlieb, W.H.; Amant, F.; Advani, S.; Goswami, C.; Hirte, H.; Provencher, D.; Somani, N.; Yamada, S.D.; Tamby, J.F.; Vergote, I. Intravenous aflibercept for treatment of recurrent symptomatic malignant ascites in patients with advanced ovarian cancer: A phase 2, randomised, double-blind, placebo-controlled study. *Lancet Oncol.* **2012**, *13*, 154–162. [CrossRef]
104. Oikawa, T.; Onozawa, C.; Sakaguchi, M.; Morita, I.; Murota, S. Three isoforms of platelet-derived growth factors all have the capability to induce angiogenesis in vivo. *Biol. Pharm. Bull.* **1994**, *17*, 1686–1688. [CrossRef] [PubMed]

105. Coxon, A.; Bready, J.; Min, H.; Kaufman, S.; Leal, J.; Yu, D.; Lee, T.A.; Sun, J.R.; Estrada, J.; Bolon, B.; et al. Context-dependent role of angiopoietin-1 inhibition in the suppression of angiogenesis and tumor growth: Implications for AMG 386, an angiopoietin-1/2-neutralizing peptibody. *Mol. Cancer Ther.* **2010**, *9*, 2641–2651. [CrossRef]
106. Monk, B.J.; Poveda, A.; Vergote, I.; Raspagliesi, F.; Fujiwara, K.; Bae, D.S.; Oaknin, A.; Ray-Coquard, I.; Provencher, D.M.; Karlan, B.Y.; et al. Final results of a phase 3 study of trebananib plus weekly paclitaxel in recurrent ovarian cancer (TRINOVA-1): Long-term survival, impact of ascites, and progression-free survival-2. *Gynecol. Oncol.* **2016**, *143*, 27–34. [CrossRef] [PubMed]
107. Vergote, I.; Scambia, G.; O'Malley, D.M.; Van Calster, B.; Park, S.Y.; Del Campo, J.M.; Meier, W.; Bamias, A.; Colombo, N.; Wenham, R.M.; et al. Trebananib or placebo plus carboplatin and paclitaxel as first-line treatment for advanced ovarian cancer (TRINOVA-3/ENGOT-ov2/GOG-3001): A randomised, double-blind, phase 3 trial. *Lancet Oncol.* **2019**, *20*, 862–876. [CrossRef]
108. Chekerov, R.; Hilpert, F.; Mahner, S.; El-Balat, A.; Harter, P.; De Gregorio, N.; Fridrich, C.; Markmann, S.; Potenberg, J.; Lorenz, R.; et al. Sorafenib plus topotecan versus placebo plus topotecan for platinum-resistant ovarian cancer (TRIAS): A multicentre, randomised, double-blind, placebo-controlled, phase 2 trial. *Lancet Oncol.* **2018**, *19*, 1247–1258. [CrossRef]
109. Lee, J.M.; Annunziata, C.M.; Hays, J.L.; Cao, L.; Choyke, P.; Yu, M.; An, D.; Turkbey, I.B.; Minasian, L.M.; Steinberg, S.M.; et al. Phase II trial of bevacizumab and sorafenib in recurrent ovarian cancer patients with or without prior-bevacizumab treatment. *Gynecol. Oncol.* **2020**, *159*, 88–94. [CrossRef] [PubMed]
110. Doebele, R.C.; Drilon, A.; Paz-Ares, L.; Siena, S.; Shaw, A.T.; Farago, A.F.; Blakely, C.M.; Seto, T.; Cho, B.C.; Tosi, D.; et al. Entrectinib in patients with advanced or metastatic NTRK fusion-positive solid tumours: Integrated analysis of three phase 1-2 trials. *Lancet Oncol.* **2020**, *21*, 271–282. [CrossRef]
111. Wilhelm, S.M.; Carter, C.; Tang, L.; Wilkie, D.; McNabola, A.; Rong, H.; Chen, C.; Zhang, X.; Vincent, P.; McHugh, M.; et al. BAY 43-9006 exhibits broad spectrum oral antitumor activity and targets the RAF/MEK/ERK pathway and receptor tyrosine kinases involved in tumor progression and angiogenesis. *Cancer Res.* **2004**, *64*, 7099–7109. [CrossRef]
112. Guida, T.; Anaganti, S.; Provitera, L.; Gedrich, R.; Sullivan, E.; Wilhelm, S.M.; Santoro, M.; Carlomagno, F. Sorafenib inhibits imatinib-resistant KIT and platelet-derived growth factor receptor beta gatekeeper mutants. *Clin. Cancer Res.* **2007**, *13*, 3363–3369. [CrossRef]
113. U.S. Food and Drug Administration (FDA). NEXAVAR Safely and Effectively. 2018. Available online: https://www.accessdata.fda.gov/drugsatfda_docs/label/2018/021923s020lbl.pdf (accessed on 7 December 2021).
114. Matei, D.; Sill, M.W.; Lankes, H.A.; DeGeest, K.; Bristow, R.E.; Mutch, D.; Yamada, S.D.; Cohn, D.; Calvert, V.; Farley, J.; et al. Activity of sorafenib in recurrent ovarian cancer and primary peritoneal carcinomatosis: A gynecologic oncology group trial. *J. Clin. Oncol.* **2011**, *29*, 69–75. [CrossRef] [PubMed]
115. Russo, N.; Russo, M.; Daino, D.; Bucci, F.; Pluchino, N.; Casarosa, E.; Artini, P.G.; Cela, V.; Luisi, M.; Genazzani, A.R. Polycystic ovary syndrome: Brain-derived neurotrophic factor (BDNF) plasma and follicular fluid levels. *Gynecol. Endocrinol.* **2012**, *28*, 241–244. [CrossRef] [PubMed]
116. Dissen, G.A.; Garcia-Rudaz, C.; Paredes, A.; Mayer, C.; Mayerhofer, A.; Ojeda, S.R. Excessive ovarian production of nerve growth factor facilitates development of cystic ovarian morphology in mice and is a feature of polycystic ovarian syndrome in humans. *Endocrinology* **2009**, *150*, 2906–2914. [CrossRef] [PubMed]
117. Garrido, M.P.; Hurtado, I.; Valenzuela-Valderrama, M.; Salvatierra, R.; Hernandez, A.; Vega, M.; Selman, A.; Quest, A.F.G.; Romero, C. NGF-Enhanced Vasculogenic Properties of Epithelial Ovarian Cancer Cells Is Reduced by Inhibition of the COX-2/PGE2 Signaling Axis. *Cancers* **2019**, *11*, 1970. [CrossRef] [PubMed]
118. Maness, L.M.; Weber, J.T.; Banks, W.A.; Beckman, B.S.; Zadina, J.E. The neurotrophins and their receptors: Structure, function, and neuropathology. *Neurosci. Biobehav. Rev.* **1994**, *18*, 143–159. [CrossRef]
119. Yu, X.; Liu, Z.; Hou, R.; Nie, Y.; Chen, R. Nerve growth factor and its receptors on onset and diagnosis of ovarian cancer. *Oncol. Lett.* **2017**, *14*, 2864–2868. [CrossRef] [PubMed]
120. Laetsch, T.W.; Hong, D.S. Tropomyosin Receptor Kinase Inhibitors for the Treatment of TRK Fusion Cancer. *Clin. Cancer Res.* **2021**, *27*, 4974–4982. [CrossRef]
121. Jiang, T.; Wang, G.; Liu, Y.; Feng, L.; Wang, M.; Liu, J.; Chen, Y.; Ouyang, L. Development of small-molecule tropomyosin receptor kinase (TRK) inhibitors for NTRK fusion cancers. *Acta. Pharm. Sin. B.* **2021**, *11*, 355–372. [CrossRef]
122. U.S. Food and Drug Administration (FDA). FDA Approves Larotrectinib for Solid Tumors with NTRK Gene Fusions. 2018. Available online: https://www.fda.gov/drugs/fda-approves-larotrectinib-solid-tumors-ntrk-gene-fusions (accessed on 7 December 2021).
123. U.S. Food and Drug Administration (FDA). FDA Approves Entrectinib for NTRK Solid Tumors and ROS-1 NSCLC. 2019. Available online: https://www.fda.gov/drugs/resources-information-approved-drugs/fda-approves-entrectinib-ntrk-solid-tumors-and-ros-1-nsclc (accessed on 7 December 2021).
124. Blake, J.F.; Kolakowski, G.R.; Tuch, B.B.; Ebata, K.; Brandhuber, B.J.; Winski, S.L.; Bouhana, K.S.; Nanda, N.; Wu, W.-I.; Parker, A.; et al. The development of LOXO-195, a second generation TRK kinase inhibitor that overcomes acquired resistance to 1st generation inhibitors observed in patients with TRK-fusion cancers. *Eur. J. Cancer* **2016**, *69*, S144–S145. [CrossRef]
125. Vignali, D.A.; Collison, L.W.; Workman, C.J. How regulatory T cells work. *Nat. Rev. Immunol.* **2008**, *8*, 523–532. [CrossRef]
126. Buchbinder, E.I.; Desai, A. CTLA-4 and PD-1 Pathways: Similarities, Differences, and Implications of Their Inhibition. *Am. J. Clin. Oncol.* **2016**, *39*, 98–106. [CrossRef]

127. Messerschmidt, J.L.; Prendergast, G.C.; Messerschmidt, G.L. How Cancers Escape Immune Destruction and Mechanisms of Action for the New Significantly Active Immune Therapies: Helping Nonimmunologists Decipher Recent Advances. *Oncologist* **2016**, *21*, 233–243. [CrossRef] [PubMed]
128. Zheng, Y.; Zhu, J.; Zhang, H.; Liu, Y.; Sun, H. Metformin inhibits ovarian cancer growth and migration in vitro and in vivo by enhancing cisplatin cytotoxicity. *Am. J. Transl. Res.* **2018**, *10*, 3086–3098.
129. Hamilton, E.; O'Malley, D.M.; O'Cearbhaill, R.; Cristea, M.; Fleming, G.F.; Tariq, B.; Fong, A.; French, D.; Rossi, M.; Brickman, D.; et al. Tamrintamab pamozirine (SC-003) in patients with platinum-resistant/refractory ovarian cancer: Findings of a phase 1 study. *Gynecol. Oncol.* **2020**, *158*, 640–645. [CrossRef] [PubMed]
130. Varga, A.; Piha-Paul, S.; Ott, P.A.; Mehnert, J.M.; Berton-Rigaud, D.; Morosky, A.; Yang, P.; Ruman, J.; Matei, D. Pembrolizumab in patients with programmed death ligand 1-positive advanced ovarian cancer: Analysis of KEYNOTE-028. *Gynecol. Oncol.* **2019**, *152*, 243–250. [CrossRef]
131. Matulonis, U.A.; Shapira-Frommer, R.; Santin, A.D.; Lisyanskaya, A.S.; Pignata, S.; Vergote, I.; Raspagliesi, F.; Sonke, G.S.; Birrer, M.; Provencher, D.M.; et al. Antitumor activity and safety of pembrolizumab in patients with advanced recurrent ovarian cancer: Results from the phase II KEYNOTE-100 study. *Ann. Oncol.* **2019**, *30*, 1080–1087. [CrossRef] [PubMed]
132. Sanborn, R.E.; Pishvaian, M.J.; Kluger, H.M.; Callahan, M.K.; Weise, A.M.; Lutzky, J.; Yellin, M.J.; Rawls, T.; Vitale, L.; Halim, A.; et al. Clinical results with combination of anti-CD27 agonist antibody, varlilumab, with anti-PD1 antibody nivolumab in advanced cancer patients. *J. Clin. Oncol.* **2017**, *35*, 3007. [CrossRef]
133. Sanborn, R.E.; Pishvaian, M.J.; Callahan, M.K.; Weise, A.M.; Sikic, B.I.; Rahma, O.E.; Cho, D.C.; Rizvi, N.A.; Bitting, R.L.; Starodub, A.; et al. Anti-CD27 agonist antibody varlilumab (varli) with nivolumab (nivo) for colorectal (CRC) and ovarian (OVA) cancer: Phase (Ph) 1/2 clinical trial results. *J. Clin. Oncol.* **2018**, *36*, 3001. [CrossRef]
134. Zamarin, D.; Burger, R.A.; Sill, M.W.; Powell, D.J., Jr.; Lankes, H.A.; Feldman, M.D.; Zivanovic, O.; Gunderson, C.; Ko, E.; Mathews, C.; et al. Randomized Phase II Trial of Nivolumab Versus Nivolumab and Ipilimumab for Recurrent or Persistent Ovarian Cancer: An NRG Oncology Study. *J. Clin. Oncol.* **2020**, *38*, 1814–1823. [CrossRef]
135. Bashey, A.; Medina, B.; Corringham, S.; Pasek, M.; Carrier, E.; Vrooman, L.; Lowy, I.; Solomon, S.R.; Morris, L.E.; Holland, H.K.; et al. CTLA4 blockade with ipilimumab to treat relapse of malignancy after allogeneic hematopoietic cell transplantation. *Blood* **2009**, *113*, 1581–1588. [CrossRef] [PubMed]
136. Weidemann, S.; Gagelmann, P.; Gorbokon, N.; Lennartz, M.; Menz, A.; Luebke, A.M.; Kluth, M.; Hube-Magg, C.; Blessin, N.C.; Fraune, C.; et al. Mesothelin Expression in Human Tumors: A Tissue Microarray Study on 12,679 Tumors. *Biomedicines* **2021**, *9*, 397. [CrossRef] [PubMed]
137. Luke, J.J.; Barlesi, F.; Chung, K.; Tolcher, A.W.; Kelly, K.; Hollebecque, A.; Le Tourneau, C.; Subbiah, V.; Tsai, F.; Kao, S.; et al. Phase I study of ABBV-428, a mesothelin-CD40 bispecific, in patients with advanced solid tumors. *J. Immunother. Cancer* **2021**, *9*, e002015. [CrossRef]
138. Soong, R.S.; Song, L.; Trieu, J.; Lee, S.Y.; He, L.; Tsai, Y.C.; Wu, T.C.; Hung, C.F. Direct T cell activation via CD40 ligand generates high avidity CD8+ T cells capable of breaking immunological tolerance for the control of tumors. *PLoS ONE* **2014**, *9*, e93162. [CrossRef]
139. Berinstein, N.L.; Karkada, M.; Oza, A.M.; Odunsi, K.; Villella, J.A.; Nemunaitis, J.J.; Morse, M.A.; Pejovic, T.; Bentley, J.; Buyse, M.; et al. Survivin-targeted immunotherapy drives robust polyfunctional T cell generation and differentiation in advanced ovarian cancer patients. *Oncoimmunology* **2015**, *4*, e1026529. [CrossRef]
140. Dorigo, O.; Tanyi, J.L.; Strauss, J.; Oza, A.M.; Pejovic, T.; Ghatage, P.; Villella, J.A.; Fiset, S.; MacDonald, L.D.; Leopold, L.; et al. Clinical data from the DeCidE1 trial: Assessing the first combination of DPX-Survivac, low dose cyclophosphamide (CPA), and epacadostat (INCB024360) in subjects with stage IIc-IV recurrent epithelial ovarian cancer. *J. Clin. Oncol.* **2018**, *36*, 5510. [CrossRef]
141. Lee, W.S.; Yang, H.; Chon, H.J.; Kim, C. Combination of anti-angiogenic therapy and immune checkpoint blockade normalizes vascular-immune crosstalk to potentiate cancer immunity. *Exp. Mol. Med.* **2020**, *52*, 1475–1485. [CrossRef]
142. Peyraud, F.; Italiano, A. Combined PARP Inhibition and Immune Checkpoint Therapy in Solid Tumors. *Cancers* **2020**, *12*, 1502. [CrossRef] [PubMed]
143. Meng, J.; Peng, J.; Feng, J.; Maurer, J.; Li, X.; Li, Y.; Yao, S.; Chu, R.; Pan, X.; Li, J.; et al. Niraparib exhibits a synergistic anti-tumor effect with PD-L1 blockade by inducing an immune response in ovarian cancer. *J. Transl. Med.* **2021**, *19*, 415. [CrossRef]
144. Lee, E.K.; Konstantinopoulos, P.A. PARP inhibition and immune modulation: Scientific rationale and perspectives for the treatment of gynecologic cancers. *Ther. Adv. Med. Oncol.* **2020**, *12*, 1758835920944116. [CrossRef] [PubMed]
145. Wen, W.X.; Leong, C.O. Association of BRCA1- and BRCA2-deficiency with mutation burden, expression of PD-L1/PD-1, immune infiltrates, and T cell-inflamed signature in breast cancer. *PLoS ONE* **2019**, *14*, e0215381. [CrossRef]
146. McAlpine, J.N.; Porter, H.; Kobel, M.; Nelson, B.H.; Prentice, L.M.; Kalloger, S.E.; Senz, J.; Milne, K.; Ding, J.; Shah, S.P.; et al. BRCA1 and BRCA2 mutations correlate with TP53 abnormalities and presence of immune cell infiltrates in ovarian high-grade serous carcinoma. *Mod. Pathol.* **2012**, *25*, 740–750. [CrossRef] [PubMed]
147. Jiao, S.; Xia, W.; Yamaguchi, H.; Wei, Y.; Chen, M.K.; Hsu, J.M.; Hsu, J.L.; Yu, W.H.; Du, Y.; Lee, H.H.; et al. PARP Inhibitor Upregulates PD-L1 Expression and Enhances Cancer-Associated Immunosuppression. *Clin. Cancer. Res.* **2017**, *23*, 3711–3720. [CrossRef] [PubMed]

148. Lee, J.M.; Annunziata, C.M.; Houston, N.; Kohn, E.C.; Lipkowitz, S.; Minasian, L.; Nichols, E.; Trepel, J.; Trewhitt, K.; Zia, F.; et al. 936PD—A phase II study of durvalumab, a PD-L1 inhibitor and olaparib in recurrent ovarian cancer (OvCa). *Ann. Oncol.* **2018**, *29*, viii334. [CrossRef]
149. Adams, S.F.; Rixe, O.; Lee, J.-H.; McCance, D.J.; Westgate, S.; Eberhardt, S.C.; Rutledge, T.; Muller, C. Phase I study combining olaparib and tremelimumab for the treatment of women with BRCA-deficient recurrent ovarian cancer. *J. Clin. Oncol.* **2017**, *35*, e17052. [CrossRef]
150. Sleire, L.; Forde, H.E.; Netland, I.A.; Leiss, L.; Skeie, B.S.; Enger, P.O. Drug repurposing in cancer. *Pharm. Res.* **2017**, *124*, 74–91. [CrossRef] [PubMed]
151. Antoszczak, M.; Markowska, A.; Markowska, J.; Huczynski, A. Old wine in new bottles: Drug repurposing in oncology. *Eur. J. Pharm.* **2020**, *866*, 172784. [CrossRef]
152. Hwang, J.R.; Kim, W.Y.; Cho, Y.J.; Ryu, J.Y.; Choi, J.J.; Jeong, S.Y.; Kim, M.S.; Kim, J.H.; Paik, E.S.; Lee, Y.Y.; et al. Chloroquine reverses chemoresistance via upregulation of p21(WAF1/CIP1) and autophagy inhibition in ovarian cancer. *Cell Death Dis.* **2020**, *11*, 1034. [CrossRef]
153. Madariaga, A.; Marastoni, S.; Colombo, I.; Mandilaras, V.; Cabanero, M.; Bruce, J.; Garg, S.; Wang, L.; Gill, S.; Dhani, N.C.; et al. Phase I/II trial assessing hydroxychloroquine and itraconazole in women with advanced platinum-resistant epithelial ovarian cancer (EOC) (HYDRA-01). *J. Clin. Oncol.* **2020**, *38*, 6049. [CrossRef]
154. Kodama, M.; Kodama, T.; Newberg, J.Y.; Katayama, H.; Kobayashi, M.; Hanash, S.M.; Yoshihara, K.; Wei, Z.; Tien, J.C.; Rangel, R.; et al. In vivo loss-of-function screens identify KPNB1 as a new druggable oncogene in epithelial ovarian cancer. *Proc. Natl. Acad. Sci. USA* **2017**, *114*, E7301–E7310. [CrossRef]
155. Zhang, X.; Qin, T.; Zhu, Z.; Hong, F.; Xu, Y.; Zhang, X.; Xu, X.; Ma, A. Ivermectin Augments the In Vitro and In Vivo Efficacy of Cisplatin in Epithelial Ovarian Cancer by Suppressing Akt/mTOR Signaling. *Am. J. Med. Sci.* **2020**, *359*, 123–129. [CrossRef]
156. Irvin, S.; Clarke, M.A.; Trabert, B.; Wentzensen, N. Systematic review and meta-analysis of studies assessing the relationship between statin use and risk of ovarian cancer. *Cancer Causes Control* **2020**, *31*, 869–879. [CrossRef] [PubMed]
157. Abdullah, M.I.; Abed, M.N.; Richardson, A. Inhibition of the mevalonate pathway augments the activity of pitavastatin against ovarian cancer cells. *Sci. Rep.* **2017**, *7*, 8090. [CrossRef]
158. Gobel, A.; Zinna, V.M.; Dell'Endice, S.; Jaschke, N.; Kuhlmann, J.D.; Wimberger, P.; Rachner, T.D. Anti-tumor effects of mevalonate pathway inhibition in ovarian cancer. *BMC Cancer* **2020**, *20*, 703. [CrossRef] [PubMed]
159. Landen, C.N., Jr.; Goodman, B.; Katre, A.A.; Steg, A.D.; Nick, A.M.; Stone, R.L.; Miller, L.D.; Mejia, P.V.; Jennings, N.B.; Gershenson, D.M.; et al. Targeting aldehyde dehydrogenase cancer stem cells in ovarian cancer. *Mol. Cancer* **2010**, *9*, 3186–3199. [CrossRef]
160. Guo, F.; Yang, Z.; Kulbe, H.; Albers, A.E.; Sehouli, J.; Kaufmann, A.M. Inhibitory effect on ovarian cancer ALDH+ stem-like cells by Disulfiram and Copper treatment through ALDH and ROS modulation. *Biomed. Pharm.* **2019**, *118*, 109371. [CrossRef] [PubMed]
161. Xu, J.; Shen, Y.; Wang, C.; Tang, S.; Hong, S.; Lu, W.; Xie, X.; Cheng, X. Arsenic compound sensitizes homologous recombination proficient ovarian cancer to PARP inhibitors. *Cell Death Discov.* **2021**, *7*, 259. [CrossRef]
162. Byun, J.M.; Lee, D.S.; Landen, C.N.; Kim, D.H.; Kim, Y.N.; Lee, K.B.; Sung, M.S.; Park, S.G.; Jeong, D.H. Arsenic trioxide and tetraarsenic oxide induce cytotoxicity and have a synergistic effect with cisplatin in paclitaxel-resistant ovarian cancer cells. *Acta Oncol.* **2019**, *58*, 1594–1602. [CrossRef]
163. Romero, I.L.; McCormick, A.; McEwen, K.A.; Park, S.; Karrison, T.; Yamada, S.D.; Pannain, S.; Lengyel, E. Relationship of type II diabetes and metformin use to ovarian cancer progression, survival, and chemosensitivity. *Obs. Gynecol.* **2012**, *119*, 61–67. [CrossRef]
164. Tseng, C.H. Metformin reduces ovarian cancer risk in Taiwanese women with type 2 diabetes mellitus. *Diabetes Metab. Res. Rev.* **2015**, *31*, 619–626. [CrossRef]
165. Brown, J.R.; Chan, D.K.; Shank, J.J.; Griffith, K.A.; Fan, H.; Szulawski, R.; Yang, K.; Reynolds, R.K.; Johnston, C.; McLean, K.; et al. Phase II clinical trial of metformin as a cancer stem cell-targeting agent in ovarian cancer. *JCI Insight* **2020**, *5*, e133247. [CrossRef]
166. Kurtova, A.V.; Xiao, J.; Mo, Q.; Pazhanisamy, S.; Krasnow, R.; Lerner, S.P.; Chen, F.; Roh, T.T.; Lay, E.; Ho, P.L.; et al. Blocking PGE2-induced tumour repopulation abrogates bladder cancer chemoresistance. *Nature* **2015**, *517*, 209–213. [CrossRef]
167. Kashiwagi, E.; Inoue, S.; Mizushima, T.; Chen, J.; Ide, H.; Kawahara, T.; Reis, L.O.; Baras, A.S.; Netto, G.J.; Miyamoto, H. Prostaglandin receptors induce urothelial tumourigenesis as well as bladder cancer progression and cisplatin resistance presumably via modulating PTEN expression. *Br. J. Cancer* **2018**, *118*, 213–223. [CrossRef]
168. Wang, C.; Guan, W.; Peng, J.; Chen, Y.; Xu, G.; Dou, H. Gene/paclitaxel co-delivering nanocarriers prepared by framework-induced self-assembly for the inhibition of highly drug-resistant tumors. *Acta Biomater.* **2020**, *103*, 247–258. [CrossRef]
169. Mizushima, N.; Levine, B.; Cuervo, A.M.; Klionsky, D.J. Autophagy fights disease through cellular self-digestion. *Nature* **2008**, *451*, 1069–1075. [CrossRef] [PubMed]
170. Sun, Y.; Liu, J.H.; Jin, L.; Sui, Y.X.; Han, L.L.; Huang, Y. Effect of autophagy-related beclin1 on sensitivity of cisplatin-resistant ovarian cancer cells to chemotherapeutic agents. *Asian Pac. J. Cancer Prev.* **2015**, *16*, 2785–2791. [CrossRef] [PubMed]
171. Bao, L.; Jaramillo, M.C.; Zhang, Z.; Zheng, Y.; Yao, M.; Zhang, D.D.; Yi, X. Induction of autophagy contributes to cisplatin resistance in human ovarian cancer cells. *Mol. Med. Rep.* **2015**, *11*, 91–98. [CrossRef]

172. Karsli-Uzunbas, G.; Guo, J.Y.; Price, S.; Teng, X.; Laddha, S.V.; Khor, S.; Kalaany, N.Y.; Jacks, T.; Chan, C.S.; Rabinowitz, J.D.; et al. Autophagy is required for glucose homeostasis and lung tumor maintenance. *Cancer Discov.* **2014**, *4*, 914–927. [CrossRef]
173. Qu, X.; Yu, J.; Bhagat, G.; Furuya, N.; Hibshoosh, H.; Troxel, A.; Rosen, J.; Eskelinen, E.L.; Mizushima, N.; Ohsumi, Y.; et al. Promotion of tumorigenesis by heterozygous disruption of the beclin 1 autophagy gene. *J. Clin. Invest.* **2003**, *112*, 1809–1820. [CrossRef]
174. Sit, K.H.; Paramanantham, R.; Bay, B.H.; Chan, H.L.; Wong, K.P.; Thong, P.; Watt, F. Sequestration of mitotic (M-phase) chromosomes in autophagosomes: Mitotic programmed cell death in human Chang liver cells induced by an OH* burst from vanadyl(4). *Anat Rec* **1996**, *245*, 1–8. [CrossRef]
175. Kaminskyy, V.; Abdi, A.; Zhivotovsky, B. A quantitative assay for the monitoring of autophagosome accumulation in different phases of the cell cycle. *Autophagy* **2011**, *7*, 83–90. [CrossRef] [PubMed]
176. Liu, M.; Jiang, L.; Fu, X.; Wang, W.; Ma, J.; Tian, T.; Nan, K.; Liang, X. Cytoplasmic liver kinase B1 promotes the growth of human lung adenocarcinoma by enhancing autophagy. *Cancer Sci.* **2018**, *109*, 3055–3067. [CrossRef] [PubMed]
177. Degenhardt, K.; Mathew, R.; Beaudoin, B.; Bray, K.; Anderson, D.; Chen, G.; Mukherjee, C.; Shi, Y.; Gelinas, C.; Fan, Y.; et al. Autophagy promotes tumor cell survival and restricts necrosis, inflammation, and tumorigenesis. *Cancer Cell* **2006**, *10*, 51–64. [CrossRef] [PubMed]
178. Rosenfeldt, M.T.; Ryan, K.M. The multiple roles of autophagy in cancer. *Carcinogenesis* **2011**, *32*, 955–963. [CrossRef] [PubMed]
179. Hu, Y.L.; Jahangiri, A.; Delay, M.; Aghi, M.K. Tumor cell autophagy as an adaptive response mediating resistance to treatments such as antiangiogenic therapy. *Cancer Res.* **2012**, *72*, 4294–4299. [CrossRef]
180. Zou, Z.; Yuan, Z.; Zhang, Q.; Long, Z.; Chen, J.; Tang, Z.; Zhu, Y.; Chen, S.; Xu, J.; Yan, M.; et al. Aurora kinase A inhibition-induced autophagy triggers drug resistance in breast cancer cells. *Autophagy* **2012**, *8*, 1798–1810. [CrossRef]
181. Wang, J.; Wu, G.S. Role of autophagy in cisplatin resistance in ovarian cancer cells. *J. Biol. Chem.* **2014**, *289*, 17163–17173. [CrossRef]
182. Zhang, Y.; Cheng, Y.; Ren, X.; Zhang, L.; Yap, K.L.; Wu, H.; Patel, R.; Liu, D.; Qin, Z.H.; Shih, I.M.; et al. NAC1 modulates sensitivity of ovarian cancer cells to cisplatin by altering the HMGB1-mediated autophagic response. *Oncogene* **2012**, *31*, 1055–1064. [CrossRef]
183. Mauthe, M.; Orhon, I.; Rocchi, C.; Zhou, X.; Luhr, M.; Hijlkema, K.J.; Coppes, R.P.; Engedal, N.; Mari, M.; Reggiori, F. Chloroquine inhibits autophagic flux by decreasing autophagosome-lysosome fusion. *Autophagy* **2018**, *14*, 1435–1455. [CrossRef]
184. Cadena, I.; Werth, V.P.; Levine, P.; Yang, A.; Downey, A.; Curtin, J.; Muggia, F. Lasting pathologic complete response to chemotherapy for ovarian cancer after receiving antimalarials for dermatomyositis. *Ecancermedicalscience* **2018**, *12*, 837. [CrossRef]
185. Liu, L.Q.; Wang, S.B.; Shao, Y.F.; Shi, J.N.; Wang, W.; Chen, W.Y.; Ye, Z.Q.; Jiang, J.Y.; Fang, Q.X.; Zhang, G.B.; et al. Hydroxychloroquine potentiates the anti-cancer effect of bevacizumab on glioblastoma via the inhibition of autophagy. *Biomed. Pharm.* **2019**, *118*, 109339. [CrossRef]
186. Wang, K.; Gao, W.; Dou, Q.; Chen, H.; Li, Q.; Nice, E.C.; Huang, C. Ivermectin induces PAK1-mediated cytostatic autophagy in breast cancer. *Autophagy* **2016**, *12*, 2498–2499. [CrossRef]
187. Li, N.; Zhan, X. Anti-parasite drug ivermectin can suppress ovarian cancer by regulating lncRNA-EIF4A3-mRNA axes. *EPMA J.* **2020**, *11*, 289–309. [CrossRef] [PubMed]
188. Stancu, C.; Sima, A. Statins: Mechanism of action and effects. *J. Cell Mol. Med.* **2001**, *5*, 378–387. [CrossRef] [PubMed]
189. Nielsen, S.F.; Nordestgaard, B.G.; Bojesen, S.E. Statin use and reduced cancer-related mortality. *N. Engl. J. Med.* **2012**, *367*, 1792–1802. [CrossRef] [PubMed]
190. Liu, Y.; Qin, A.; Li, T.; Qin, X.; Li, S. Effect of statin on risk of gynecologic cancers: A meta-analysis of observational studies and randomized controlled trials. *Gynecol. Oncol.* **2014**, *133*, 647–655. [CrossRef] [PubMed]
191. Desai, P.; Wallace, R.; Anderson, M.L.; Howard, B.V.; Ray, R.M.; Wu, C.; Safford, M.; Martin, L.W.; Rohan, T.; Manson, J.E.; et al. An analysis of the association between statin use and risk of endometrial and ovarian cancers in the Women's Health Initiative. *Gynecol. Oncol.* **2018**, *148*, 540–546. [CrossRef]
192. Yu, O.; Boudreau, D.M.; Buist, D.S.; Miglioretti, D.L. Statin use and female reproductive organ cancer risk in a large population-based setting. *Cancer Causes Control* **2009**, *20*, 609–616. [CrossRef]
193. Liu, H.; Liang, S.L.; Kumar, S.; Weyman, C.M.; Liu, W.; Zhou, A. Statins induce apoptosis in ovarian cancer cells through activation of JNK and enhancement of Bim expression. *Cancer Chemother. Pharm.* **2009**, *63*, 997–1005. [CrossRef]
194. Jones, H.M.; Fang, Z.; Sun, W.; Clark, L.H.; Stine, J.E.; Tran, A.Q.; Sullivan, S.A.; Gilliam, T.P.; Zhou, C.; Bae-Jump, V.L. Atorvastatin exhibits anti-tumorigenic and anti-metastatic effects in ovarian cancer in vitro. *Am. J. Cancer Res.* **2017**, *7*, 2478–2490.
195. Rao, P.S.; Rao, U.S. Statins decrease the expression of c-Myc protein in cancer cell lines. *Mol. Cell Biochem.* **2021**, *476*, 743–755. [CrossRef]
196. Drake, M.T.; Clarke, B.L.; Khosla, S. Bisphosphonates: Mechanism of action and role in clinical practice. *Mayo Clin. Proc.* **2008**, *83*, 1032–1045. [CrossRef]
197. Dunford, J.E.; Thompson, K.; Coxon, F.P.; Luckman, S.P.; Hahn, F.M.; Poulter, C.D.; Ebetino, F.H.; Rogers, M.J. Structure-activity relationships for inhibition of farnesyl diphosphate synthase in vitro and inhibition of bone resorption in vivo by nitrogen-containing bisphosphonates. *J. Pharmacol. Exp. Ther.* **2001**, *296*, 235–242.

198. Kavanagh, K.L.; Guo, K.; Dunford, J.E.; Wu, X.; Knapp, S.; Ebetino, F.H.; Rogers, M.J.; Russell, R.G.; Oppermann, U. The molecular mechanism of nitrogen-containing bisphosphonates as antiosteoporosis drugs. *Proc. Natl. Acad. Sci. USA* **2006**, *103*, 7829–7834. [CrossRef]
199. Hirata, J.; Kikuchi, Y.; Kudoh, K.; Kita, T.; Seto, H. Inhibitory effects of bisphosphonates on the proliferation of human ovarian cancer cell lines and the mechanism. *Med. Chem.* **2006**, *2*, 223–226. [CrossRef]
200. Yancik, R. Ovarian cancer. Age contrasts in incidence, histology, disease stage at diagnosis, and mortality. *Cancer* **1993**, *71*, 517–523. [CrossRef]
201. Barrett, J.A.; Baron, J.A.; Karagas, M.R.; Beach, M.L. Fracture risk in the U.S. Medicare population. *J. Clin. Epidemiol.* **1999**, *52*, 243–249. [CrossRef]
202. Ji, M.X.; Yu, Q. Primary osteoporosis in postmenopausal women. *Chronic. Dis. Transl. Med.* **2015**, *1*, 9–13. [CrossRef]
203. Stokes, M.; Abdijadid, S. Disulfiram. In *StatPearls*; StatPearls Publishing: Treasure Island, FL, USA, 2021.
204. Deng, S.; Yang, X.; Lassus, H.; Liang, S.; Kaur, S.; Ye, Q.; Li, C.; Wang, L.P.; Roby, K.F.; Orsulic, S.; et al. Distinct expression levels and patterns of stem cell marker, aldehyde dehydrogenase isoform 1 (ALDH1), in human epithelial cancers. *PLoS ONE* **2010**, *5*, e10277. [CrossRef]
205. Li, Y.; Chen, T.; Zhu, J.; Zhang, H.; Jiang, H.; Sun, H. High ALDH activity defines ovarian cancer stem-like cells with enhanced invasiveness and EMT progress which are responsible for tumor invasion. *Biochem. Biophys. Res. Commun.* **2018**, *495*, 1081–1088. [CrossRef]
206. Papaioannou, M.; Mylonas, I.; Kast, R.E.; Bruning, A. Disulfiram/copper causes redox-related proteotoxicity and concomitant heat shock response in ovarian cancer cells that is augmented by auranofin-mediated thioredoxin inhibition. *Oncoscience* **2014**, *1*, 21–29. [CrossRef]
207. Alimoghaddam, K. A review of arsenic trioxide and acute promyelocytic leukemia. *Int. J. Hematol. Oncol. Stem Cell Res.* **2014**, *8*, 44–54.
208. Zhang, J.; Wang, B. Arsenic trioxide (As_2O_3) inhibits peritoneal invasion of ovarian carcinoma cells in vitro and in vivo. *Gynecol. Oncol.* **2006**, *103*, 199–206. [CrossRef]
209. Luo, D.; Zhang, X.; Du, R.; Gao, W.; Luo, N.; Zhao, S.; Li, Y.; Chen, R.; Wang, H.; Bao, Y.; et al. Low dosage of arsenic trioxide (As_2O_3) inhibits angiogenesis in epithelial ovarian cancer without cell apoptosis. *J. Biol. Inorg. Chem.* **2018**, *23*, 939–947. [CrossRef]
210. Askar, N.; Cirpan, T.; Toprak, E.; Karabulut, B.; Selvi, N.; Terek, M.C.; Uslu, R.; Sanli, U.A.; Goker, E. Arsenic trioxide exposure to ovarian carcinoma cells leads to decreased level of topoisomerase II and cytotoxicity. *Int. J. Gynecol. Cancer* **2006**, *16*, 1552–1556. [CrossRef]
211. Zhang, N.; Wu, Z.M.; McGowan, E.; Shi, J.; Hong, Z.B.; Ding, C.W.; Xia, P.; Di, W. Arsenic trioxide and cisplatin synergism increase cytotoxicity in human ovarian cancer cells: Therapeutic potential for ovarian cancer. *Cancer Sci.* **2009**, *100*, 2459–2464. [CrossRef]
212. Bornstein, J.; Sagi, S.; Haj, A.; Harroch, J.; Fares, F. Arsenic Trioxide inhibits the growth of human ovarian carcinoma cell line. *Gynecol. Oncol.* **2005**, *99*, 726–729. [CrossRef]
213. Porta, C.; Paglino, C.; Mosca, A. Targeting PI3K/Akt/mTOR Signaling in Cancer. *Front. Oncol.* **2014**, *4*, 64. [CrossRef]
214. Tian, T.; Li, X.; Zhang, J. mTOR Signaling in Cancer and mTOR Inhibitors in Solid Tumor Targeting Therapy. *Int. J. Mol. Sci.* **2019**, *20*, 755. [CrossRef]
215. Choi, C.H.; Ryu, J.Y.; Cho, Y.J.; Jeon, H.K.; Choi, J.J.; Ylaya, K.; Lee, Y.Y.; Kim, T.J.; Chung, J.Y.; Hewitt, S.M.; et al. The anti-cancer effects of itraconazole in epithelial ovarian cancer. *Sci. Rep.* **2017**, *7*, 6552. [CrossRef]
216. Day, C.; Bailey, C.J. Biguanides. In *xPharm: The Comprehensive Pharmacology Reference*; Enna, S.J., Bylund, D.B., Eds.; Elsevier: New York, NY, USA, 2007; pp. 1–3.
217. Jackson, A.L.; Sun, W.; Kilgore, J.; Guo, H.; Fang, Z.; Yin, Y.; Jones, H.M.; Gilliam, T.P.; Zhou, C.; Bae-Jump, V.L. Phenformin has anti-tumorigenic effects in human ovarian cancer cells and in an orthotopic mouse model of serous ovarian cancer. *Oncotarget* **2017**, *8*, 100113–100127. [CrossRef]
218. Garrido, M.P.; Vega, M.; Romero, C. Antitumoral Effects of Metformin in Ovarian Cancer. In *Metformin*; IntechOpen: London, UK, 2019. [CrossRef]
219. Evans, J.M.; Donnelly, L.A.; Emslie-Smith, A.M.; Alessi, D.R.; Morris, A.D. Metformin and reduced risk of cancer in diabetic patients. *BMJ* **2005**, *330*, 1304–1305. [CrossRef]
220. Lv, Z.; Guo, Y. Metformin and Its Benefits for Various Diseases. *Front. Endocrinol. (Lausanne)* **2020**, *11*, 191. [CrossRef]
221. Hardie, D.G.; Ross, F.A.; Hawley, S.A. AMPK: A nutrient and energy sensor that maintains energy homeostasis. *Nat. Rev. Mol. Cell Biol.* **2012**, *13*, 251–262. [CrossRef]
222. Zou, Z.; Tao, T.; Li, H.; Zhu, X. mTOR signaling pathway and mTOR inhibitors in cancer: Progress and challenges. *Cell Biosci.* **2020**, *10*, 31. [CrossRef]
223. Rattan, R.; Giri, S.; Hartmann, L.C.; Shridhar, V. Metformin attenuates ovarian cancer cell growth in an AMP-kinase dispensable manner. *J. Cell Mol. Med.* **2011**, *15*, 166–178. [CrossRef]
224. Ben Sahra, I.; Laurent, K.; Loubat, A.; Giorgetti-Peraldi, S.; Colosetti, P.; Auberger, P.; Tanti, J.F.; Le Marchand-Brustel, Y.; Bost, F. The antidiabetic drug metformin exerts an antitumoral effect in vitro and in vivo through a decrease of cyclin D1 level. *Oncogene* **2008**, *27*, 3576–3586. [CrossRef]

225. Hodeib, M.; Ogrodzinski, M.; Vergnes, L.; Reuek, K.; Lunt, S.; Walsh, C.; Karlan, B.Y.; Aspuria, P.J. Metformin and phenformin inhibit cell proliferation and alter metabolism in high-grade serous ovarian cancer(HGSC). *Gynecol. Oncol.* **2017**, *145*, 119. [CrossRef]
226. Garrido, M.P.; Vera, C.; Vega, M.; Quest, A.F.G.; Romero, C. Metformin prevents nerve growth factor-dependent proliferative and proangiogenic effects in epithelial ovarian cancer cells and endothelial cells. *Ther. Adv. Med. Oncol.* **2018**, *10*, 1758835918770984. [CrossRef]
227. Dos Santos Guimaraes, I.; Ladislau-Magescky, T.; Tessarollo, N.G.; Dos Santos, D.Z.; Gimba, E.R.P.; Sternberg, C.; Silva, I.V.; Rangel, L.B.A. Chemosensitizing effects of metformin on cisplatin- and paclitaxel-resistant ovarian cancer cell lines. *Pharm. Rep.* **2018**, *70*, 409–417. [CrossRef]
228. Garrido, M.P.; Salvatierra, R.; Valenzuela-Valderrama, M.; Vallejos, C.; Bruneau, N.; Hernandez, A.; Vega, M.; Selman, A.; Quest, A.F.G.; Romero, C. Metformin Reduces NGF-Induced Tumour Promoter Effects in Epithelial Ovarian Cancer Cells. *Pharmaceuticals* **2020**, *13*, 315. [CrossRef] [PubMed]
229. Blandino, G.; Valerio, M.; Cioce, M.; Mori, F.; Casadei, L.; Pulito, C.; Sacconi, A.; Biagioni, F.; Cortese, G.; Galanti, S.; et al. Metformin elicits anticancer effects through the sequential modulation of DICER and c-MYC. *Nat. Commun.* **2012**, *3*, 865. [CrossRef] [PubMed]
230. Anastasiou, D. Tumour microenvironment factors shaping the cancer metabolism landscape. *Br. J. Cancer* **2017**, *116*, 277–286. [CrossRef] [PubMed]
231. Zhang, R.; Zhang, P.; Wang, H.; Hou, D.; Li, W.; Xiao, G.; Li, C. Inhibitory effects of metformin at low concentration on epithelial-mesenchymal transition of CD44(+)CD117(+) ovarian cancer stem cells. *Stem Cell Res. Ther.* **2015**, *6*, 262. [CrossRef] [PubMed]
232. Hirsch, H.A.; Iliopoulos, D.; Tsichlis, P.N.; Struhl, K. Metformin selectively targets cancer stem cells, and acts together with chemotherapy to block tumor growth and prolong remission. *Cancer Res.* **2009**, *69*, 7507–7511. [CrossRef]
233. Iliopoulos, D.; Hirsch, H.A.; Struhl, K. Metformin decreases the dose of chemotherapy for prolonging tumor remission in mouse xenografts involving multiple cancer cell types. *Cancer Res.* **2011**, *71*, 3196–3201. [CrossRef] [PubMed]
234. Shank, J.J.; Yang, K.; Ghannam, J.; Cabrera, L.; Johnston, C.J.; Reynolds, R.K.; Buckanovich, R.J. Metformin targets ovarian cancer stem cells in vitro and in vivo. *Gynecol. Oncol.* **2012**, *127*, 390–397. [CrossRef] [PubMed]
235. Steg, A.D.; Bevis, K.S.; Katre, A.A.; Ziebarth, A.; Dobbin, Z.C.; Alvarez, R.D.; Zhang, K.; Conner, M.; Landen, C.N. Stem cell pathways contribute to clinical chemoresistance in ovarian cancer. *Clin. Cancer Res.* **2012**, *18*, 869–881. [CrossRef]
236. Buckanovich, R.J.; Brown, J.; Shank, J.; Griffith, K.A.; Reynolds, R.K.; Johnston, C.; McLean, K.; Uppal, S.; Liu, J.R.; Cabrera, L.; et al. A phase II clinical trial of metformin as a cancer stem cell targeting agent in stage IIc/III/IV ovarian, fallopian tube, and primary peritoneal cancer. *J. Clin. Oncol.* **2017**, *35*, 5556. [CrossRef]
237. Wang, Q.; Lopez-Ozuna, V.M.; Baloch, T.; Bithras, J.; Amin, O.; Kessous, R.; Kogan, L.; Laskov, I.; Yasmeen, A. Biguanides in combination with olaparib limits tumorigenesis of drug-resistant ovarian cancer cells through inhibition of Snail. *Cancer Med.* **2020**, *9*, 1307–1320. [CrossRef]
238. Schulten, H.J. Pleiotropic Effects of Metformin on Cancer. *Int. J. Mol. Sci.* **2018**, *19*, 2850. [CrossRef] [PubMed]
239. Ghlichloo, I.; Gerriets, V. Nonsteroidal Anti-inflammatory Drugs (NSAIDs). In *StatPearls*; StatPearls Publishing: Treasure Island, FL, USA, 2021.
240. Kune, G. Commentary: Aspirin and cancer prevention. *Int. J. Epidemiol.* **2007**, *36*, 957–959. [CrossRef]
241. Friis, S.; Riis, A.H.; Erichsen, R.; Baron, J.A.; Sorensen, H.T. Low-Dose Aspirin or Nonsteroidal Anti-inflammatory Drug Use and Colorectal Cancer Risk: A Population-Based, Case-Control Study. *Ann. Intern. Med.* **2015**, *163*, 347–355. [CrossRef]
242. Kim, S.; Shore, D.L.; Wilson, L.E.; Sanniez, E.I.; Kim, J.H.; Taylor, J.A.; Sandler, D.P. Lifetime use of nonsteroidal anti-inflammatory drugs and breast cancer risk: Results from a prospective study of women with a sister with breast cancer. *BMC Cancer* **2015**, *15*, 960. [CrossRef]
243. Hilovska, L.; Jendzelovsky, R.; Fedorocko, P. Potency of non-steroidal anti-inflammatory drugs in chemotherapy. *Mol. Clin. Oncol.* **2015**, *3*, 3–12. [CrossRef]
244. Lau, L.; Hansford, L.M.; Cheng, L.S.; Hang, M.; Baruchel, S.; Kaplan, D.R.; Irwin, M.S. Cyclooxygenase inhibitors modulate the p53/HDM2 pathway and enhance chemotherapy-induced apoptosis in neuroblastoma. *Oncogene* **2007**, *26*, 1920–1931. [CrossRef] [PubMed]
245. Lee, J.P.; Hahn, H.S.; Hwang, S.J.; Choi, J.Y.; Park, J.S.; Lee, I.H.; Kim, T.J. Selective cyclooxygenase inhibitors increase paclitaxel sensitivity in taxane-resistant ovarian cancer by suppressing P-glycoprotein expression. *J. Gynecol. Oncol.* **2013**, *24*, 273–279. [CrossRef] [PubMed]
246. Hanahan, D.; Weinberg, R.A. Hallmarks of cancer: The next generation. *Cell* **2011**, *144*, 646–674. [CrossRef] [PubMed]
247. Rabinowitz, J.D.; Enerback, S. Lactate: The ugly duckling of energy metabolism. *Nat. Metab.* **2020**, *2*, 566–571. [CrossRef]
248. Choi, S.Y.; Collins, C.C.; Gout, P.W.; Wang, Y. Cancer-generated lactic acid: A regulatory, immunosuppressive metabolite? *J. Pathol.* **2013**, *230*, 350–355. [CrossRef]
249. Sonveaux, P.; Vegran, F.; Schroeder, T.; Wergin, M.C.; Verrax, J.; Rabbani, Z.N.; De Saedeleer, C.J.; Kennedy, K.M.; Diepart, C.; Jordan, B.F.; et al. Targeting lactate-fueled respiration selectively kills hypoxic tumor cells in mice. *J. Clin. Invest.* **2008**, *118*, 3930–3942. [CrossRef] [PubMed]

250. Sasaki, S.; Futagi, Y.; Ideno, M.; Kobayashi, M.; Narumi, K.; Furugen, A.; Iseki, K. Effect of diclofenac on SLC16A3/MCT4 by the Caco-2 cell line. *Drug Metab. Pharm.* **2016**, *31*, 218–223. [CrossRef] [PubMed]
251. Soudyab, M.; Iranpour, M.; Ghafouri-Fard, S. The Role of Long Non-Coding RNAs in Breast Cancer. *Arch. Iran. Med.* **2016**, *19*, 508–517. [PubMed]
252. Slack, F.J.; Chinnaiyan, A.M. The Role of Non-coding RNAs in Oncology. *Cell* **2019**, *179*, 1033–1055. [CrossRef]
253. Han Li, C.; Chen, Y. Small and Long Non-Coding RNAs: Novel Targets in Perspective Cancer Therapy. *Curr. Genom.* **2015**, *16*, 319–326. [CrossRef]
254. Chen, S.N.; Chang, R.; Lin, L.T.; Chern, C.U.; Tsai, H.W.; Wen, Z.H.; Li, Y.H.; Li, C.J.; Tsui, K.H. MicroRNA in Ovarian Cancer: Biology, Pathogenesis, and Therapeutic Opportunities. *Int. J. Environ. Res. Public Health* **2019**, *16*, 1510. [CrossRef]
255. Macfarlane, L.A.; Murphy, P.R. MicroRNA: Biogenesis, Function and Role in Cancer. *Curr. Genom.* **2010**, *11*, 537–561. [CrossRef]
256. Retamales-Ortega, R.; Orostica, L.; Vera, C.; Cuevas, P.; Hernandez, A.; Hurtado, I.; Vega, M.; Romero, C. Role of Nerve Growth Factor (NGF) and miRNAs in Epithelial Ovarian Cancer. *Int. J. Mol. Sci.* **2017**, *18*, 507. [CrossRef]
257. Garrido, M.P.; Torres, I.; Avila, A.; Chnaiderman, J.; Valenzuela-Valderrama, M.; Aramburo, J.; Orostica, L.; Duran-Jara, E.; Lobos-Gonzalez, L.; Romero, C. NGF/TRKA Decrease miR-145-5p Levels in Epithelial Ovarian Cancer Cells. *Int. J. Mol. Sci.* **2020**, *21*, 7657. [CrossRef]
258. Minami, K.; Taniguchi, K.; Sugito, N.; Kuranaga, Y.; Inamoto, T.; Takahara, K.; Takai, T.; Yoshikawa, Y.; Kiyama, S.; Akao, Y.; et al. MiR-145 negatively regulates Warburg effect by silencing KLF4 and PTBP1 in bladder cancer cells. *Oncotarget* **2017**, *8*, 33064–33077. [CrossRef]
259. Zhao, S.; Zhang, Y.; Pei, M.; Wu, L.; Li, J. miR-145 inhibits mitochondrial function of ovarian cancer by targeting ARL5B. *J. Ovarian. Res.* **2021**, *14*, 8. [CrossRef] [PubMed]
260. Sheng, Q.; Zhang, Y.; Wang, Z.; Ding, J.; Song, Y.; Zhao, W. Cisplatin-mediated down-regulation of miR-145 contributes to up-regulation of PD-L1 via the c-Myc transcription factor in cisplatin-resistant ovarian carcinoma cells. *Clin. Exp. Immunol.* **2020**, *200*, 45–52. [CrossRef]
261. Fernandes, J.C.R.; Acuna, S.M.; Aoki, J.I.; Floeter-Winter, L.M.; Muxel, S.M. Long Non-Coding RNAs in the Regulation of Gene Expression: Physiology and Disease. *Noncoding RNA* **2019**, *5*, 17. [CrossRef]
262. Bayoumi, A.S.; Sayed, A.; Broskova, Z.; Teoh, J.P.; Wilson, J.; Su, H.; Tang, Y.L.; Kim, I.M. Crosstalk between Long Noncoding RNAs and MicroRNAs in Health and Disease. *Int. J. Mol. Sci.* **2016**, *17*, 356. [CrossRef]
263. Zhang, H.M.; Yang, F.Q.; Chen, S.J.; Che, J.; Zheng, J.H. Upregulation of long non-coding RNA MALAT1 correlates with tumor progression and poor prognosis in clear cell renal cell carcinoma. *Tumour Biol.* **2015**, *36*, 2947–2955. [CrossRef]
264. Jiang, Y.; Li, Y.; Fang, S.; Jiang, B.; Qin, C.; Xie, P.; Zhou, G.; Li, G. The role of MALAT1 correlates with HPV in cervical cancer. *Oncol. Lett.* **2014**, *7*, 2135–2141. [CrossRef]
265. Wang, Y.; Wang, X.; Han, L.; Hu, D. LncRNA MALAT1 Regulates the Progression and Cisplatin Resistance of Ovarian Cancer Cells via Modulating miR-1271-5p/E2F5 Axis. *Cancer Manag. Res.* **2020**, *12*, 9999–10010. [CrossRef] [PubMed]
266. Zou, A.; Liu, R.; Wu, X. Long non-coding RNA MALAT1 is up-regulated in ovarian cancer tissue and promotes SK-OV-3 cell proliferation and invasion. *Neoplasma* **2016**, *63*, 865–872. [CrossRef] [PubMed]
267. Jin, Y.; Feng, S.J.; Qiu, S.; Shao, N.; Zheng, J.H. LncRNA MALAT1 promotes proliferation and metastasis in epithelial ovarian cancer via the PI3K-AKT pathway. *Eur. Rev. Med. Pharm. Sci.* **2017**, *21*, 3176–3184.
268. Zhang, D.; Fang, C.; Li, H.; Lu, C.; Huang, J.; Pan, J.; Yang, Z.; Liang, E.; Liu, Z.; Zhou, X.; et al. Long ncRNA MALAT1 promotes cell proliferation, migration, and invasion in prostate cancer via sponging miR-145. *Transl. Androl. Urol.* **2021**, *10*, 2307–2319. [CrossRef] [PubMed]
269. Barani, M.; Bilal, M.; Sabir, F.; Rahdar, A.; Kyzas, G.Z. Nanotechnology in ovarian cancer: Diagnosis and treatment. *Life Sci.* **2021**, *266*, 118914. [CrossRef] [PubMed]
270. Zahedi, P.; Yoganathan, R.; Piquette-Miller, M.; Allen, C. Recent advances in drug delivery strategies for treatment of ovarian cancer. *Expert Opin. Drug Deliv.* **2012**, *9*, 567–583. [CrossRef] [PubMed]
271. Udomprasert, A.; Kangsamaksin, T. DNA origami applications in cancer therapy. *Cancer Sci.* **2017**, *108*, 1535–1543. [CrossRef] [PubMed]
272. Aghebati-Maleki, A.; Dolati, S.; Ahmadi, M.; Baghbanzhadeh, A.; Asadi, M.; Fotouhi, A.; Yousefi, M.; Aghebati-Maleki, L. Nanoparticles and cancer therapy: Perspectives for application of nanoparticles in the treatment of cancers. *J. Cell Physiol.* **2020**, *235*, 1962–1972. [CrossRef] [PubMed]
273. Byeon, Y.; Lee, J.W.; Choi, W.S.; Won, J.E.; Kim, G.H.; Kim, M.G.; Wi, T.I.; Lee, J.M.; Kang, T.H.; Jung, I.D.; et al. CD44-Targeting PLGA Nanoparticles Incorporating Paclitaxel and FAK siRNA Overcome Chemoresistance in Epithelial Ovarian Cancer. *Cancer Res.* **2018**, *78*, 6247–6256. [CrossRef] [PubMed]
274. Vangijzegem, T.; Stanicki, D.; Laurent, S. Magnetic iron oxide nanoparticles for drug delivery: Applications and characteristics. *Expert Opin. Drug Deliv.* **2019**, *16*, 69–78. [CrossRef]
275. de Toledo, L.A.S.; Rosseto, H.C.; Bruschi, M.L. Iron oxide magnetic nanoparticles as antimicrobials for therapeutics. *Pharm. Dev. Technol.* **2018**, *23*, 316–323. [CrossRef]
276. Zhao, S.; Yu, X.; Qian, Y.; Chen, W.; Shen, J. Multifunctional magnetic iron oxide nanoparticles: An advanced platform for cancer theranostics. *Theranostics* **2020**, *10*, 6278–6309. [CrossRef]

277. Ramalingam, V.; Harshavardhan, M.; Dinesh Kumar, S.; Malathi devi, S. Wet chemical mediated hematite α-Fe2O3 nanoparticles synthesis: Preparation, characterization and anticancer activity against human metastatic ovarian cancer. *J. Alloy. Compd.* **2020**, *834*, 155118. [CrossRef]
278. Lee, J.; Cho, Y.J.; Lee, J.W.; Ahn, H.J. KSP siRNA/paclitaxel-loaded PEGylated cationic liposomes for overcoming resistance to KSP inhibitors: Synergistic antitumor effects in drug-resistant ovarian cancer. *J. Control. Release* **2020**, *321*, 184–197. [CrossRef]
279. Risnayanti, C.; Jang, Y.S.; Lee, J.; Ahn, H.J. PLGA nanoparticles co-delivering MDR1 and BCL2 siRNA for overcoming resistance of paclitaxel and cisplatin in recurrent or advanced ovarian cancer. *Sci. Rep.* **2018**, *8*, 7498. [CrossRef]
280. Zou, S.; Cao, N.; Cheng, D.; Zheng, R.; Wang, J.; Zhu, K.; Shuai, X. Enhanced apoptosis of ovarian cancer cells via nanocarrier-mediated codelivery of siRNA and doxorubicin. *Int J. Nanomedicine* **2012**, *7*, 3823–3835. [CrossRef] [PubMed]
281. Valadi, H.; Ekstrom, K.; Bossios, A.; Sjostrand, M.; Lee, J.J.; Lotvall, J.O. Exosome-mediated transfer of mRNAs and microRNAs is a novel mechanism of genetic exchange between cells. *Nat. Cell Biol.* **2007**, *9*, 654–659. [CrossRef] [PubMed]
282. Kosaka, N.; Kogure, A.; Yamamoto, T.; Urabe, F.; Usuba, W.; Prieto-Vila, M.; Ochiya, T. Exploiting the message from cancer: The diagnostic value of extracellular vesicles for clinical applications. *Exp. Mol. Med.* **2019**, *51*, 1–9. [CrossRef] [PubMed]
283. Tian, F.; Zhang, S.; Liu, C.; Han, Z.; Liu, Y.; Deng, J.; Li, Y.; Wu, X.; Cai, L.; Qin, L.; et al. Protein analysis of extracellular vesicles to monitor and predict therapeutic response in metastatic breast cancer. *Nat. Commun.* **2021**, *12*, 2536. [CrossRef]
284. Fontana, F.; Carollo, E.; Melling, G.E.; Carter, D.R.F. Extracellular Vesicles: Emerging Modulators of Cancer Drug Resistance. *Cancers* **2021**, *13*, 749. [CrossRef]
285. Liu, C.; Lin, X.; Su, C. Extracellular Vesicles: "Stealth Transport Aircrafts" for Drugs. *Theranostics An. Old Concept New Cloth.* **2020**. [CrossRef]
286. Garcia-Manrique, P.; Matos, M.; Gutierrez, G.; Pazos, C.; Blanco-Lopez, M.C. Therapeutic biomaterials based on extracellular vesicles: Classification of bio-engineering and mimetic preparation routes. *J. Extracell. Vesicles* **2018**, *7*, 1422676. [CrossRef] [PubMed]
287. Li, P.; Xin, H.; Lu, L. Extracellular vesicle-encapsulated microRNA-424 exerts inhibitory function in ovarian cancer by targeting MYB. *J. Transl. Med.* **2021**, *19*, 4. [CrossRef] [PubMed]
288. Yong, T.; Zhang, X.; Bie, N.; Zhang, H.; Zhang, X.; Li, F.; Hakeem, A.; Hu, J.; Gan, L.; Santos, H.A.; et al. Tumor exosome-based nanoparticles are efficient drug carriers for chemotherapy. *Nat. Commun.* **2019**, *10*, 3838. [CrossRef]
289. Liu, H.; Shen, M.; Zhao, D.; Ru, D.; Duan, Y.; Ding, C.; Li, H. The Effect of Triptolide-Loaded Exosomes on the Proliferation and Apoptosis of Human Ovarian Cancer SKOV3 Cells. *Biomed. Res. Int.* **2019**, *2019*, 2595801. [CrossRef] [PubMed]

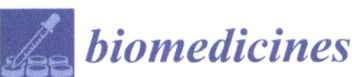

Review

Endometrial Carcinoma: Immune Microenvironment and Emerging Treatments in Immuno-Oncology

Sandrine Rousset-Rouviere [1,2,3], Philippe Rochigneux [1,3,4], Anne-Sophie Chrétien [1,3,5], Stéphane Fattori [1,3,5], Laurent Gorvel [1,3,5], Magali Provansal [4], Eric Lambaudie [1,2,3], Daniel Olive [1,3,5] and Renaud Sabatier [1,3,4,*]

1. Immunomonitoring Department, Institut Paoli-Calmettes, 13009 Marseille, France; roussetrouvieres@ipc.unicancer.fr (S.R.-R.); rochigneuxp@ipc.unicancer.fr (P.R.); anne-sophie.chretien@inserm.fr (A.-S.C.); stephane.fattori@inserm.fr (S.F.); laurent.gorvel@inserm.fr (L.G.); lambaudiee@ipc.unicancer.fr (E.L.); daniel.olive@inserm.fr (D.O.)
2. Department of Surgical Oncology, Institut Paoli-Calmettes, 13009 Marseille, France
3. Predictive Oncology Laboratory, CRCM, Inserm U1068, CNRS U7258, Institut Paoli-Calmettes, Aix Marseille University, 13009 Marseille, France
4. Department of Medical Oncology, Institut Paoli-Calmettes, 13009 Marseille, France; provansalm@ipc.unicancer.fr
5. Team Immunity and Cancer, CRCM, Inserm U1068, CNRS U7258, Institut Paoli-Calmettes, Aix Marseille University, 13009 Marseille, France
* Correspondence: sabatierr@ipc.unicancer.fr; Tel.: +33-4-9122-3537

Citation: Rousset-Rouviere, S.; Rochigneux, P.; Chrétien, A.-S.; Fattori, S.; Gorvel, L.; Provansal, M.; Lambaudie, E.; Olive, D.; Sabatier, R. Endometrial Carcinoma: Immune Microenvironment and Emerging Treatments in Immuno-Oncology. *Biomedicines* **2021**, *9*, 632. https://doi.org/10.3390/biomedicines9060632

Academic Editor: Naomi Nakayama

Received: 13 May 2021
Accepted: 31 May 2021
Published: 2 June 2021

Publisher's Note: MDPI stays neutral with regard to jurisdictional claims in published maps and institutional affiliations.

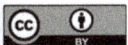

Copyright: © 2021 by the authors. Licensee MDPI, Basel, Switzerland. This article is an open access article distributed under the terms and conditions of the Creative Commons Attribution (CC BY) license (https:// creativecommons.org/licenses/by/ 4.0/).

Abstract: Endometrial cancer (EC) can easily be cured when diagnosed at an early stage. However, advanced and metastatic EC is a common disease, affecting more than 15,000 patients per year in the United Sates. Only limited treatment options were available until recently, with a taxane–platinum combination as the gold standard in first-line setting and no efficient second-line chemotherapy or hormone therapy. EC can be split into four molecular subtypes, including hypermutated cases with POLE mutations and 25–30% harboring a microsatellite instability (MSI) phenotype with mismatch repair deficiency (dMMR). These tumors display a high load of frameshift mutations, leading to increased expression of neoantigens that can be targeted by the immune system, including (but not limited) to T-cell response. Recent data have demonstrated this impact of programmed death 1 and programmed death ligand 1 (PD-1/PD-L1) inhibitors on chemo-resistant metastatic EC. The uncontrolled KEYNOTE-158 and GARNET trials have shown high response rates with pembrolizumab and dostarlimab in chemoresistant MSI-high tumors. Most responders experiment long responses that last more than one year. Similar, encouraging results were obtained for MMR proficient (MMRp) cases treated with a combination of pembrolizumab and the angiogenesis inhibitor lenvatinib. Approvals have, thus, been obtained or are underway for EC with immune checkpoint inhibitors (ICI) used as monotherapy, and in combination with antiangiogenic agents. Combinations with other targeted therapies are under evaluation and randomized studies are ongoing to explore the impact of ICI-chemotherapy triplets in first-line setting. We summarize in this review the current knowledge of the immune environment of EC, both for MMRd and MMRp tumors. We also detail the main clinical data regarding PD-1/PD-L1 inhibitors and discuss the next steps of development for immunotherapy, including various ICI-based combinations planned to limit resistance to immunotherapy.

Keywords: endometrial carcinoma; immune micro-environment; immune checkpoints inhibitors; microsatellite instability; mismatch repair deficiency

1. Introduction

In 2020, endometrial cancer (EC) was the fourth most common cancer in women, with an incidence of 382,069 new cases and 89,929 deaths worldwide in 2018 [1,2]. EC mostly affects post-menopausal women (68 years of age, on average). In industrialized countries, most patients are diagnosed in a localized stage, with a favorable prognosis (5-year overall survival: 80%) and are treated with a hysterectomy, with or without adjuvant therapy [3]. However, for patients with advanced disease, with lymph node invasion or metastasis (peritoneal or visceral), the 5-year overall survival is only 50% and 20%, respectively [4]. In advanced endometrial cancer, therapeutic options are limited: in first-line setting, a taxane–platinum combination is the gold standard, but no standard second-line treatment (chemotherapy or endocrine therapy) is available [5]. Furthermore, systemic chemotherapies are not always feasible due to patient comorbidities and performance status after platinum failure.

Endometrial cancers are broadly classified into two groups: type I endometrioid tumors are linked to estrogen excess, obesity, hormone-receptor positivity, and favorable prognosis compared with type II, primarily serous, tumors that are more common in older, non-obese women and have a worse outcome [6–8]. Moreover, the FIGO stage, the histological type, the pathological grade (both gathered in the old-fashioned type 1/type 2 classification), hormone receptors expression, and the presence of vascular emboli stratify prognostic groups and guide complementary treatments (classification ESMO–ESGO–ESTRO) [3]. However, the prognostic value of these classifications remains suboptimal, in particular due to the heterogeneity of tumors grouped together within the same histological type.

Molecular classification of EC based on The Cancer Genome Atlas Project (TCGA) [9], called the Proactive Molecular Risk classification tool for endometrial cancers (ProMisE) identified four classes of EC based on genomic characterization [10]: (i) ultramutated EC (harboring somatic mutations in the proofreading exonuclease domain of the DNA replicase POLE) are tumors with the highest rate of mutations and neo-antigens and the best prognosis; (ii) microsatellite instability-high (MSI-H) genotype (hypermutated) present a defect in the mismatch repair (MMR) pathway: the insertion or deletion of repeated units during DNA replication are no longer corrected by the proteins MLH1, MSH2, MSH6, and PMS2; (iii) copy number low tumors (most low grade endometrioid) have a moderate rate of mutations and exhibit both a low somatic copy number variation number (SCNAs) and a wild typeTP53 gene; (iv) copy number high tumors (serous-like) have TP53 mutations and present the lowest rate of mutations and a very large number of SCNAs.

This molecular classification was very recently incorporated into the ESGO recommendations [11]. However, this molecular classification alone does not explain the different responses to systemic therapies. A better description of the tumor immune micro-environment could refine the prognosis and help define new targets for immuno-oncological therapies [11].

2. Rationale for Targeting the Immune Microenvironment in Endometrial Cancer

2.1. Tumor-Infiltrating Lymphocytes According to Molecular Subtypes

Similarly to many tumor types (melanoma, lung, and colorectal carcinoma), the frequency of lymphocytes infiltrating tumor and peritumoral areas is correlated with the risk of recurrence in endometrial cancer. Kondratiev et al. demonstrated by immunohistochemistry (IHC) that a number of CD8 + LTs > 10 per field (at ×40 magnification) found in the peritumoral zone is an independent prognostic factor associated with improved survival [12]. However, the immune infiltrate differs among molecular subtypes of EC.

Interestingly, tumor-infiltrating CD8+ T lymphocytes within cancer cell nests are particularly abundant in MSI tumors (30% of 123 EC samples analyzed by IHC) [13]. These findings were confirmed by another study by Pakish et al. in MSI-high tumors ($n = 60$) demonstrating that immune cells were more present in stroma of MSI-H EC compared with microsatellite stable (MSS) cases, including granzyme B+ cells, activated T-cells (CD8+ granzyme B+), and PD-L1+ cells [14]. Specifically, inherited Lynch syndrome MSI-H EC had increased CD8+ cells and activated T-cells in stroma, with reduced macrophages in stroma and tumor compared with sporadic MSI-H EC [14].

Within the MSI-H subtype, immunotherapy response is associated with higher rates of tumor infiltrating immune cells, both in EC and other MSI-H tumors types [15]. MSI-H and non-MSI-H colorectal tumors exhibited distinct levels of infiltration and immune phenotypes. Surprisingly, there was no significant difference between MSI-H and non-

MSI-H endometrial tumors. Regardless of cancer type, the abundance of tumor infiltrating immune cells was an independent prognostic factor, with better accuracy than MSI-H status. The authors conclude that the study of immune infiltrate is a fundamental biomarker for predicting response to immunotherapy treatments.

POLE hypermutated tumors (7–12% of EC) also had an important TILs infiltration, with an overexpression of genes involved in the cytotoxic functions of TILs, in particular T-bet, Eomes, interferon γ (IFNγ), perforin, and granzyme B, and markers of exhaustion markers on TILS, consistent with chronic exposure to neo-antigens [16]. In silico analysis confirmed that POLE-mutant cancers are predicted to display more antigenic neoepitopes than other EC, providing a potential rational for POLE immunogenicity [16].

2.2. The PD1/PD-L1 Axis in Endometrial Cancer

Endometrial cancer cells and tumor microenvironment are able to modulate the immune response. Among gynecological cancers, EC displays the highest overexpression of programmed cell death 1 (PD-1, CD279) and programmed cell death ligand-1 (PD-L1, CD274): 40–80% for endometrioid cancers, 10–68% for serous tumors, 23–69% for clear cells tumors, respectively [17,18]. PD-1 is a cell surface protein encoded by the *PDCD1* gene and expressed in particular on the surface of activated B and T lymphocytes [19]. The PD-1 pathway is a negative feedback system that controls the cytotoxic activity of lymphocytes in order to prevent autoimmune reactions (Figure 1).

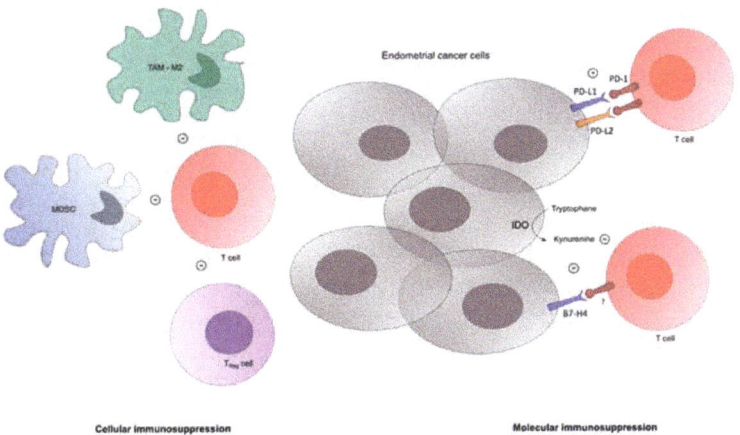

Figure 1. Immunosuppression in tumor microenvironment of endometrial cancer. MDSC: myeloid derived suppressor cell, Treg: T regulator lymphocyte, IDO: indoleamine-2,3-dioxygenase, TAM: tumor associated macrophage.

Its major ligand PD-L1 is constitutively expressed at a low level on antigen-presenting cells (dendritic cells, macrophages and B cells) and is upregulated in these cells after their activation as well as in activated T cells and in various cancer cells [20–22]. PD-L1 is regulated by many inflammatory cytokines, including IFNγ, GM-CSF, LPS, IL-4, and IL-10 [23,24]. In tumors, PD-L1 expression has been abundantly detected and is often associated with a poor prognosis [25,26]. The upregulation of PD-L1 is modulated by CD8 + T cells and IFNγ. Therefore, PD-L1 expression could be viewed as a negative feedback loop dependent on an infiltrating immune response [27]. PD-L1 is expressed in 92% of endometrial cancers. High PD-L1 expression is associated with advanced tumor stage and poor tumor differentiation; however, unlike what is usually observed in other solid tumors, PD-L1 does not appear as a prognostic factor in endometrial cancers [28].

On the other hand, the PD-L2 expression is much more restricted. It is mainly expressed on antigen presenting cells but expression can be induced on several other immune and non-immune cells depending on environmental stimuli [26]. PD-L2 has moderate-to-high expression in triple negative breast cancer and gastric cancer and low expression in renal carcinoma [29]. PD-L2 is expressed at low levels within endometrial tumors, but at higher rates in serous tumors. More data are needed to better understand its role in immune response before confirming it can be considered a good candidate to target in this tumor type [30,31].

Modulation of the immune response thus appears to be different within molecular subtypes. Willvonseder et al. demonstrated greater infiltration by TILs in high-grade tumors compared to low-grade tumors, as well as in the POLE and MSI-H subgroups [32]. The greater infiltration of ultramutated POLE and MSI-H tumors is accompanied by overexpression of PD-1 and PD-L1 [33]. Likewise, the immune microenvironment of MSI-H endometrial tumors harbors more activated CD8 + T-cells and PD-L1 + cells in MSI-H vs. MSS [14]. In a large cohort of 183 EC, Kim et al. showed that a high level of PD-L1 + T-cells was significantly associated with a shorter PFS predominantly in MSS tumors [34].

2.3. Other Immune-Response Related Features in Endometrial Cancer

Cytotoxic T lymphocyte antigen-4 (CTLA-4), lymphocyte activation gene-3 (LAG-3), and IDO may also be upregulated in POLE tumors. In mutated TP53 tumors, infiltration by regulatory T lymphocytes is an independent prognostic factor. Analysis of immune populations by multiplexed IHC in 460 endometrial cancers stratified according to the four molecular subtypes showed a profound variation in the immune response between the molecular subtypes of endometrial cancer, but also within them [35]. Even though POLE and MSI-H tumors are the most immune-responsive, some serous-like and copy-number low tumors (defined according to IHC) also harbored strong immune responses. Besides regulatory T-cells, myeloid-derived suppressor cells (MDSCs) are also differentially expressed in EC. MDSCs are immature myeloid cells with immune suppressive action based on L-arginine depletion in the tumor microenvironment, causing T-cell receptor down-regulation [36]. MDSC levels are higher in EC than in normal endometrium [30], increase with advanced stage disease, and are associated with poor prognosis and poor response to cytotoxic treatments [37]. Tumor-associated macrophages (TAMs) are also involved in EC immune escape. EC cells expressing CD47 interact with the SIRPα macrophages-inhibiting signal. TAMs identified in EC are predominantly M2 macrophages with reduced phagocytosis properties contributing to EC progression and immune-suppression [38,39].

These points suggest that patient selection for immunomodulatory treatments may not be limited to MMRd to achieve the highest sensitivity and specificity. However, MMRd analysis by IHC remains easier to achieve and a cheaper way to predict PD1/PD-L1-inhibitors efficacy in EC, and has been widely used in recent clinical trials evaluating these drugs.

3. Immune Checkpoint Inhibitors in EC. PD-(L)1 Inhibitors as Backbone of all Strategies under Investigation

Until recently, cytotoxic chemotherapies were the gold standard for metastatic endometrial cancer treatment, whatever the line of treatment. The first-line regimen for advanced EC is still the combination of carboplatin and paclitaxel with overall response rates (ORR) of 50 to 60%, median progression-free survival of one year, and a median overall survival slightly of above three years [40,41]. After platinum failure, mono-chemotherapies are routinely used with poor results. For instance, doxorubicin and paclitaxel, the most prescribed second-line regimen, only offers a 4-month median PFS and a 12-month median OS [42]. Therefore, recurrent EC is a relevant clinical need and new therapies with innovative mechanisms of action have been explored to improve the outcome of patients with advanced EC. Among them, immunotherapy seems to be the most promising.

3.1. Clinical Trials Exploring PD-(L)1 Inhibitors as Monotherapy for Recurrent EC

As shown above, an MMRd phenotype/MSI-H genotype or POLE mutations can be predictive factors of ICI efficacy. Several research programs have thus explored the impact of ICI in these subsets. We can split trials in two categories. Studies that included less than 100 patients with metastatic or advanced endometrial cancer, mainly assessing PD-L1 inhibitors impact; and those with more than 100 patients, focused on PD-1 inhibitor large evaluations (Table 1). PD-1 inhibiting monoclonal antibodies limit the interaction of PD1 expressed by T-cells with its ligands (PD-L1 and PD-L2) upregulated in cancer cells. This inhibits the negative feedback loop resulting in the activation of anti-tumor immune response. PD-L1 specific antibodies only avoid PD-1/PD-L1 combination, resulting in a similar immune effect, but might induce less immune toxicity, notably pneumonitis.

Atezolizumab was administered, in a multi-cohort phase 1 study, to 15 patients with advanced/recurrent uterine cancer naive of anti-PD-(L)1 therapies [43]. After a dose escalation part, patients received atezolizumab at the dose of 15 mg/kg or the fixed dose of 1200 mg IV every three weeks for 16 cycles (one year) or until progression, unacceptable toxicity, or withdrawal. Treatment efficacy was analyzed according to PD-L1 expression on immune cells as defined by the Ventana PD-L1 SP142 IHC assay. Patients with less than 5% of positive IC (IC0 or IC1) and patients with 5% or more positive IC (IC2 and IC3) were separated. Overall response rate (ORR) was 13% (two responders out of 15 patients). These two responders were IC2/3 (among five cases). None of the ten IC0/1 patients had objective responses. It is worth noting that one responder had a MHI-high/TMB-high tumor (the other was not evaluable) whereas none of the non-responders had microsatellite instability or high tumor mutational burden. Median PFS was 4.2 months in the IC2/3 group vs. 1.4 months in the IC0/1 subset. Statistical evaluation of the significance of these results could not be performed due to the very small sample size.

Nivolumab (240 mg IV every 2 weeks until progression or unacceptable toxicity) was explored in a Japanese phase 2 multicohort open-label trial, including 23 unselected EC [44]. Results have been presented at the ASCO meeting in 2020. ORR was 23%, with a median PFS of 3.4 months and a 12-month OS of 42%. PD-L1 expression was not predictive of response and both patients with MSI-H tumors displayed partial response.

A non-randomized phase 2 trial enrolled previously treated recurrent EC in two cohorts exploring avelumab efficacy [45]. A dMMR/POLEmut cohort of 15 patients and a pMMR/non-POLEmut cohort of 16 patients. They received avelumab at the dose of 10 mg/kg IV every two weeks for a maximum of 24 months. Most of objective responses were observed in the dMMR cohort (26.7%) with one complete response (CR) and three partial responses (PR). The median PFS was 4.4 months in this subset with a 6-month PFS rate of 40%. Only one patient responded in the pMMR cohort, for a 6-month PFS rate of 6.3%. Exploratory analyses did not identify a predictive biomarker. Among the 25 tumors with PD-L1 expression evaluated using the tumor proportion score (considered positive if TPS $\geq$ 1%), seven (28%) were PD-L1 positive. However, all patients with objective responses in both dMMR and pMMR cohorts had PD-L1–negative tumors. Tumor mutational burden and tumor infiltrating lymphocytes were also not correlated to response.

The phase 2 non-randomized PHAEDRA study enrolled 71 patients (36 dMMR and 35 pMMR) with advanced EC [46]. They received durvalumab 1500 mg IV every 4 weeks. Patients with dMMR tumors should have received less than four prior lines of treatment but could have been treatment naïve in the metastatic setting, whereas patients with pMMR disease had to be pre-treated. ORR was 47% in the dMMR population (6 CR plus 11 PR) vs. 3% in the pMMR subgroup. Median PFS was 5.5 months for dMMR cases with a 1-year overall survival rate of 71% vs. 1.8 months and a 51% 1-year survival rate for pMMR cases. Sensitivity to durvalumab seemed to be higher for treatment-naïve patients with a 57% ORR when durvalumab was given as first-line treatment vs. 38% when the PD-L1 inhibitor was administered in the second-line setting. The PD-L1 combined positive score (22C3 antibody) was negative in most responders.

Table 1. Prospective clinical studies with results available.

Drugs	ICI Target	Schemes	N	ORR (%)	Median PFS (Months)	Median OS (Months)	Reference
Monotherapy (all for pretreated advanced EC)							
Atezolizumab	PD-L1	15 mg/kg or 1200 mg IV Q3W	15	13.3	1.4 (4.2 for IC2/3 cases)	9.6	[43]
Nivolumab	PD-1	240 mg IV Q2W	23	23	3.4	NA	[44]
Avelumab	PD-L1	10 mg/kg IV Q2W	15 dMMR 16 pMMR	26.7 6.25	4.4 6.25	Not reached 6.6	[45]
Durvalumab	PD-L1	1500 mg IV Q4W	36 dMMR 35 pMMR	47 3	5.5 1.8	Not reached 11.5	[46]
Pembrolizumab	PD-1	10 mg/kg IV Q2W	24 PDL1+	13	1.8	Not reached	[47]
		200 mg IV Q3W	107 unselected 49 MSI-H	11.2 57.1	NA 26.0	NA Not reached	[48,49]
Dostarlimab	PD-1	500 mg IV Q3W for 4 doses then 1000 mg IV Q6W	103 dMMR 142 pMMR	44.7 13.4	NA NA	NA NA	[50]
Combinations							
Pembrolizumab + lenvatinib	PD-1	200 mg IV Q3W + 20 mg orally once per day Single-arm ph2 in pretreated EC	94 pMMR 11 dMMR	24 W-ORR 36.2% 63.6%	7.4 for the whole set	16.7 for the whole set	[51]
		200 mg IV Q3W + 20 mg orally once per day Randomized ph3 vs. chemo in pretreated EC	697 pMMR 130 dMMR	NA	6.6 vs. 3.8 for pMMR HR = 0.60 (95CI 0.50–0.72)	17.4 vs. 12.0 for pMMR HR = 0.68 (95CI 0.56–0.84)	[52]
Nivolumab ± cabozantinib	PD-1	240 mg IV Q2W ± 40 mg orally once per day Ph 2 randomized study	36 nivo + cabo 18 nivo	25.0 16.7	5.3 1.9 $p = 0.07$ (significant)	NA	[53]
Avelumab + talazoparib	PD-L1	1200 mg IV Q3W +1 mg orally once per day Single-arm ph2 for pretreated EC	35 pMMR	8.6	6m-PFS = 25.8%	NA	[54]

Abbreviations: ICI, immune-checkpoint inhibitor; ORR, overall response rate; PFS, progression-free survival; OS, overall survival; EC, endometrial cancer; IC, tumor-infiltrating immune cell; dMMR, MMR deficient pMMR, MMR proficient; MSI-H, microsatellite instability-high; NA, not available.

Pembrolizumab (anti-PD-1) impact was first assessed in a cohort of the multitumor phase I KEYNOTE-028 trial [47]. Twenty-four patients with PD-L1 positive EC received pembrolizumab alone. Three of them (13%) had objective responses, including one case with POLE mutation. The Keynote-158 trial was a multi-cohort phase 2 study that enrolled patients with previously treated metastatic solid tumors. Patients with EC could be included in two cohorts: cohort D (N = 107) with all EC and cohort K with MSI-H solid tumors [48,49]. Forty-nine MSI-H cases (21% of the whole study population) were enrolled in both cohorts. Patients received pembrolizumab (PD-1 inhibitor) every three weeks for a maximum of 35 cycles. ORR was 11.2% in cohort D and 57.1% for MSI-H tumors (45.5% of 11 patients in cohort D and 60.5% of 38 patients in cohort K). Among MSI-H cases, less than 25% (11 cases) displayed progression as best responses. Median duration of response was not reached with 89% of responders still in response at one year. One-year PFS and OS rates were 58.4% and 73.5%, respectively. According to these results, and that of other cohorts of this study, pembrolizumab obtained FDA approval for all unresectable or metastatic dMMR/MSI-H solid tumors, irrespective of localization, with progression following treatment, and for which there were no satisfactory alternative treatment options [55]. Response according to PD-L1 expression was not described.

The GARNET trial is an open-label uncontrolled multi-cohorts phase 1 trial exploring the impact of dostarlimab (PD-1 inhibitor) in various tumor types. The A1 (dMMR) and A2 (pMMR) cohorts of the expansion phase enrolled patients with previously treated EC [50,56]. They receive dostarlimab at the dose of 500 mg IV every 3 weeks for four doses, then 1000 mg IV every 6 weeks until disease progression. Efficacy data have been presented for 103 dMMR and 142 pMMR EC. ORR were 44.7% and 13.4% in dMMR and pMMR cohorts, respectively. Disease control rate was 57.3% and 35.2% in each cohort. Median duration of response has not been reached in both cohort, with 89% of responders still in response in the dMMR subgroup. PFS and OS data are not yet available for this trial, as well as efficacy according to PD-L1 expression. FDA and EMA approvals for dMMR recurrent EC were obtained in April 2021.

No new safety signal was identified in these trials, without any treatment-related death. Eleven to nineteen grade 3 treatment-related adverse events were observed. Immune related adverse events (AEs) were mainly dysthyroidism and digestive disorders.

3.2. PD-(L)1 Inhibitors-Based Combinations

Due to the complexity of immune response activation and the various mechanisms leading to resistance to PD-(L)1 inhibitors, combination strategies were developed to obtain synergistic benefits or to reduce primary or secondary resistance. In order to inhibit other immune checkpoints, combos with CTLA-4, TIGIT, IDO, and PVRIG are under early clinical evaluations (NCT03015129, NCT04570839, NCT04106414, NCT03667716) [57], and future data will provide insights about their clinical utilities in this setting.

The most advanced combinations explore angiogenesis and PARP inhibitors in the recurrent setting, and chemotherapy in the first-line setting.

3.2.1. Angiogenesis Inhibitors

Angiogenesis-inhibiting drugs are described as having a synergistic effect with ICI, by decreasing hypoxia, which is correlated with myeloid cell activation; enhancing T cells spreading to the tumor microenvironment; and favoring lymphocyte activation [58,59]. Combinations with ICI have, thus, been developed to limit primary resistance to immunotherapy.

Lenvatinib is an oral multityrosine kinase inhibitor targeting VEGFR among other proteins. Firstly developed as monotherapy in thyroid cancer and hepatocellular carcinoma, it is currently widely explored in other solid tumors in combinations with ICI. Concerning EC, the first evidence of activity has been observed in association with pembrolizumab in the KEYNOTE-146 study, a phase Ib/II multicohort trial [51]. One hundred and eight previously treated patients with EC were enrolled, including 11 with dMMR tumor and

94 MMRp cases. They received pembrolizumab 200 mg every 3 weeks and lenvatinib 200 mg once daily. ORR at week 24 (primary endpoint) was 38% in the whole population, 36.2% for MSS tumors, and 63.6% in the MSI-H subset. Seven (7.3%) patients experienced complete responses and 28 (29.8%) partial responses in the MSS cohort. Responses were observed in all histologic subtypes. Median duration of response was not reached in this cohort. Outcome seemed better than in historical cohorts with 7.4 months and 16.4 months of median PFS and OS, respectively. PD-L1 status was determined by the 22C3 assay, with 49% of PD-L1 positive tumors. Treatment efficacy did not depend on PD-L1 expression, as 35.8% of patients with PD-L1-positive tumors and 39.5% of patients with PD-L1-negative tumors had objective responses, respectively. Concerning safety, the combination led to more adverse events than pembrolizumab alone with grade 3–4 AEs for 66.9% of patients. Immune-related AEs were observed for more than half (57.3%) of the patients, but mostly concerned dysthyroidism (47.6%). Angiogenesis inhibition-related toxicities were frequent with 32.4% grade 3–4 hypertension. Twenty-two patients (17.7%) discontinued at least one of the drugs because of AEs, and dose interruptions were necessary for 70.2%. These results led the FDA to grant accelerated approval for this combination for the treatment of patients with MSS/MMRp advanced endometrial carcinoma, who have disease progression following prior systemic therapy, but are not candidates for curative surgery or radiation. A phase trial assessing this combination to physician's choice chemotherapy (paclitaxel or doxorubicin) in the same setting is ongoing ([52], NCT03517449). Patients are stratified according to their MMR status; and MMRp cases are stratified according to ECOG performance status, geographic region, and priori history of pelvic radiation. Interim results of co-primary endpoints (PFS and OS) have been presented very recently [Makker V, et al. Abstract 11512. Society of Gynecologic Oncology Annual Meeting on Women's Cancer; 2021]. Median PFS was 7.2 months for the combination versus 3.8 months in the chemotherapy arm in the whole population (HR = 0.56 (95CI 0.47–0.66), $p < 0.0001$) and 6.6 versus 3.8 in the MMRp subset (HR = 0.50 (95CI 0.40–0.72), $p < 0.0001$). Results were similar concerning OS with more than 5 months of median OS improvement in the experimental arm for MMRp tumors (17.4 vs. 12.0 months; HR = 0.68 (95CI 0.56–0.84), $p = 0.0001$). Moreover, the pembrolizumab–lenvatinib combination is also explored in the first-line setting in the ongoing ENGOT-en9 phase III study [60]. Newly diagnosed stage III–IV EC are randomized (1:1 ratio) between the combo and the carboplatin-paclitaxel regimen. Co-primary endpoints are PFS and OS (Table 2).

In a 2/1 ratio randomized phase II study for pretreated advanced EC, 76 patients (with only two MSI-H cases) received nivolumab alone or in combination with cabozantinib [53]. Median PFS was statistically higher in the combination arm: 5.3 months versus 1.9 months with nivolumab alone. An exploratory cohort with 9 carcinosarcoma and 20 patients previously treated with ICI was also presented. Only one patient with carcinosarcoma responded to treatment and six in the prior ICI subgroup. Digestive disorders (47.2%), transaminases increase (44.4%, and fatigue (8.9%) were the most frequent adverse events in the cabozantinib arm.

Others multikinase angiogenesis inhibitors (lucitanib, anlotinib) are under investigation in association with anti-PD-1 agents in a single-arm phase II trials for pretreated EC (NCT04042116, NCT04157491).

Efficacy of bevacizumab, a well described VEGFR inhibiting monoclonal antibody, has been widely assessed for EC treatment in the last 10 years. Used as monotherapy after platinum-failure, only few (13%) objective responses were observed, with a 6-month PFS of 40% [64]. Similar results were obtained in combination with the mTOR-inhibitor temsirolimus [65]. In the first-line setting, addition of bevacizumab to the standard carboplatin-paclitaxel regimen did not bring any survival benefits compared to chemotherapy alone [66]. Nevertheless, due to the potential synergistic effect of this drug in combination with ICI, bevacizumab is currently explored in combination with atezolizumab in a phase II single-arm trial planned to enroll 55 patients with previously treated advanced EC (NCT03526432).

Table 2. Ongoing prospective clinical studies with combinations including immune checkpoints inhibitors.

Drugs	Study Design	N	Primary Objectives	Reference, NCT
	First-line setting			
Pembrolizumab–lenvatinib vs. carboplatin–paclitaxel	Randomized ph 3	875	PFS + OS	EnGOT-en9 [57] NCT03884101
Carboplatin–paclitaxel + pembrolizumab/placebo	Randomized ph 3	220 dMMR 590 pMMR	PFS	NRG-GY018 NCT03914612
Carboplatin–paclitaxel + atezolizumab/placebo	Randomized ph 3	550	PFS + OS	AtTEND [61] NCT03603184
Carboplatin–paclitaxel + dostarlimab/placebo	Randomized ph 3	470	PFS	RUBY [62] NCT03981796
Carboplatin–paclitaxel + avelumab/placebo	Randomized ph 2	120	PFS	MITO END-3 NCT03503786
Carboplatin–paclitaxel + durvalumab/placebo + olaparib/placebo	Randomized ph 3	699	PFS	DUO-E [63] NCT04269200
	Pretreated advanced EC			
Lucitanib + nivolumab	Multicohort non-randomized ph 2	227 not limited to EC	ORR	NCT04042116
Anlotinib + anti-PD-1	Non-randomized phase 2	23	ORR	NCT04157491
Atezolizumab + bevacizumab	Non-randomized phase 2	55	ORR	NCT03526432
Atezolizumab + bevacizumab + rucaparib	Non-randomized phase 2	30	ORR	ENDOBARR NCT03694262
Dostarlimab + niraparib	Non-randomized phase 2	44	CBR	NCT03016338
Durvalumab + tremelimumab + olaparib	Multicohort non-randomized ph 2 limited to HRD solid tumors	270 not limited to EC	PFS	GUIDE2REPAIR NCT04169841
Pembrolizumab + hypo-fractioned radiotherapy + immunomodulatory cocktail	Randomized phase 2	43 uterine cancer	26W-ORR	PRIMMO NCT03192059
NP137 + pembrolizumab and/or carboplatin/paclitaxel	Non-randomized phase 1b/2	240 uterine carcinoma	ORR	GYNET NCT04652076
Ataluren + pembrolizumab	Non-randomized phase 1b/2	47 EC or CCR	ORR	NCT04014530
Mirvetuximab soravtansine + pembrolizumab	Non-randomized phase 2	35 pMMR	ORR + PFS	NCT03835819

Abbreviations: PFS, progression-free survival; OS, overall survival; ORR, overall response rate; CBR, clinical benefit rate; EC, endometrial cancer; HRD, homologous recombination deficiency.

3.2.2. PARP Inhibitors

PARP inhibitors were developed in the last years, mainly in several tumor types with homologous recombination deficiency, notably with BRCA1/2 mutations [67–74]. These drugs are thought to be able to enhance ICI activity via various pathways [75]. By altering DNA repair mechanisms in cancer cells, they probably enhance the number of genomic alterations (also known as tumor mutation burden) that is a surrogate marker of ICI efficacy [76]. Moreover, double-strand breaks repair decrease also leads to the ATM–ATR–Chk1 pathway, resulting in PD-L1 upregulation, which may make higher the impact of PD-L1 blockades [77]. Cancer development is frequently associated with chronic inflammation driven by interferon (IFN) production. However, PARP inhibitors also enhance IFN production via the cGAS–STING pathway [78]. This pathway is activated by the accumulation of cytoplasmic double-strand DNA. STING activation induces type I IFN synthesis TBK1 and IRF3. As type I IFN is involved in regulation of multiple immune cell types, including DCs, NK cells, and T cells, this could enhance ICI impact. Some early phase studies were launched during the last years to explore these hypotheses.

The Dana–Farber Institute is currently sponsoring a phase II multicohort trial, including 35 MSS cases receiving avelumab (PD-L1 inhibitor) in association with the PARP inhibitor talazoparib (NCT02912572). Preliminary results of this cohort were presented at the 2020 ESMO meeting [54]. Thirty-five patients with pretreated advanced EC have been included. Only three of them had partial response (ORR = 8.6%) including one of 12 serous tumors. Six-month PFS was 25.8%. Most common grade 3–4 toxicities were hematological disorders with anemia (45.7%), thrombocytopenia (28.6%), and neutropenia (11.4%). Following the same biological basis, another PARP inhibitor (niraparib) is explored in combination with dostarlimab in a Canadian cohort of 44 pretreated advanced EC (NCT03016338).

In the non-randomized phase II ENDOBAAR trial, 30 patients with previously treated advanced EC are receiving a triplet with bevacizumab, atezolizumab, and the PARP inhibitor rucaparib (NCT03694262). Efficacy of the combination will be assessed by estimating the ORR.

Patients with advanced EC harboring homologous recombination genes mutations are currently enrolled in the multicohort GUIDE2REPAIR trial [79]. This non-randomized phase II study will explore the combination of dual blockade with durvalumab and the CTLA-4 inhibitor tremelimumab with olaparib (PARP inhibitor).

3.2.3. Chemotherapy

Cytotoxic agents are the corner stone of cancer treatment since the 1950s with huge successes for chemosensitive diseases, such as testicular cancer. However, despite administration of multidrug regimen or use of high-dose treatments, chemotherapy only brings a short survival improvement in most metastatic solid malignancies. Chemotherapy action is based on cell-cycle arrest induced by DNA alterations by replication or nucleotides synthesis inhibition or by mitosis inhibition. However, primary and secondary resistances nearly always occur because of emergence of new genetic and epigenetic alterations or upregulation of multidrug transporters. New paradigms appear to combine cytotoxic chemotherapies to other anticancer treatments. Concerning immunotherapy, several observations have been made suggesting that chemotherapy may enhance ICI efficacy. First, some cytotoxic drugs can induce immunogenic cell death. For instance, apoptosis resulting from the action of platinum and alkylating agents seems to be the best candidate for CD8 T lymphocytes activation via various mechanisms that are detailed elsewhere [80]. Secondly, chemotherapy can help to deplete immune response inhibiting cells, such as Tregs, MDCSs, and protumoral macrophages [61–63]. Third, chemotherapy may induce a homeostatic proliferation of T cells by inducing lymphopenia [81]. Lymphotoxic chemotherapy may help reshape the T-cells repertoire by favoring differentiation to tumor-killing T cells. Finally, chemotherapy can help reduce the tumor burden. Tumor volume is indeed correlated with immune response efficacy. Large tumor masses are more immunosuppressive than small cancers, and antitumor immune response is likely to be more effective on small volume tumors [82].

No relevant preliminary data have been published so far concerning the associations of immunotherapy and chemotherapy for advanced EC. However, several phase III trials are ongoing for patients treated in the first-line setting (Table 2). The NRG-GY018 study is comparing carboplatin (AUC5-6 every 3 weeks), plus paclitaxel (175 mg/m^2 every 3 weeks), plus placebo to the same chemotherapy regimen with pembrolizumab (NCT03914612). It is of note that pembrolizumab may be continued until 5 years after inclusion. The control arm of the AtTEnd/ENGOT-en7 study is the same as above, and is compared to the combination of chemotherapy and atezolizumab (NCT03603184) [83]. Patients included in the RUBY study are treated with the same chemotherapy regimen plus dostarlimab (NCT03981796) [84]. We can also cite the Italian MITO END-3 phase 2 randomized study evaluating the same chemotherapy regimen associated with avelumab or placebo (NCT03503786). Finally, DUO-E is a phase 3 randomized trial assessing the combination of carboplatin–paclitaxel chemotherapy plus durvalumab or placebo and olaparib or placebo (NCT04269200) [85].

3.2.4. Other Associations

Immune-checkpoint inhibitors are also under investigation with other anticancer therapeutics used in EC, such as radiation therapy and innovative targeted therapies. Activation of antitumor immune response by radiotherapy is an old myth known for decades as the abscopal effect [86]. There is increasing evidence that the association of radiotherapy with immunotherapy may help to boost immune response, at the irradiated site, but also in a distant manner [87,88]. Several preclinical and clinical studies are ongoing to explore efficacy and safety issues related to this combination. Concerning EC, some dedicated clinical trials have been initiated in both early stage and advanced disease. Pembrolizumab is assessed in combination with radiotherapy in dMMR high intermediate risk early stage EC in a multicenter phase III randomized study (NCT04214067). The PRIMMO study is an ongoing randomized phase II trial evaluating pembrolizumab plus hypo-fractioned radiotherapy, plus an immunomodulatory cocktail (vitamin D, curcumin, lansoprazole, aspirin, and low-dose cyclophosphamide) in patients with pretreated advanced uterine tumors (cervix or endometrial carcinoma and uterine sarcoma) [89]. Primary endpoint is ORR at week 26.

Netrin-1 is a protein overexpressed in over 80% of uterine tumors. Netrin-1 up-regulation is a mechanism to allow escape from apoptosis [90]. In early clinical studies, NP137, a monoclonal antibody that targets this protein, showed promising response rates in a not yet published first in a human study (NCT02977195). Moreover, some preclinical data suggest that it may decrease resistance to chemotherapy and ICI [91]. A phase Ib/II study was recently initiated to assess the combination of NP137 with pembrolizumab and/or chemotherapy in pretreated patients with locally advanced/metastatic endometrial carcinoma or cervix carcinoma (NCT04652076). Other combinations with investigational treatments (ataluren, mirvetuximab soravtansine) are currently evaluated in early phase trials (NCT04014530, NCT03835819).

4. Conclusions

There is now strong evidence that immune microenvironment modifications and immune response activation are of high importance for EC. Mismatch repair status has to be determined for all our patients. Despite its limits to perfectly identify responders to immune checkpoints inhibitors, MMR deficiency is a recognized theranostic marker for clinical management of advanced EC. Pembrolizumab and dostarlimab have shown impressive results in MMR deficient cases, and the association of pembrolizumab and lenvatinib is becoming a standard of care for pretreated recurrent MMR proficient EC. However, further advances are needed to understand primary and secondary mechanisms of resistance to immunotherapy and to implement ICI in the first-line metastatic setting and in early stage tumors.

Author Contributions: All authors contributed to the design, writing, and review of the article. All authors have read and agreed to the published version of the manuscript.

Funding: This research received no external funding.

Conflicts of Interest: P.R., A.-S.C., M.P., S.F., L.G. and E.L. have no COI to declare related to this work. D.O. is cofounder and shareholder of ImCheck Therapeutics, Emergence Therapeutics, and Alderaan Biotechnology. R.S. received research grants from ESAI and AstraZeneca; report consulting or advisory roles for GSK, Pfizer, Roche, and Novartis; and received non-financial support from Pfizer, Roche, GSK, Novartis, and AstraZeneca.

References

1. Bray, F.; Ferlay, J.; Soerjomataram, I.; Siegel, R.L.; Torre, L.A.; Jemal, A. Global cancer statistics 2018: GLOBOCAN estimates of incidence and mortality worldwide for 36 cancers in 185 countries. *CA Cancer J. Clin.* **2018**, *68*, 394–424. [CrossRef]
2. Siegel, R.L.; Miller, K.D.; Jemal, A. Cancer statistics, 2020. *CA Cancer J. Clin.* **2020**, *70*, 7–30. [CrossRef] [PubMed]
3. Colombo, N.; Creutzberg, C.; Amant, F.; Bosse, T.; González-Martín, A.; Ledermann, J.; Marth, C.; Nout, R.A.; Querleu, D.; Mirza, M.R.; et al. ESMO-ESGO-ESTRO Consensus Conference on Endometrial Cancer: Diagnosis, Treatment and Follow-up. *Int. J. Gynecol. Cancer* **2016**, *26*, 2–30. [CrossRef] [PubMed]
4. Brinton, L.A.; Lacey, J.V.; Trimble, E.L. Hormones and endometrial cancer—New data from the Million Women Study. *Lancet* **2005**, *365*, 1517–1518. [CrossRef]
5. Colombo, N.; Preti, E.; Landoni, F.; Carinelli, S.; Colombo, A.; Marini, C.; Sessa, C.; Colombo, N. Endometrial cancer: ESMO Clinical Practice Guidelines for diagnosis, treatment and follow-up. *Ann. Oncol.* **2013**, *24* (Suppl. S6), vi33–vi38. [CrossRef]
6. Morice, P.; Leary, A.; Creutzberg, C.; Abu-Rustum, N.; Darai, E. Endometrial cancer. *Lancet* **2016**, *387*, 1094–1108. [CrossRef]
7. Doll, A.; Abal, M.; Rigau, M.; Monge, M.; Gonzalez, M.; Demajo, S.; Colás, E.; Llauradó, M.; Alazzouzi, H.; Planagumá, J.; et al. Novel molecular profiles of endometrial cancer—New light through old windows. *J. Steroid Biochem. Mol. Biol.* **2008**, *108*, 221–229. [CrossRef] [PubMed]
8. Albertini, A.-F.; Devouassoux-Shisheboran, M.; Genestie, C. Anatomopathologie des cancers de l'endomètre. *Bull. Cancer* **2012**, *99*, 7–12. [CrossRef]
9. Kandoth, C.; Schultz, N.; Cherniack, A.D.; Akbani, R.; Liu, Y.; Shen, H.; Robertson, A.G.; Pashtan, I.; Shen, R.; Cancer Genome Atlas Research Network; et al. Integrated genomic characterization of endometrial carcinoma. *Nature* **2013**, *497*, 67–73. [CrossRef]
10. Genestie, C.; Leary, A.; Devouassoux, M.; Auguste, A. Classification histologique et moléculaire des cancers de l'endomètre et leurs implications dans la thérapeutique. *Bull. Cancer* **2017**, *104*, 1001–1012. [CrossRef]
11. Concin, N.; Matias-Guiu, X.; Vergote, I.; Cibula, D.; Mirza, M.R.; Marnitz, S.; Ledermann, J.; Bosse, T.; Chargari, C.; Fagotti, A.; et al. ESGO/ESTRO/ESP guidelines for the management of patients with endometrial carcinoma. *Radiother. Oncol.* **2021**, *154*, 327–353. [CrossRef]
12. Kondratiev, S.; Sabo, E.; Yakirevich, E.; Lavie, O.; Resnick, M.B. Intratumoral CD8+ T Lymphocytes as a Prognostic Factor of Survival in Endometrial Carcinoma. *Clin. Cancer Res.* **2004**, *10*, 4450–4456. [CrossRef]
13. Suemori, T.; Susumu, N.; Iwata, T.; Banno, K.; Yamagami, W.; Hirasawa, A.; Sugano, K.; Matsumoto, E.; Aoki, D. Intratumoral CD8+ Lymphocyte Infiltration as a Prognostic Factor and Its Relationship with Cyclooxygenase 2 Expression and Microsatellite Instability in Endometrial Cancer. *Int. J. Gynecol. Cancer* **2015**, *25*, 1165–1172. [CrossRef] [PubMed]
14. Pakish, J.B.; Zhang, Q.; Chen, Z.; Liang, H.; Chisholm, G.B.; Yuan, Y.; Mok, S.C.; Broaddus, R.R.; Lu, K.H.; Yates, M.S. Immune Microenvironment in Microsatellite-Instable Endometrial Cancers: Hereditary or Sporadic Origin Matters. *Clin. Cancer Res.* **2017**, *23*, 4473–4481. [CrossRef] [PubMed]
15. Zhang, P.; Liu, M.; Cui, Y.; Zheng, P.; Liu, Y. Microsatellite instability status differentially associates with intratumoral immune microenvironment in human cancers. *Brief. Bioinform.* **2020**, *22*, bbaa180. [CrossRef] [PubMed]
16. Van Gool, I.C.; Eggink, F.A.; Freeman-Mills, L.; Stelloo, E.; Marchi, E.; de Bruyn, M.; Palles, C.; Nout, R.A.; de Kroon, C.D.; Osse, E.M.; et al. POLE Proofreading Mutations Elicit an Antitumor Immune Response in Endometrial Cancer. *Clin. Cancer Res.* **2015**, *21*, 3347–3355. [CrossRef] [PubMed]
17. Vanderstraeten, A.; Tuyaerts, S.; Amant, F. The immune system in the normal endometrium and implications for endometrial cancer development. *J. Reprod. Immunol.* **2015**, *109*, 7–16. [CrossRef]
18. Brahmer, J.R.; Tykodi, S.S.; Chow, L.Q.M.; Hwu, W.-J.; Topalian, S.L.; Hwu, P.; Drake, C.G.; Camacho, L.H.; Kauh, J.; Odunsi, K.; et al. Safety and Activity of Anti–PD-L1 Antibody in Patients with Advanced Cancer. *N. Engl. J. Med.* **2012**, *366*, 2455–2465. [CrossRef]
19. Chen, L. Co-inhibitory molecules of the B7–CD28 family in the control of T-cell immunity. *Nat. Rev. Immunol.* **2004**, *4*, 336–347. [CrossRef]
20. Taube, J.M.; Klein, A.; Brahmer, J.R.; Xu, H.; Pan, X.; Kim, J.H.; Chen, L.; Pardoll, D.M.; Topalian, S.L.; Anders, R.A. Association of PD-1, PD-1 Ligands, and Other Features of the Tumor Immune Microenvironment with Response to Anti–PD-1 Therapy. *Clin. Cancer Res.* **2014**, *20*, 5064–5074. [CrossRef] [PubMed]
21. Boussiotis, V.A.; Chatterjee, P.; Li, L. Biochemical Signaling of PD-1 on T Cells and Its Functional Implications. *Cancer J.* **2014**, *20*, 265–271. [CrossRef] [PubMed]
22. Sheppard, K.-A.; Fitz, L.J.; Lee, J.M.; Benander, C.; George, J.A.; Wooters, J.; Qiu, Y.; Jussif, J.M.; Carter, L.L.; Wood, C.R.; et al. PD-1 inhibits T-cell receptor induced phosphorylation of the ZAP70/CD3ζ signalosome and downstream signaling to PKCθ. *FEBS Lett.* **2004**, *574*, 37–41. [CrossRef] [PubMed]
23. Mu, C.-Y.; Huang, J.-A.; Chen, Y.; Chen, C.; Zhang, X.-G. High expression of PD-L1 in lung cancer may contribute to poor prognosis and tumor cells immune escape through suppressing tumor infiltrating dendritic cells maturation. *Med. Oncol.* **2011**, *28*, 682–688. [CrossRef]
24. Huang, W.; Ran, R.; Shao, B.; Li, H. Prognostic and clinicopathological value of PD-L1 expression in primary breast cancer: A meta-analysis. *Breast Cancer Res. Treat.* **2019**, *178*, 17–33. [CrossRef]
25. Blank, C.; Gajewski, T.F.; Mackensen, A. Interaction of PD-L1 on tumor cells with PD-1 on tumor-specific T cells as a mechanism of immune evasion: Implications for tumor immunotherapy. *Cancer Immunol. Immunother.* **2005**, *54*, 307–314. [CrossRef] [PubMed]

26. Fife, B.T.; Bluestone, J.A. Control of peripheral T-cell tolerance and autoimmunity via the CTLA-4 and PD-1 pathways. *Immunol. Rev.* **2008**, *224*, 166–182. [CrossRef]
27. Spranger, S.; Spaapen, R.M.; Zha, Y.; Williams, J.; Meng, Y.; Ha, T.T.; Gajewski, T.F. Up-Regulation of PD-L1, IDO, and Tregs in the Melanoma Tumor Microenvironment Is Driven by CD8+ T Cells. *Sci. Transl. Med.* **2013**, *5*, 200ra116. [CrossRef]
28. Lu, L.; Li, Y.; Luo, R.; Xu, J.; Feng, Z.; Wang, M. Prognostic and Clinicopathological Role of PD-L1 in Endometrial Cancer: A Meta-Analysis. *Front. Oncol.* **2020**, *10*, 632. [CrossRef]
29. Yearley, J.H.; Gibson, C.; Yu, N.; Moon, C.; Murphy, E.; Juco, J.; Lunceford, J.; Cheng, J.; Chow, L.Q.; Seiwert, T.Y.; et al. PD-L2 Expression in Human Tumors: Relevance to Anti-PD-1 Therapy in Cancer. *Clin. Cancer Res.* **2017**, *23*, 3158–3167. [CrossRef] [PubMed]
30. Vanderstraeten, A.; Luyten, C.; Verbist, G.; Tuyaerts, S.; Amant, F. Mapping the immunosuppressive environment in uterine tumors: Implications for immunotherapy. *Cancer Immunol. Immunother.* **2014**, *63*, 545–557. [CrossRef] [PubMed]
31. Marinelli, O.; Annibali, D.; Morelli, M.B.; Zeppa, L.; Tuyaerts, S.; Aguzzi, C.; Amantini, C.; Maggi, F.; Ferretti, B.; Santoni, G.; et al. Biological Function of PD-L2 and Correlation with Overall Survival in Type II Endometrial Cancer. *Front. Oncol.* **2020**, *10*, 538064. [CrossRef]
32. Willvonseder, B.; Stögbauer, F.; Steiger, K.; Jesinghaus, M.; Kuhn, P.-H.; Brambs, C.; Engel, J.; Bronger, H.; Schmidt, G.P.; Haller, B.; et al. The immunologic tumor microenvironment in endometrioid endometrial cancer in the morphomolecular context: Mutual correlations and prognostic impact depending on molecular alterations. *Cancer Immunol. Immunother.* **2020**, *70*, 1679–1689. [CrossRef]
33. Howitt, B.E.; Shukla, S.A.; Sholl, L.M.; Ritterhouse, L.L.; Watkins, J.C.; Rodig, S.J.; Stover, E.H.; Strickland, K.; D'Andrea, A.D.; Wu, C.J.; et al. Association of Polymerase e–Mutated and Microsatellite-Instable Endometrial Cancers with Neoantigen Load, Number of Tumor-Infiltrating Lymphocytes, and Expression of PD-1 and PD-L1. *JAMA Oncol.* **2015**, *1*, 1319–1323. [CrossRef] [PubMed]
34. Kim, J.; Kim, S.; Lee, H.S.; Yang, W.; Cho, H.; Chay, D.B.; Cho, S.J.; Hong, S.; Kim, J.-H. Prognostic implication of programmed cell death 1 protein and its ligand expressions in endometrial cancer. *Gynecol. Oncol.* **2018**, *149*, 381–387. [CrossRef] [PubMed]
35. Talhouk, A.; DeRocher, H.; Schmidt, P.; Leung, S.; Milne, K.; Gilks, C.B.; Anglesio, M.S.; Nelson, B.H.; McAlpine, J.N. Molecular Subtype Not Immune Response Drives Outcomes in Endometrial Carcinoma. *Clin. Cancer Res.* **2019**, *25*, 2537–2548. [CrossRef]
36. Munder, M. Arginase: An emerging key player in the mammalian immune system. *Br. J. Pharmacol.* **2009**, *158*, 638–651. [CrossRef] [PubMed]
37. Mabuchi, S.; Sasano, T. Myeloid-Derived Suppressor Cells as Therapeutic Targets in Uterine Cervical and Endometrial Cancers. *Cells* **2021**, *10*, 1073. [CrossRef] [PubMed]
38. Gu, S.; Ni, T.; Wang, J.; Liu, Y.; Fan, Q.; Wang, Y.; Huang, T.; Chu, Y.; Sun, X.; Wang, Y. CD47 Blockade Inhibits Tumor Progression through Promoting Phagocytosis of Tumor Cells by M2 Polarized Macrophages in Endometrial Cancer. *J. Immunol. Res.* **2018**, *2018*, 1–12. [CrossRef] [PubMed]
39. Krishnan, V.; Schaar, B.; Tallapragada, S.; Dorigo, O. Tumor associated macrophages in gynecologic cancers. *Gynecol. Oncol.* **2018**, *149*, 205–213. [CrossRef] [PubMed]
40. Miller, D.S.; Filiaci, V.L.; Mannel, R.S.; Cohn, D.E.; Matsumoto, T.; Tewari, K.S.; DiSilvestro, P.; Pearl, M.L.; Argenta, P.A.; Powell, M.A.; et al. Carboplatin and Paclitaxel for Advanced Endometrial Cancer: Final Overall Survival and Adverse Event Analysis of a Phase III Trial (NRG Oncology/GOG0209). *J. Clin. Oncol.* **2020**, *38*, 3841–3850. [CrossRef]
41. Nomura, H.; Aoki, D.; Takahashi, F.; Katsumata, N.; Watanabe, Y.; Konishi, I.; Jobo, T.; Hatae, M.; Hiura, M.; Yaegashi, N. Randomized phase II study comparing docetaxel plus cisplatin, docetaxel plus carboplatin, and paclitaxel plus carboplatin in patients with advanced or recurrent endometrial carcinoma: A Japanese Gynecologic Oncology Group study (JGOG2041). *Ann. Oncol.* **2011**, *22*, 636–642. [CrossRef] [PubMed]
42. McMeekin, S.; Dizon, D.; Barter, J.; Scambia, G.; Manzyuk, L.; Lisyanskaya, A.; Oaknin, A.; Ringuette, S.; Mukhopadhyay, P.; Rosenberg, J.; et al. Phase III randomized trial of second-line ixabepilone versus paclitaxel or doxorubicin in women with advanced endometrial cancer. *Gynecol. Oncol.* **2015**, *138*, 18–23. [CrossRef] [PubMed]
43. Liu, J.F.; Gordon, M.; Veneris, J.; Braiteh, F.; Balmanoukian, A.; Eder, J.P.; Oaknin, A.; Hamilton, E.; Wang, Y.; Sarkar, I.; et al. Safety, clinical activity and biomarker assessments of atezolizumab from a Phase I study in advanced/recurrent ovarian and uterine cancers. *Gynecol. Oncol.* **2019**, *154*, 314–322. [CrossRef] [PubMed]
44. Hasegawa, K.; Tamura, K.; Katsumata, N.; Matsumoto, K.; Takahashi, S.; Mukai, H.; Nomura, H.; Minami, H. Efficacy and safety of nivolumab (Nivo) in patients (pts) with advanced or recurrent uterine cervical or corpus cancers. *J. Clin. Oncol.* **2018**, *36*, 5594. [CrossRef]
45. Konstantinopoulos, P.A.; Luo, W.; Liu, J.F.; Gulhan, D.C.; Krasner, C.; Ishizuka, J.J.; Gockley, A.A.; Buss, M.; Growdon, W.B.; Crowe, H.; et al. Phase II Study of Avelumab in Patients with Mismatch Repair Deficient and Mismatch Repair Proficient Recurrent/Persistent Endometrial Cancer. *J. Clin. Oncol.* **2019**, *37*, 2786–2794. [CrossRef]
46. Antill, Y.; Kok, P.; Stockler, M.; Robledo, K.; Yip, S.; Parry, M.; Smith, D.; Spurdle, A.; Barnes, E.; Friedlander, M.; et al. Updated results of activity of durvalumab in advanced endometrial cancer (AEC) according to mismatch repair (MMR) status: The phase II PHAEDRA trial (ANZGOG1601). *Ann. Oncol.* **2019**, *30*, ix192. [CrossRef]

47. Ott, P.A.; Bang, Y.-J.; Berton-Rigaud, D.; Elez, E.; Pishvaian, M.J.; Rugo, H.S.; Puzanov, I.; Mehnert, J.M.; Aung, K.L.; Lopez, J.; et al. Safety and Antitumor Activity of Pembrolizumab in Advanced Programmed Death Ligand 1–Positive Endometrial Cancer: Results From the KEYNOTE-028 Study. *J. Clin. Oncol.* **2017**, *35*, 2535–2541. [CrossRef]
48. Marabelle, A.; Le, D.T.; Ascierto, P.A.; Di Giacomo, A.M.; De Jesus-Acosta, A.; Delord, J.-P.; Geva, R.; Gottfried, M.; Penel, N.; Hansen, A.R.; et al. Efficacy of Pembrolizumab in Patients with Noncolorectal High Microsatellite Instability/Mismatch Repair–Deficient Cancer: Results from the Phase II KEYNOTE-158 Study. *J. Clin. Oncol.* **2019**, *38*, 1–10. [CrossRef] [PubMed]
49. O'Malley, D.; Marabelle, A.; De Jesus-Acosta, A.; Piha-Paul, S.; Arkhipov, A.; Longo, F.; Motola-Kuba, D.; Shapira-Frommer, R.; Geva, R.; Rimel, B.; et al. Pembrolizumab in patients with MSI-H advanced endometrial cancer from the KEYNOTE-158 study. *Ann. Oncol.* **2019**, *30*, v425–v426. [CrossRef]
50. Oaknin, A.; Tinker, A.V.; Gilbert, L.; Samouëlian, V.; Mathews, C.; Brown, J.; Barretina-Ginesta, M.-P.; Moreno, V.; Gravina, A.; Abdeddaim, C.; et al. Clinical Activity and Safety of the Anti–Programmed Death 1 Monoclonal Antibody Dostarlimab for Patients with Recurrent or Advanced Mismatch Repair–Deficient Endometrial Cancer: A Nonrandomized Phase 1 Clinical Trial. *JAMA Oncol.* **2020**, *6*, 1766–1772. [CrossRef]
51. Makker, V.; Taylor, M.H.; Aghajanian, C.; Oaknin, A.; Mier, J.; Cohn, A.L.; Romeo, M.; Bratos, R.; Brose, M.S.; DiSimone, C.; et al. Lenvatinib Plus Pembrolizumab in Patients with Advanced Endometrial Cancer. *J. Clin. Oncol.* **2020**, *38*, 2981–2992. [CrossRef] [PubMed]
52. Makker, V.; Casado Herraez, A.; Aghajanian, C.; Fujiwara, K.; Pignata, S.; Penson, R.T.; Dutcus, C.E.; Guo, M.; Dutta, L.; Orlowski, R.; et al. A phase 3 trial evaluating efficacy and safety of lenvatinib in combination with pembrolizumab in patients with advanced endometrial cancer. *J. Clin. Oncol.* **2019**, *37*, TPS5607. [CrossRef]
53. Lheureux, S.; Matei, D.; Konstantinopoulos, P.A.; Block, M.S.; Jewell, A.; Gaillard, S.; McHale, M.S.; McCourt, C.K.; Temkin, S.; Girda, E.; et al. A randomized phase II study of cabozantinib and nivolumab versus nivolumab in recurrent endometrial cancer. *J. Clin. Oncol.* **2020**, *38*, 6010. [CrossRef]
54. Konstantinopoulos, P.; Gockley, N.; Xiong, N.; Tayob, N.; Krasner, C.; Buss, M.; Campos, S.; Schumer, S.; Wright, A.; Liu, J.; et al. LBA35 Phase II study of PARP inhibitor talazoparib and PD-L1 inhibitor avelumab in patients (pts) with microsatellite stable (MSS) recurrent/persistent endometrial cancer. *Ann. Oncol.* **2020**, *31*, S1165. [CrossRef]
55. Marcus, L.; Lemery, S.J.; Keegan, P.; Pazdur, R. FDA Approval Summary: Pembrolizumab for the Treatment of Microsatellite Instability-High Solid Tumors. *Clin. Cancer Res.* **2019**, *25*, 3753–3758. [CrossRef]
56. Oaknin, A.; Gilbert, L.; Tinker, A.; Sabatier, R.; Boni, V.; O'Malley, D.; Ghamande, S.; Duska, L.; Ghatage, P.; Guo, W.; et al. LBA36 Safety and antitumor activity of dostarlimab in patients (pts) with advanced or recurrent DNA mismatch repair deficient (dMMR) or proficient (MMRp) endometrial cancer (EC): Results from GARNET. *Ann. Oncol.* **2020**, *31*, S1166. [CrossRef]
57. Musacchio, L.; Boccia, S.M.; Caruso, G.; Santangelo, G.; Fischetti, M.; Tomao, F.; Perniola, G.; Palaia, I.; Muzii, L.; Pignata, S.; et al. Immune Checkpoint Inhibitors: A Promising Choice for Endometrial Cancer Patients? *J. Clin. Med.* **2020**, *9*, 1721. [CrossRef] [PubMed]
58. Labiano, S.; Palazon, A.; Melero, I. Immune Response Regulation in the Tumor Microenvironment by Hypoxia. *Semin. Oncol.* **2015**, *42*, 378–386. [CrossRef]
59. Fukumura, D.; Kloepper, J.; Amoozgar, Z.; Duda, D.G.; Jain, R.K. Enhancing cancer immunotherapy using antiangiogenics: Opportunities and challenges. *Nat. Rev. Clin. Oncol.* **2018**, *15*, 325–340. [CrossRef]
60. Marth, C.; Vulsteke, C.; Rubio Pérez, M.J.; Makker, V.; Braicu, E.I.; McNeish, I.A.; Madry, R.; Ayhan, A.; Hasegawa, K.; Wu, X.; et al. ENGOT-en9/LEAP-001: A phase III study of first-line pembrolizumab plus lenvatinib versus chemotherapy in advanced or recurrent endometrial cancer. *J. Clin. Oncol.* **2020**, *38*, TPS6106. [CrossRef]
61. Sakaguchi, S.; Mikami, N.; Wing, J.B.; Tanaka, A.; Ichiyama, K.; Ohkura, N. Regulatory T Cells and Human Disease. *Annu. Rev. Immunol.* **2020**, *38*, 541–566. [CrossRef] [PubMed]
62. Gabrilovich, D.I. Myeloid-Derived Suppressor Cells. *Cancer Immunol. Res.* **2017**, *5*, 3–8. [CrossRef] [PubMed]
63. Buhtoiarov, I.N.; Sondel, P.M.; Wigginton, J.M.; Buhtoiarova, T.N.; Yanke, E.M.; Mahvi, D.A.; Rakhmilevich, A.L. Anti-tumour synergy of cytotoxic chemotherapy and anti-CD40 plus CpG-ODN immunotherapy through repolarization of tumour-associated macrophages. *Immunology* **2011**, *132*, 226–239. [CrossRef] [PubMed]
64. Aghajanian, C.; Sill, M.W.; Darcy, K.M.; Greer, B.; McMeekin, D.S.; Rose, P.G.; Rotmensch, J.; Barnes, M.N.; Hanjani, P.; Leslie, K.K. Phase II Trial of Bevacizumab in Recurrent or Persistent Endometrial Cancer: A Gynecologic Oncology Group Study. *J. Clin. Oncol.* **2011**, *29*, 2259–2265. [CrossRef] [PubMed]
65. Alvarez, E.A.; Brady, W.E.; Walker, J.L.; Rotmensch, J.; Zhou, X.C.; Kendrick, J.E.; Yamada, S.D.; Schilder, J.M.; Cohn, D.; Harrison, C.R.; et al. Phase II trial of combination bevacizumab and temsirolimus in the treatment of recurrent or persistent endometrial carcinoma: A Gynecologic Oncology Group study. *Gynecol. Oncol.* **2013**, *129*, 22–27. [CrossRef] [PubMed]
66. Lorusso, D.; Ferrandina, G.; Colombo, N.; Pignata, S.; Pietragalla, A.; Sonetto, C.; Pisano, C.; Lapresa, M.; Savarese, A.; Tagliaferri, P.; et al. Carboplatin-paclitaxel compared to Carboplatin-Paclitaxel-Bevacizumab in advanced or recurrent endometrial cancer: MITO END-2—A randomized phase II trial. *Gynecol. Oncol.* **2019**, *155*, 406–412. [CrossRef]
67. Ray-Coquard, I.; Pautier, P.; Pignata, S.; Pérol, D.; González-Martín, A.; Berger, R.; Fujiwara, K.; Vergote, I.; Colombo, N.; Mäenpää, J.; et al. Olaparib plus Bevacizumab as First-Line Maintenance in Ovarian Cancer. *N. Engl. J. Med.* **2019**, *381*, 2416–2428. [CrossRef]

68. Moore, K.; Colombo, N.; Scambia, G.; Kim, B.-G.; Oaknin, A.; Friedlander, M.; Lisyanskaya, A.; Floquet, A.; Leary, A.; Sonke, G.S.; et al. Maintenance Olaparib in Patients with Newly Diagnosed Advanced Ovarian Cancer. *N. Engl. J. Med.* **2018**, *379*, 2495–2505. [CrossRef]
69. González-Martín, A.; Pothuri, B.; Vergote, I.; DePont Christensen, R.; Graybill, W.; Mirza, M.R.; McCormick, C.; Lorusso, D.; Hoskins, P.; Freyer, G.; et al. Niraparib in Patients with Newly Diagnosed Advanced Ovarian Cancer. *N. Engl. J. Med.* **2019**, *381*, 2391–2402. [CrossRef]
70. Coleman, R.L.; Oza, A.M.; Lorusso, D.; Aghajanian, C.; Oaknin, A.; Dean, A.; Colombo, N.; Weberpals, J.I.; Clamp, A.; Scambia, G.; et al. Rucaparib maintenance treatment for recurrent ovarian carcinoma after response to platinum therapy (ARIEL3): A randomised, double-blind, placebo-controlled, phase 3 trial. *Lancet* **2017**, *390*, 1949–1961. [CrossRef]
71. Litton, J.; Hurvitz, S.; Mina, L.; Rugo, H.; Lee, K.-H.; Gonçalves, A.; Diab, S.; Woodward, N.; Goodwin, A.; Yerushalmi, R.; et al. Talazoparib versus chemotherapy in patients with germline BRCA1/2-mutated HER2-negative advanced breast cancer: Final overall survival results from the EMBRACA trial. *Ann. Oncol.* **2020**, *31*, 1526–1535. [CrossRef]
72. Robson, M.; Tung, N.; Conte, P.; Im, S.-A.; Senkus, E.; Xu, B.; Masuda, N.; Delaloge, S.; Li, W.; Armstrong, A.; et al. OlympiAD final overall survival and tolerability results: Olaparib versus chemotherapy treatment of physician's choice in patients with a germline BRCA mutation and HER2-negative metastatic breast cancer. *Ann. Oncol.* **2019**, *30*, 558–566. [CrossRef]
73. Hussain, M.; Mateo, J.; Fizazi, K.; Saad, F.; Shore, N.; Sandhu, S.; Chi, K.N.; Sartor, O.; Agarwal, N.; Olmos, D.; et al. Survival with Olaparib in Metastatic Castration-Resistant Prostate Cancer. *N. Engl. J. Med.* **2020**, *383*, 2345–2357. [CrossRef] [PubMed]
74. Golan, T.; Hammel, P.; Reni, M.; Van Cutsem, E.; Macarulla, T.; Hall, M.J.; Park, J.-O.; Hochhauser, D.; Arnold, D.; Oh, D.-Y.; et al. Maintenance Olaparib for Germline BRCA-Mutated Metastatic Pancreatic Cancer. *N. Engl. J. Med.* **2019**, *381*, 317–327. [CrossRef] [PubMed]
75. Li, A.; Yi, M.; Qin, S.; Chu, Q.; Luo, S.; Wu, K. Prospects for combining immune checkpoint blockade with PARP inhibition. *J. Hematol. Oncol.* **2019**, *12*, 1–12. [CrossRef] [PubMed]
76. Pilié, P.G.; Gay, C.M.; Byers, L.A.; O'Connor, M.J.; Yap, T.A. PARP Inhibitors: Extending Benefit Beyond BRCA-Mutant Cancers. *Clin. Cancer Res.* **2019**, *25*, 3759–3771. [CrossRef]
77. Sato, H.; Niimi, A.; Yasuhara, T.; Permata, T.B.M.; Hagiwara, Y.; Isono, M.; Nuryadi, E.; Sekine, R.; Oike, T.; Kakoti, S.; et al. DNA double-strand break repair pathway regulates PD-L1 expression in cancer cells. *Nat. Commun.* **2017**, *8*, 1–11. [CrossRef] [PubMed]
78. Barber, G.N. STING: Infection, inflammation and cancer. *Nat. Rev. Immunol.* **2015**, *15*, 760–770. [CrossRef]
79. Fumet, J.-D.; Limagne, E.; Thibaudin, M.; Truntzer, C.; Bertaut, A.; Rederstorff, E.; Ghiringhelli, F. Precision medicine phase II study evaluating the efficacy of a double immunotherapy by durvalumab and tremelimumab combined with olaparib in patients with solid cancers and carriers of homologous recombination repair genes mutation in response or stable after olaparib treatment. *BMC Cancer* **2020**, *20*, 1–10. [CrossRef]
80. Salas-Benito, D.; Pérez-Gracia, J.L.; Ponz-Sarvisé, M.; Rodriguez-Ruiz, M.E.; Martínez-Forero, I.; Castañón, E.; López-Picazo, J.M.; Sanmamed, M.F.; Melero, I. Paradigms on Immunotherapy Combinations with Chemotherapy. *Cancer Discov.* **2021**, *11*, 1–15. [CrossRef]
81. Gattinoni, L.; Finkelstein, S.E.; Klebanoff, C.A.; Antony, P.A.; Palmer, D.C.; Spiess, P.J.; Hwang, L.N.; Yu, Z.; Wrzesinski, C.; Heimann, D.M.; et al. Removal of homeostatic cytokine sinks by lymphodepletion enhances the efficacy of adoptively transferred tumor-specific CD8+ T cells. *J. Exp. Med.* **2005**, *202*, 907–912. [CrossRef]
82. Rabinovich, G.A.; Gabrilovich, D.; Sotomayor, E.M. Immunosuppressive Strategies that are Mediated by Tumor Cells. *Annu. Rev. Immunol.* **2007**, *25*, 267–296. [CrossRef]
83. Colombo, N.; Barretina-Ginesta, M.P.; Beale, P.J.; Harano, K.; Hudson, E.; Marmé, F.; Marth, C.; Radaglio, M.; Secord, A.A.; Fossati, R.; et al. AtTEnd/ENGOT-en7: A multicenter phase III double-blind randomized controlled trial of atezolizumab in combination with paclitaxel and carboplatin in women with advanced/recurrent endometrial cancer. *J. Clin. Oncol.* **2019**, *37*, TPS5608. [CrossRef]
84. Mirza, M.R.; Coleman, R.L.; Hanker, L.C.; Slomovitz, B.M.; Valabrega, G.; Im, E.; Walker, M.; Guo, W.; Powell, M.A. ENGOT-EN6/NSGO-RUBY: A phase III, randomized, double-blind, multicenter study of dostarlimab + carboplatin-paclitaxel versus placebo + carboplatin-paclitaxel in recurrent or primary advanced endometrial cancer (EC). *J. Clin. Oncol.* **2020**, *38*, TPS6107. [CrossRef]
85. Westin, S.N.; Moore, K.N.; Van Nieuwenhuysen, E.; Oza, A.M.; Mileshkin, L.R.; Okamoto, A.; Suzuki, A.; Meyer, K.; Barker, L.; Rhee, J.; et al. DUO-E/GOG-3041/ENGOT-EN10: A randomized phase III trial of first-line carboplatin (carb) and paclitaxel (pac) in combination with durvalumab (durva), followed by maintenance durva with or without olaparib (ola), in patients (pts) with newly diagnosed (nd) advanced or recurrent endometrial cancer (EC). *J. Clin. Oncol.* **2020**, *38*, TPS6108. [CrossRef]
86. Ngwa, W.; Irabor, O.C.; Schoenfeld, J.D.; Hesser, J.; DeMaria, S.; Formenti, S.C. Using immunotherapy to boost the abscopal effect. *Nat. Rev. Cancer* **2018**, *18*, 313–322. [CrossRef] [PubMed]
87. Lee, L.; Matulonis, U. Immunotherapy and radiation combinatorial trials in gynecologic cancer: A potential synergy? *Gynecol. Oncol.* **2019**, *154*, 236–245. [CrossRef]
88. Walle, T.; Martinez Monge, R.; Cerwenka, A.; Ajona, D.; Melero, I.; Lecanda, F. Radiation effects on antitumor immune responses: Current perspectives and challenges. *Ther. Adv. Med. Oncol.* **2018**, *10*, 1758834017742575. [CrossRef]

89. Tuyaerts, S.; Van Nuffel, A.M.T.; Naert, E.; Van Dam, P.A.; Vuylsteke, P.; De Caluwé, A.; Aspeslagh, S.; Dirix, P.; Lippens, L.; De Jaeghere, E.; et al. PRIMMO study protocol: A phase II study combining PD-1 blockade, radiation and immunomodulation to tackle cervical and uterine cancer. *BMC Cancer* **2019**, *19*, 1–10. [CrossRef]
90. Grandin, M.; Meier, M.; Delcros, J.G.; Nikodemus, D.; Reuten, R.; Patel, T.R.; Goldschneider, D.; Orriss, G.; Krahn, N.; Boussouar, A.; et al. Structural Decoding of the Netrin-1/UNC5 Interaction and its Therapeutic Implications in Cancers. *Cancer Cell* **2016**, *29*, 173–185. [CrossRef]
91. Paradisi, A.; Creveaux, M.; Gibert, B.; Devailly, G.; Redoulez, E.; Neves, D.; Cleyssac, E.; Treilleux, I.; Klein, C.; Niederfellner, G.; et al. Combining chemotherapeutic agents and netrin-1 interference potentiates cancer cell death. *EMBO Mol. Med.* **2013**, *5*, 1821–1834. [CrossRef] [PubMed]

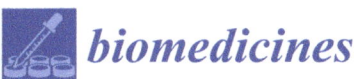

Review

Vulvar and Vaginal Melanomas—The Darker Shades of Gynecological Cancers

Elena-Codruța Dobrică [1,2,†], Cristina Vâjâitu [2,3,†], Carmen Elena Condrat [4], Dragoș Crețoiu [4,5], Ileana Popa [6], Bogdan Severus Gaspar [7,8], Nicolae Suciu [4,9], Sanda Maria Crețoiu [5,*] and Valentin Nicolae Varlas [10,11]

1. Department of Pathophysiology, University of Medicine and Pharmacy of Craiova, 200349 Craiova, Romania; codrutadobrica@gmail.com
2. Department of Dermatology and Allergology, "Elias" Emergency University Hospital, 011461 Bucharest, Romania; cristina.vajaitu@gmail.com
3. Dermatology Department, Carol Davila University of Medicine and Pharmacy, 050474 Bucharest, Romania
4. Alessandrescu-Rusescu National Institute for Mother and Child Health, Fetal Medicine Excellence Research Center, 11062 Bucharest, Romania; drcarmencondrat@gmail.com (C.E.C.); dragos.cretoiu@umfcd.ro (D.C.); nsuciu54@yahoo.com (N.S.)
5. Department of Cell and Molecular Biology and Histology, Carol Davila University of Medicine and Pharmacy, 050474 Bucharest, Romania
6. Department of Anatomopathology, Colțea Clinical Hospital, 030167 Bucharest, Romania; ileanapopa2004@gmail.com
7. Surgery Department, Carol Davila University of Medicine and Pharmacy, 050474 Bucharest, Romania; bogdan.gaspar@umfcd.ro
8. Surgery Clinic, Bucharest Emergency Clinical Hospital, 014461 Bucharest, Romania
9. Division of Obstetrics, Gynecology and Neonatology, Carol Davila University of Medicine and Pharmacy, 050474 Bucharest, Romania
10. Department of Obstetrics and Gynecology, Filantropia Clinical Hospital, 011132 Bucharest, Romania; valentin.varlas@umfcd.ro
11. Faculty of Dental Medicine, Carol Davila University of Medicine and Pharmacy, 050474 Bucharest, Romania
* Correspondence: sanda@cretoiu.ro
† Equal contribution to this paper.

Abstract: Melanomas of the skin are poorly circumscribed lesions, very frequently asymptomatic but unfortunately with a continuous growing incidence. In this landscape, one can distinguish melanomas originating in the mucous membranes and located in areas not exposed to the sun, namely the vulvo-vaginal melanomas. By contrast with cutaneous melanomas, the incidence of these types of melanomas is constant, being diagnosed in females in their late sixties. While hairy skin and glabrous skin melanomas of the vulva account for 5% of all cancers located in the vulva, melanomas of the vagina and urethra are particularly rare conditions. The location in areas less accessible to periodic inspection determines their diagnosis in advanced stages, often metastatic. Moreover, despite the large number of drugs newly approved in recent decades for the treatment of cutaneous melanoma, especially in the category of biological drugs, the mortality of vulvo-vaginal melanomas has remained almost constant. This, together with the absence of specific treatment guidelines due to the lack of a sufficient number of cases to conduct randomized clinical trials, makes melanomas with this localization a discouraging diagnosis, associated with a very poor prognosis. Our aim is therefore to draw attention to this oftentimes overlooked entity in order to encourage the community to employ various strategies meant to increase research in this area. By highlighting the main risk factors of vulvar and vaginal melanomas, as well as the clinical manifestations and molecular changes underlying these neoplasms, ideally novel therapeutic schemes will, in time, be brought into effect.

Keywords: vulvar melanoma; vaginal melanoma; targeted therapy; gynecological cancer; melanoma treatment

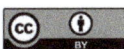

1. Introduction

Melanoma is an extremely aggressive tumor with a high metastatic rate, whose diagnosis in advanced stages was associated, until a decade ago, with minimal chances of survival [1]. It is a tumor originating in melanocyte cells which are formed during embryogenesis from the neural crest of the trunk [2]. Melanocytes come from progenitor cells with a high migration capacity. This migratory capacity explains why they are distributed and present at the level of a large number of structures: the skin—the basal layer of the epidermis (with an important role in the uniform pigmentation by forming epidermal–melanin units)—the inner ear, gastrointestinal tract and the nerve structures [3]. The incidence of melanoma has seen a spectacular increase in the last two decades, with over 300,000 new cases in 2018, the most affected countries being Australia and New Zealand (over 33 cases/100,000 inhabitants), the average age of onset of melanoma being 65 years old [4,5]. Regarding the distribution according to sex, in the case of melanomas discovered in adulthood, there is a predominance of cases in males, with a reversal of the phenomenon for melanomas diagnosed between 15–39 years, over 60% of cases appearing in the female population [6,7]. An interesting phenomenon was observed in the young population diagnosed with melanoma, the cases experiencing an alarming increase between 1999–2006, with a decrease in the next 10 years, dynamics overlapping with the increasing popularity of photoprotection methods and awareness of the danger posed by tanning beds exposure [6,8]. Due to the poorly associated prognosis determined mainly by the discovery of melanoma in advanced stages, melanoma remains the skin cancer with the highest mortality, the 5-year survival rate being less than 80% and depending on the degree of local tumor extension, lymphatic invasion, and presence of metastases [9,10]. Although dermatoscopic evaluation has become essential in pigmentary lesions screening, the diagnosis of melanoma is difficult even for experienced dermatologists, the clinical and dermatoscopic appearance presenting a great variability and sometimes even possessing misleading histological aspects that can lead to false-negative results [9,11,12].

Melanomas with genital location are included in the category of rare neoplasms, vulvar and vaginal melanomas totaling less than 1–2% of all melanomas diagnosed in females [13,14]. Vulvar melanoma represents approximately 5% of all cancers located in the vulva, being more common in adulthood (average age is 68 years) [15,16]. Between 2.5 and 4.5 patients/100,000 inhabitants are affected each year by vulvar cancer, melanoma with this location being among the top four most common vulvar cancers, the most frequent being squamous cell carcinoma (over 75% of cases versus 5.6% for melanoma) [17,18].

On the other hand, vaginal melanoma is even a rarer condition, accounting for less than 0.05–0.1% of genital neoplasms [19]. The average age of onset is lower than in the case of vulvar melanoma (57 years), and the prognosis is much worse, less than a third of patients surviving 5 years after diagnosis, despite the correct instituted treatment [20]. In a study performed on 1400 patients with vulvar melanoma and 463 with vaginal melanoma, Wohlmuth et al. highlight the occurrence of the former at a significantly younger age ($p < 0.001$) [21].

Unlike cutaneous melanoma, which is much more common in Caucasians, the frequency of vulvar and vaginal melanomas has very little variability related to race, but there is a slight increase in frequency in Whites (3.14 vs. 1.02: 1) [22]. This increase is statistically significant for vulvar melanoma, but not for those with vaginal localization ($p < 0.001$) [21].

Particular attention has been paid in the last years to the necessity of avoiding sun exposure using screen protective agents, periodic self-examination of pigmented lesions and periodic dermatoscopic surveillance of potentially evolving lesions, these being considered the most important methods to decrease the incidence and mortality of melanoma [23]. However, the genital area is often overlooked as a possible site of melanoma and other skin cancers, both by patients and doctors. Yet, melanoma with localization in the vulva and vagina is characterized by increased severity especially due to late diagnosis, most often in metastatic stages [18]. Moreover, the therapeutic means used in cutaneous melanomas are of little use in the treatment of melanomas with vulvar and vaginal localization, mortality having high values and not changing considerably in the last three decades (5-year survival rates vary between 10% and 63%) [17,24–26]. Thus, the present review aims to highlight the main risk factors identified in the occurrence of vulvar and vaginal melanomas, clinical manifestations, molecular changes underlying these neoplasms, as well as the main therapeutic means and their effectiveness in terms of survival.

2. Risk Factors

Melanoma, like most neoplastic pathologies, is a multifactorial disease, its occurrence being related to interactions between environmental and host factors, thus appearing as a consequence of genetic and epigenetic modifications that eventually lead to alteration of regulatory processes [27]. Although a number of risk factors involved in the etiopathogenesis of the disease have been identified for cutaneous melanoma, such as intermittent exposure with increased intensity to ultraviolet (UV) radiation, history of sunburns (more common at high latitudes), the presence of atypical nevi, specific skin phenotype (lightly pigmented skin, with light eyes, blond or reddish hair, presence of freckles), family history with specific genetic changes that alter the ultraviolets repair of melanocytes subjected to UV radiation, the use of Psoralen and Ultraviolet A therapy (PUVA) for a long time (over 15 years after exposure), the etiopathogenic mechanisms for vulvar and vaginal melanomas are not yet elucidated, and no specific factors involved in their occurrence have been identified [17,28–32]. Moreover, in a study published by Heinzelmann-Schwartzet et al., the onset of vulvar melanoma was regarded as spontaneous, de novo, with changes in a single melanocyte cell being enough to trigger the process of oncogenesis and determine the formation of melanoma [17].

However, there are studies that show a greater association between mucosal melanomas in general, and vaginal and vulvar melanomas in particular, and certain factors:

Sex. The female gender appears to be a risk factor for mucosal melanomas in general, which are twice as common as in men, compared to cutaneous melanomas whose distribution is similar between the two sexes [33].

Age. Vulvar melanoma is a disease that has an average age of onset of 68 years old, the risk of onset increasing with age (the number of cases increases from 0.11/1 million inhabitants for 15–29 years range, to 3.5/1 million inhabitants for those over 60 years old [34,35]). In contrast, cutaneous melanoma has a maximum incidence around the fourth decade of life [35].

Family history of cutaneous melanoma appears to be a risk factor for vulvar melanoma [36].

Ethnicity also seems to play an important role in the evolution of melanomas with genital localization and in their prognosis. Even if the association is not as strong as in the case of cutaneous melanomas, vulvar and vaginal melanomas are three times more common in the white race ($p < 0.001$) [22]. However, the prognosis has an inverse association, the mortality being much higher among the African population [37].

Lichen sclerosus is a precursor lesion of squamous cell carcinoma of the genital area which appears in its evolution in a percentage of approximately 5%, the causal link between the two pathologies being well known. Regarding the occurrence of vulvar melanoma in patients with lichen sclerosus, while a causal link has not been clearly established, although the number of reported cases is quite small, an increased incidence of vulvar melanoma has been observed among these patients (relative risk = 341) [38,39].

UV radiation. Though vulvar melanoma does not occur in photo-exposed areas, some studies suggest the indirect involvement of UV radiation in the pathogenesis of vulvar melanoma, through alterations of the immune response that favor modifications of the pathways involved in oncogenesis. However, it is important to note that the role of radiation in the pathogenesis of the disease is significantly lower than in skin melanoma [34].

Although the Human Papilloma Virus (HPV) is known for its roles in the development of benign (condyloma acuminata) and malignant tumors (invasive squamous cell carcinoma, anorectal cancers, penile cancers, squamous vaginal cancers) with genital localization, there is yet no mechanism to demonstrate its involvement in melanoma. There is no evidence that the HPV infection elevates the risk of vulvar or vaginal melanomas [32,40–42].

3. Clinical Manifestations

Unlike cutaneous melanoma which is most frequently distributed on photo-exposed areas (face, trunk, lower limbs) making it possible to diagnose it from early stages, vulvar and vaginal melanomas have origins that are generally overlooked by frequent inspection, the anatomical position of the lesion being the main reason for its late diagnosis and poor prognosis [43]. Melanomas of the vulvar region can occur in a variety of sites starting from the hairy skin of the labium majus to the introitus (Figure 1). The most common sites are the clitoris, the labia majora, and the labia minora, and in most cases, multiple tumors can be detected [34,44,45].

Vulvar and vaginal melanomas are pigmented lesions with variable diameters (generally over 7 mm), with macular (most frequently), papular or nodular appearance, most often asymmetrical and with an inhomogeneous appearance in terms of pigmentation [44,46,47]. There are also reports in the literature of cases with amelanotic manifestations of genital melanomas, especially at the vaginal level [20,48]. The first case of genital melanoma was described in 1861 in a 35-year-old patient who presented with multiple pigmentary lesions and evolved with neurological and digestive symptoms in the context of multiple secondary determinations and, subsequently, exitus [49]. Since then, multiple cases of vulvar and vaginal melanomas with various clinical, dermatoscopic aspects, and symptoms have been depicted in the literature (for additional details see [16,20]).

As it is a rare pathology, most of the clinical data presented in the literature are obtained from isolated case presentations or case series, most of which highlight the presence of genital bleeding, a palpable, white-gray color mass, itching, dyspareunia, yellow genital secretions, and local pain [50–54]. Cases that mention the presence of painless masses are also reported [55]. Most of the cases presented depict the tumor in the labia minora. The diagnosis is generally late, with half of the patients being diagnosed in advanced stages, with the invasion of deep structures [56].

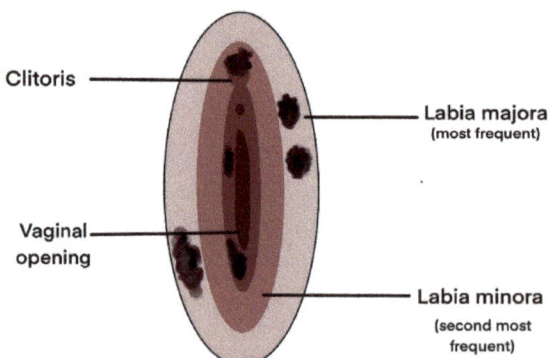

Figure 1. Most common sites for vulvar melanomas [15,36,47,57–59].

Although not so numerous and generally on small patient samples, there are prospective or retrospective clinical studies and meta-analyses that have highlighted the main clinical manifestations and the most common sites of vulvar and vaginal melanomas, which are further illustrated in Table 1.

Regarding the dermatoscopic examination, it is characterized by asymmetrical, irregular aspects, both in terms of contour and pigmentation, lacking a clear structure. In addition, multiple cases report the presence of blue-gray or white-gray areas and globular punctiform black-brown structures [45,58].

Table 1. Clinical findings in melanoma of the vulva and vagina [15,26,36,47,57–60].

Number of Patients	Tumor Localisation	Main Signs and Symptoms	Others Signs and Symptoms	References
51	Labia minora	Pain, Palpable mass, Genital bleeding, Pruritus	Dysuria, Ulceration	[57]
20	Labia majora	Genital bleeding, Pruritus, Palpable mass	Pain, Dysuria, Unhealing sore, Urinary difficulties	[36]
10	Labia majora	Pruritus	-	[47]
11	Not specified	Pruritus, Pain, Genital bleeding	-	[26]
14	Labia minora	Pruritus	-	[58]
31	Vagina	Genital bleeding, Pain, Palpable mass	Abnormal vaginal secretion, Urinary difficulties	[59]
33	Not specified	Palpable mass, Genital bleeding, Pain, Pruritus	Abnormal vaginal secretion, Dysuria, Dyspareunia, Ulceration	[60]
198	Unilateral, Clitoris	Genital bleeding, Pain, Pruritus	-	[15]

4. Histological Aspects

Melanoma may arise de novo or within an existing benign or dysplastic nevus. Lesions usually measure between 2–4 mm in thickness and are frequently ulcerated. In addition to this clinical aspect that raises the suspicion of a malignant lesion, histopathological examination is absolutely necessary to establish the diagnosis.

4.1. Macroscopic Examination

The distribution of melanomas on the skin can be at any level, therefore areas not exposed to the sun should not be neglected, which is practically the case of vulvar melanomas. Considering that vulvar melanomas often appear in older women, they should be advised to self-examine with a hand-held mirror [13]. The first step in examining pigmented nevi, moles, and brown spots and growths is to apply the ABCDEs rule and the Ugly Duckling sign (although not applicable for vulvar melanomas) [61]. As for the rest of the skin, vulvar melanomas are black or dark brown, but may also vary from white, pink, red, to other colors [13,62,63].

The ABCDE rule refers to the main macroscopical aspects taken into consideration when assessing cutaneous lesions, namely Asymmetry (the two halves of the mole are not identical), Border irregularity (edges are ragged or notched), Color variation (shades of tan, brown, or black and sometimes patches of red, blue, or white), Diameter (>6 mm or >1/4 inch) or Dermoscopic structure, and Evolution (Figure 2) [64]. The same rule can be regarded from a histological point of view, thus becoming the ABCDE(FG) rule, which refers to Asymmetry (silhouette and color imbalance), Buckshot scatter (pagetoid distribution), Cytological atypia, Deep mitosis, Enclosing lymphocytes, Fibrosis, and Gainsaying (=no) maturation [65].

Another step in the diagnosis of vulvar melanoma is dermoscopy, which facilitates early detection based on the identification of a lesion with irregular dots, multiple colors (black, blue, brown, pink, gray, and white), a blue-white veil, and atypical vessels [66]. When the lesion is assessed and determined as suspicious, the next step is to determine the most important factor for the future evolution and prognosis—the vertical depth of invasion [67]. Therefore, the most effective way to assess the local invasion is the sampling of the lesion. The evolution of melanoma depends on the correctness and accuracy of the biopsy technique. Thus, two types of biopsies of suspicious formations are described: an excisional biopsy that removes the entire lesion, and an incisional biopsy, which removes only a portion from the suspicious cutaneous lesion [68]. Excision biopsy is considered the gold standard in the correct diagnosis of melanomas, and has the advantage of providing accurate microstaging [69].

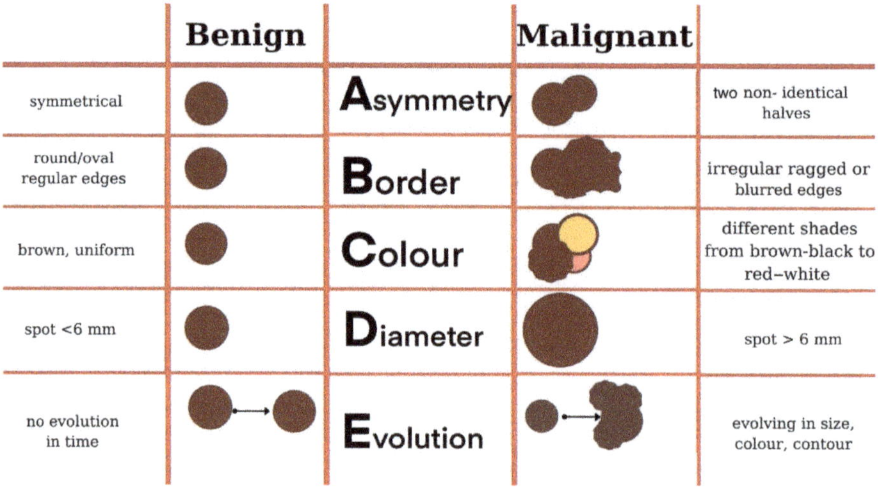

	Benign		**Malignant**	
symmetrical	●	**A**symmetry	◉	two non-identical halves
round/oval regular edges	●	**B**order	❀	irregular ragged or blurred edges
brown, uniform	●	**C**olour	◉	different shades from brown-black to red–white
spot <6 mm	●	**D**iameter	●	spot > 6 mm
no evolution in time	●→●	**E**volution	●→❀	evolving in size, colour, contour

Figure 2. ABCDE evaluation of a pigmentary skin lesion [64].

The 7th edition of The American Joint Committee on Cancer (AJCC) Cancer Staging Manual published in 2009 was the first to give up the Clark score, which was largely based on the level of anatomical invasion in the skin layers [70]. Further on, the 8th AJCC edition on melanoma staging and classification relies on the Breslow thickness in order to establish the depth of invasion, so as to accurately assign a stage based on the classical tumor, node, metastasis (TNM) scores [71]. Additionally, this latest edition specifies that tumor depth should be measured to the nearest 0.1 mm instead of 0.01 mm, in order to improve precision [72]. Although there is not yet a standardized and unanimously accepted staging of vuvar melanomas, the Gynecologic Oncology Group (GOG) recommends the use of the AJCC staging manual instead of the International Federation of Gynecology and Obstetrics (FIGO) system, in spite of the several uncertainties that still persist [18]. Specifically, while generally regarded as mucosal tumors, the molecular characteristics of vulvar melanomas differ from those of both cutaneous and mucosal melanomas in terms of mutational signatures, thus prompting some authors to consider them a unique subclass [21,73].

4.2. Microscopic Examination

From a cytological point of view, melanoma cells are of two types: epithelioid and spindle cells. The epithelioid type is characterized by large, round cells with abundant eosinophilic cytoplasm. They have vesicular nuclei with coarse irregular chromatin with peripheral condensation (pattern known as "peppered moth" nuclei). This cell type is most commonly found in nodular and superficial spreading melanomas. The stromal compartment is accompanied by a variable inflammatory infiltrate (brisk, non-brisk, absent), irregular distribution of the pigment, and dermal fibrosis.

4.3. Histological Subtypes of Melanoma

The class of tumors known as melanoma contains numerous histological subtypes that are not often considered of the utmost importance to clinicians or patients, especially in terms of prognosis [74]. Histopathological characteristics of the gynecological melanomas should be interpreted in the context of other clinical diagnostic criteria and macroscopic data.

Superficial spreading melanoma (SSM) is the most common subtype, characterized by asymmetrical proliferation of atypical melanocytes. Individual melanocyte units are distributed at the dermo-epidermal junction and are characterized by the presence of large pagetoid areas (>0.5 mm^2) [75].

Lentigo maligna melanoma (LMM) is characteristic for elderly patients repeatedly exposed to chronic sun damage. Melanocytes arranged in solitary units along the dermo-epidermal junction are organized in small nests (lentiginous pattern), sometimes the nests being horizontally confluent and variable in size and shape (nevoid/dysplastic-like pattern). Dermal invasion of atypical melanocytes is frequent, as well as the extension into the hair follicles [76].

Acral lentiginous melanoma (ALM) is more common in the Afro-Asian population, on palms and soles, and involves the eccrine glands excretory ducts [77].

Nodular melanoma (NM) is considered the most aggressive form, and grows in depth rather than in diameter, so that the ABCDE rule does not apply [78]. It is characterized by a nodular dermal proliferation of atypical melanocytes.

Regarding vulvar melanomas, a retrospective study based on 43 patients, performed by DeMatos et al., showed that most of the mucosal melanoma lesions (vulvar, vaginal, and cervical) were not classified (33%), while the rest were acral lentiginous (30%), or superficial spreading melanoma (26%). Unclassified tumors were either nodular or polypoid melanoma [79].

The most common vulvar melanomas subtypes are mucosal lentiginous and nodular melanoma. The characteristic microscopic aspects are represented by impairment of the epidermis, pagetoid spread of melanocytes, or melanocytes organized in nests (Figures 3 and 4) [80]. Usually, melanocytes are variable in size and shape, and are sometimes localized within lymphovascular spaces. Furthermore, they can frequently become confluent and lack maturation, showing atypical mitoses and increased apoptotic activity (Figures 5 and 6) [81]. The presence of an ulcerated tumor is associated with a poor prognosis.

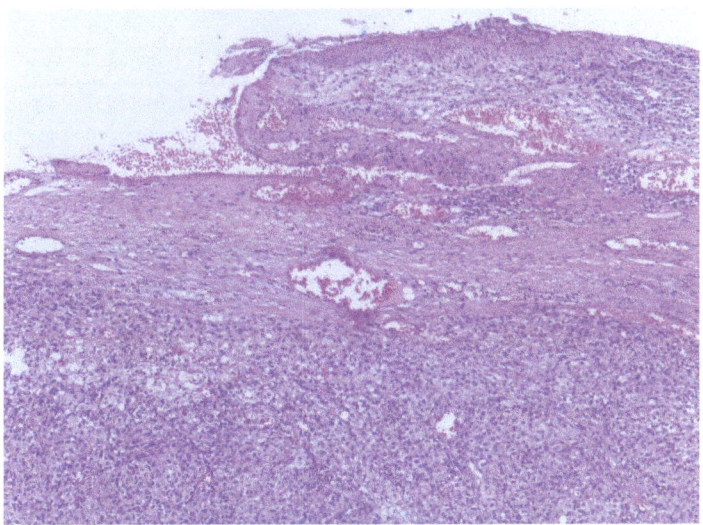

Figure 3. Vaginal melanoma. Vaginal squamous epithelium with areas of ulceration. In lamina propria one can observe tumoral cells organized in nests. Hematoxylin-eosin stain, original magnification ×4 (histological image courtesy of dr. Ileana Popa).

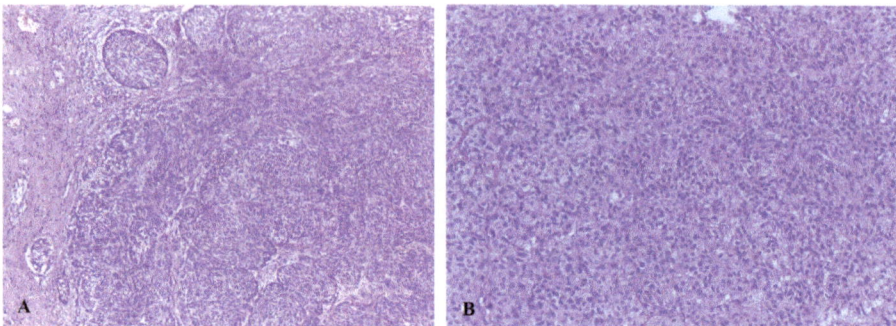

Figure 4. (**A**) Vaginal melanoma. Tumor cells organized in nests, some fusiform-looking cells (Hematoxylin-eosin stain, original magnification ×10.) (**B**) Vaginal melanoma. Epithelioid-looking malignant cells in lamina propria outlooking a nest disposition, abundant eosinophilic cytoplasm. Hematoxylin-eosin stain, original magnification ×20 (histological image courtesy of dr. Ileana Popa).

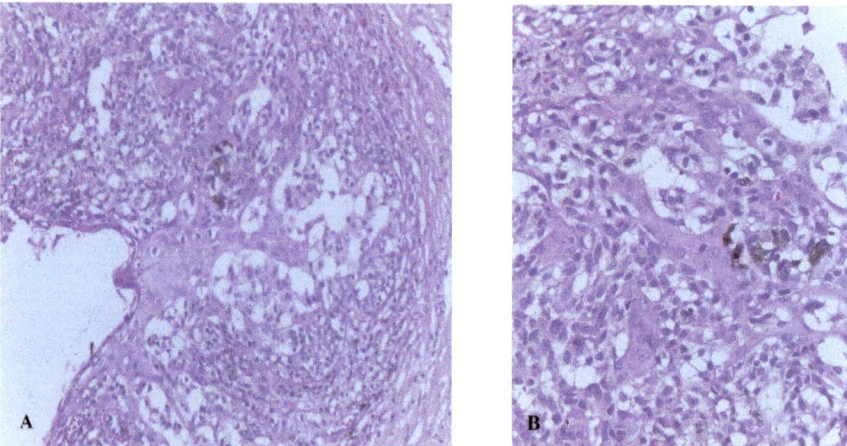

Figure 5. (**A**) Vaginal melanoma. Tumoral cells filled with melanin organized in nests at the epithelium-lamina propria junction—pathognomonic for the diagnosis, original magnification ×20. (**B**) Detail showing haphazardly distributed atypical melanocytes in lamina propria original magnification ×40 Hematoxylin-eosin stain (histological image courtesy of dr. Ileana Popa).

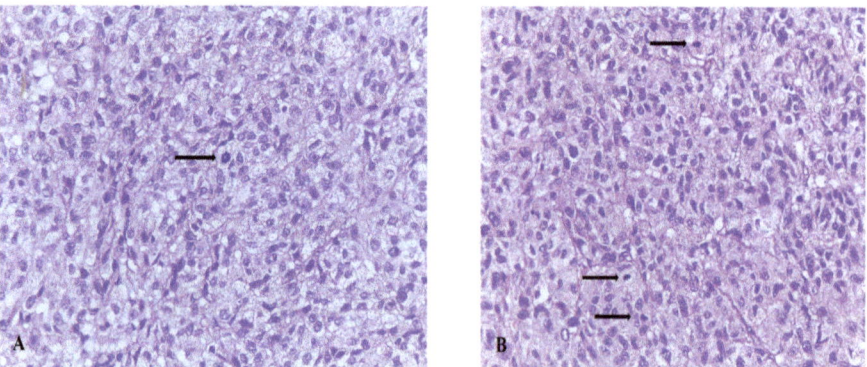

Figure 6. (**A**,**B**) Vaginal melanoma. Arrows—Nuclear mitoses—original magnification ×40. Hematoxylin-eosin stain (histological image courtesy of dr. Ileana Popa).

5. Immuno(cyto)histochemistry in the Diagnosis of Melanoma

The criteria described above are imperiled by subjective interpretations, lacking objectivity, and reproducibility. Moreover, melanomas are able to mimic a lot of other malignancies with epithelial, hematologic, mesenchymal, and neural origin, such as lymphomas, carcinomas, neuroendocrine tumors, and sarcomas [82]. Therefore, immunocytochemistry (IHC) is a step most often necessary in the correct evaluation of a melanocytic suspect lesion in patients with underlying hematological pathologies or with solid cancers with frequent skin metastasis. Immunohistochemistry can show its utility in the differential diagnosis of vulvar soft tissue lesions, i.e., Paget disease, which can mimic melanoma [83]. In addition, IHC is less expensive by comparison with electron microscopy, which can bring additional information for melanoma cells containing melanosomes and other ultrastructural particularities which are not present in Paget disease.

Melanomas are usually immunoreactive for Melanoma antigen recognized by T-cells-1 (MART-1) or melan A, S-100 protein, melanoma-specific antigen (HMB-45), tyrosinase, and Microphthalmia transcription factor (MITF) [84].

S-100 protein, a sensitive marker for melanocytic differentiation, is considered to have a sensitivity of 97–100%, but the specificity for melanoma is low since is also expressed on glial cells, Schwann cells, chondrocytes, lipocytes, dendritic cells, histiocytes [85].

One of the first specific markers that was discovered is HMB45, a marker of the cytoplasmic pre melanosomal glycoprotein gp100 [86].

Melan A is the most widely used technique for identifying basal melanocytic proliferations, having a more intense and diffuse staining than HMB45 and a specificity of 95–100% [87].

Further on, the Sry-related HMg-Box gene 10 (SOX10) nuclear transcription factor is a key player in the differentiation of pluripotent neural crest cells into melanocytes. In this regard, its use as a metastatic melanoma marker has been investigated and found to be highly specific and sensitive [88].

6. Molecular Characterization

The pathogenesis of genital tract melanomas can mimic that of cutaneous melanoma developed in areas that are sun-protected, as in the case of vulvar melanomas. Moreover, other types of mucosal melanomas (e.g., the respiratory and the gastrointestinal tract) can serve as a model for the development of vaginal or cervical melanomas. Still, there are gaps in understanding the pathogenesis of vulvar or vaginal melanomas. However, elucidating the pathways involved in melanoma genesis is a very important step towards future advanced precision treatment.

Mucosal melanomas represent a challenge in relation to treatment, since, as opposed to cutaneous melanomas, not only are they detected in more advanced stages, but they are also less responsive to immunotherapy and lack activating mutations involving dominant MAP kinases [89,90]. Mutations in KIT, NF1 and SF3B1 genes are more frequently seen in mucosal melanomas, while alterations to NRAS and BRAF genes are more common in cutaneous melanomas [91,92]. Female genital tract melanomas can sometimes contradict the pattern described above. A study involving the whole-genome analysis of 284 patients diagnosed with mucosal melanoma localized in different sites revealed 10 mutated genes (Table 2) [93].

A retrospective study performed by Rouzbachman et al. on 33 vulvar and 11 vaginal malignant melanomas identified by next-generation sequencing analysis, found that the most frequent mutations were in C-KIT and NRAS genes, while BRAF mutations were infrequent. The study did not establish a correlation with the prognosis or outcome for these patients [94].

A more recent study performed by Cai et al. on 19 melanomas of the female genital tract and paired with 25 cutaneous melanomas, 18 acral melanomas and 11 melanomas of the nasal cavity, concluded that malignant melanoma of the female genital tract harbors distinct mutation rates in the KIT, BRAF, SF3B1, KRAS, and NRAS genes. Moreover, this location of the melanoma is an entirely distinct entity from skin melanoma and melanomas of the nasal cavity, while cervix melanomas also have some particularities, and do not suffer recurrent KIT mutations, or mutations of the NRAS and SF3B1 genes [95].

Because BRAF and NRAS mutations are uncommon in non-cutaneous melanomas, we can consider that each melanoma subtype depends on a different oncogenetic pathway for its development. This leads to the idea that it will not benefit from anti-RAF treatment, although large studies are needed before considering this as a rule. However, in the era of precision medicine, the importance of driver mutations cannot be neglected, and should become part of mucosal melanoma routine clinical testing [96].

Table 2. The main mutations that occur in melanomas and their frequency of occurrence [93,97–102].

Mutated Gene	Percentage of Mutation (%)	Details
NRAS	12/67—17.9%	• codon 61—less involved in mucosal melanomas • codon 12—more involved in mucosal melanomas • more frequent in case of metastatic or recurrent melanoma [93]
BRAF	11/67—16.4%	• mostly mutations in protein tyrosine kinase domain • predominant targeting the hotspot region between amino-acids 594 and 600 [93]
NF1	11/67—16.4%	• are correlated with melanomas developed on high UV exposure areas [97] • NF-1 mutation melanomas are more frequently involving female patients, have a higher Breslow score, and can be associated with subsequent neoplasia [98]
KIT	10/67—14.9%	• are frequently screened for mutations in exons 9, 11, 13, 17, and 18 • KIT mutations are more frequently involved in vulvar melanoma than in other types of mucosal melanomas • single substitutions of an amino acid are the most frequent KIT mutations, the most common being L576P [99]
SF3B1	8/67—11.9%	• more frequently in European ancestry patients • mostly in primary melanomas [93]
TP53	6/67—8.9%	• is correlated with response to immunotherapy with CTLA-4 blockade [100]
SPRED1	5/67—7.4%	• deletion of the SPRED1 gene leads to developing resistance to MAPK inhibition, so this mutation is essential in evaluating the choice of treatment [101]
ATRX	4/67—5.9%	• ATRX works as a chromatin remodeler, thus progression of a melanoma lesion is associated with a reduced expression of ATRX gene [102]
HLA-A	4/67—5.9%	[93]
CHD8	3/67—4.4%	[93]

7. Melanoma Stage Description

Detection of a melanoma involving the vulva or vagina associates an essential step: the exclusion of any kind of metastatic dissemination in places such as mucosal membranes, skin, or the eyes [102]. Since staging approved for melanomas, in general, cannot be extended to female genital tract melanomas, there is a great need for dedicated staging.

Clark classification that stages melanomas regarding their level of invasiveness and Breslow classification regarding the vertical depth of the lesion are dedicated for cutaneous melanomas [103–105].

A new and modified Clark classification, named Chung classification, is considered specific for micro-staging of mucosal melanomas in general (Table 3) [106].

Table 3. Clark and Chung classifications comparative aspects [104–106].

Level of Invasion	Clark Classification—Level of Invasion of Cutaneous Melanoma	Chung Classification—Level of Invasion of Mucosal Melanoma
I	Lesions involving only the epidermis (in situ melanoma)	Tumor confined to the epithelium
II	Invasion of the papillary dermis—does not reach the papillary-reticular dermal interface	Tumor penetrates the basement membrane and invades at a depth of <1 mm
III	Invasion fills and expands the papillary dermis but does not extend to reticular dermis	Tumor invades at a depth of 1–2 mm
IV	Invasion into the reticular dermis but not into the subcutaneous tissue	Tumor invades at a depth of >2 mm, but without reaching the subcutaneous fat
V	Invasion through the reticular dermis into the subcutaneous tissue	Tumor penetrates the subcutaneous fat

A 25-year study that both encompasses clinical and pathological features of vulvar melanoma revealed that American Joint Committee on Cancer (AJCC) staging system is the unique prognostic factor for vulvar melanoma (Table 4) [57]. The AJCC system was revised in 2017, associating new prognostic factors [72].

Table 4. American Joint Committee—prognostic stage group for melanoma 2017 [57,72].

STAGE	T (Tumor)	N (Nodules)	M (Metastasis)
0	Tis	N0	M0
IA	T1a	N0	M0
IB	T1b, T2a	N0	M0
IIA	T2b, T3a	N0	M0
IIB	T3b, T4a	N0	M0
IIC	T4b	N0	M0
IIIA	T1a/b, T2a	N1, N2a	M0
IIIB	T0	N1b, N1c	M0
	T1a/b, T2a	N1b/c, N2b	M0
	T2b, T3a	N1a-N2b	M0
IIIC	T0	N2b/c, N3b/c	M0
	T1a-T3a	N2c, N3	M0
	T3b, T4a	N ≥ N1	M0
	T4b	N1a-N2c	M0
IIID	T4b	N3	M0
IV	Any T, Tis	Any N	M1

8. Therapeutic Approach

Melanomas with vulvar and vaginal localization represent real challenges in terms of treatment, not only due to late diagnosis in locally advanced or metastatic stages, but also due to the absence of specific therapeutic guidelines due to the small number of cases. Thus, due to the impossibility of gathering a significant number of cases to establish dedicated guidelines, the guidelines for cutaneous melanoma are often used.

The main treatment for both vulvar and vaginal melanoma is surgical excision of the tumor. Clinical experience in the last few decades has shown no significant differences in survival rates between radical excision and limited excisions with safety margins (Table 5), so limited resections are currently recommended [32,103]. Pelvic exenteration may be helpful, but only in carefully selected cases [107].

Table 5. Safety surgical margins in limited resection of vulvar and vaginal melanomas [15,103,107].

Tumor Width	Margins	Reference
<2 mm	0.5 cm	
2 mm	1 cm	[103]
>2 mm	2 cm	
<1 mm	1 cm	
1–4 mm	2 cm	[98]
invasion of subcutaneous fat/fascia, any size	>1 cm	
in situ	0.5 cm	
<2 mm	1 cm	[15]
>2 mm	2 cm	

Surgical excision may be completed in some cases by lymphadenectomy. Literature data do not provide specific information on the positive impact of lymphadenectomy in terms of survival, so it is preferred to perform the sentinel node technique in the absence of clinical involvement of regional lymph nodes, followed by lymphadenectomy in the case of a positive result [103]. In the case of clinical invasion of the regional lymph nodes, tumor extension in the adjacent structures, and/or ulceration, lymphadenectomy is recommended, not preceded by the sentinel node technique, which may or may not be followed by adjuvant treatment [108,109]. Lymphadenectomy, although a radical intervention, has no impact on long-term survival, only enabling better local control of the disease [107].

Regarding the utility of radiotherapy, chemotherapy, and immunotherapy, data presented in the literature are limited, but randomized controlled trials show minimal changes in survival [107]. Radiotherapy is generally used as neoadjuvant treatment, in case of impossibility of surgical resection, lymphatic invasion, regional extension, or as palliative treatment [103,110]. Doses of 45–55 Gy are generally used in daily sessions of 1.8–2 Gy/session [103]. The use of radiotherapy in localized forms has been associated with a decrease in survival [110,111].

Chemotherapy is mainly used as a neoadjuvant treatment or unique therapy, utilizing the same agents as those used in skin melanoma: dacarbazine and temozolomide, with dacarbazine being the first Food and Drug Administration-approved drug for melanoma treatment [103,112]. In addition, chemotherapy represents, together with surgery, the last therapeutic resource for the treatment of vulvar melanoma diagnosed in advanced stages [107].

Although on small groups of patients, there are studies showing the effectiveness of chemotherapy compared to the use of high-dose interferon for stage II vulvar melanoma [107]. Moreover, the use of temozolomide-cisplatin combination as adjuvant therapy in stages II-III showed statistically significant benefits over the use of interferon-alpha or surgery in terms of survival ($p < 0.01$) [109]. The carboplatin–paclitaxel–bevacizumab combination has been shown to be effective in decreasing tumor volume, thus allowing surgical resection without the need for further grafting [113]. Chemotherapy is used mainly in regionally advanced forms or with distant metastases, but the benefits are minimal, the use of chemotherapy is generally associated with a decrease in overall survival and recurrence-free survival [110,113]. Up until 2011, only four drugs had been approved for the treatment of melanoma; currently, their number has reached 30, and this increase is based mainly on newly emerged molecules from the class of immunotherapeutics or biological drugs [112].

The class of immunotherapeutics includes molecules that interfere with the immune cascade of carcinogenesis, such as interferon α-2b (IFN α-2b), peginterferon α-2b (PegIFN α-2b), interleukin 2 (IL-2), inhibitor of death protein 1 (PD-L1 blockade)–nivolumab, regulatory T lymphocyte inhibitors, monoclonal antibodies against cytotoxic T cell antigen 4 (CTLA-4)–ipilimumab [112]. These are especially used in advanced stages (stage III-IV) of cutaneous melanoma, but for vulvar melanoma, there are not enough clinical data to demonstrate efficacy in terms of overall survival or disease-free survival. However, their use doubled in the period 2012–2015 compared to the corresponding previous period ($p < 0.01$), most frequently for regionally advanced forms and those with distant metastases [110]. IFN α-2b appeared to lead to an increase in disease-free survival in a randomized clinical trial, while no effects on survival after the use of IL-2 alone or in combination with peptide vaccines were observed [107]. Albert et al. observed in a study on 1917 patients with vulvar melanoma (3/4 with localized disease) that the combination of immunotherapy with local surgery was associated with an increase in overall survival, although statistically insignificant [110]. On the other hand, the use of immunotherapy in combination with chemotherapy and biological therapy was associated with a decrease in overall survival and recurrence-free survival in a study on 48 patients with vulvar and vaginal melanomas [113]. The same data were supported by Tcheung et al. who did not find significant differences in overall survival in patients treated with immunotherapy and chemotherapy [114].

Although targeted therapy has evolved in the last years and significantly improved the prognosis of patients with cutaneous melanoma, its use in vulvar and vaginal melanomas is still limited by the different mutagenic profiles involving fewer BRAF mutations and more c-KIT, NF1 and SF3B1 mutations [91,112]. Thus, monoclonal antibodies such as imatinib, sunitinib, dasatinib, nilotinib (for c-kit mutations) could have been a promising option due to a large number of c-kit mutations, but the results are not as good as in the case of cutaneous melanoma. Imatinib has been shown to reduce tumor size and PET uptake, as well as the disappearance of metastases in a patient with recurrent vulvar melanoma and c-kit mutation in exon 13 [115]. There are phase II studies with promising results for the use of imatinib and dasatinib in patients with mucosal melanomas with c-kit mutations [107,116]. Cocorocchio et al. also mention a positive response to avapritinib therapy in a patient with advanced vulvar melanoma with a c-kit mutation in exon 17, who had a previous negative response to the ipilimumab–nivolumab combination [117].

The prognosis is generally poor, characterized by frequent recurrences (up to 70%), with a low overall survival (average survival between 15–78 months), and with a recurrence disease-free interval of up to 64 months [113,114,118–121] (Table 6). The main prognostic factors are tumor size, lymphatic invasion, Breslow depth, and the presence of ulcerated lesions [114,122].

Vaginal melanoma is characterized by higher recurrence rates and lower average survival, requiring wider excisions with complete lymphadenectomy and even pelvic exenteration [113,121,123,124]. Along with the surgical excision, adjuvant chemotherapy (dacarbazine) or the combination of targeted therapy (ipilimumab)–radiotherapy have been mentioned in the literature in isolated case presentations or case series, with favorable results [113,121]. In the case of the combination of ipilimumab–radiotherapy, it was found that the administration of radiotherapy in doses of 3000 cGy in 5 fractions was accompanied by the absence of recurrences compared to radiotherapy in doses of 6020 cGy in 28 fractions (for isolated cases, no statistical significance was demonstrated in randomized clinical trials) [113].

Table 6. Survival rates according to type of treatment [110,114–116,118].

Number of Patients	Mean Depth Invasion	Management	Median Survival (Months)	Reccurence	Reference
13	Not provided	Not provided	15	Not provided	[119]
7	8 mm	Wide local excision	31	71%	[118]
14	3.23 mm	13% Radical surgery and lymphadenectomy 27% Wide local excision and lymph node evaluation 53% Wide local excision	Not provided	42%	[122]
9	4 mm	Radical surgery and lymphadenectomy	78	32–43% (in situ)	[120]
85	3.2 mm	12.9% Chemotherapy 24.7% Immunotherapy (IL-2, IFN, vaccine trials) 2.35% Chemotherapy and Immunotherapy 15.29% Radiotherapy 78.8% Surgery	62.4	Not provided	[114]
48	>3 mm	29.58% Wide local excision and lymphadenectomy 21.42% Radical surgery (8% pelvic exenteration)	39.6	Not provided	[113]
1917	Not provided	95.044% Surgery 10.38% Radiation 9.99% Immunotherapy 5.32% Chemotherapy	Not provided	Not provided	[110]

9. Conclusions

Vulvar and vaginal melanomas are rare neoplasms, with aggressive evolution, most often diagnosed in advanced stages. Gynecological melanomas currently represent a discouraging diagnosis due to the absence of specific therapeutic guidelines and management measures with satisfactory results. Despite the significant development of targeted therapy that has brought major benefits in the prognosis of cutaneous melanoma, vulvar and vaginal melanoma have a low response to these therapies due to the presence of different mutagenic profiles. Thus, despite the use in various clinical trials of many types of targeted therapies, or combinations of chemotherapy and immunotherapy, surgical excision within safe limits remains the therapeutic approach with the best survival rate. The molecular mechanisms of the vulvar and vaginal melanomas are not yet fully understood, these types of melanomas being considered an independent subcategory of melanoma. As new mechanisms are discovered, new targeted therapies may appear to improve the prognosis and subsequently, the survival rates.

Author Contributions: Conceptualization, E.-C.D., C.E.C., B.S.G. and S.M.C.; methodology, E.-C.D.; software, E.-C.D., C.V., S.M.C. and D.C.; validation, E.-C.D., C.V., S.M.C. and D.C.; formal analysis, E.-C.D., C.V., S.M.C., N.S. and D.C.; investigation E.-C.D., C.E.C., S.M.C. and V.N.V.; resources, E.-C.D., C.V., S.M.C., I.P. and D.C.; data curation, E.-C.D., C.V., N.S. and S.M.C.; writing—original draft preparation, E.-C.D., C.V., I.P. and S.M.C.; writing—review and editing, E.-C.D., B.S.G., C.E.C., S.M.C. and V.N.V.; visualization, E.-C.D., C.E.C. and S.M.C.; supervision, B.S.G.; S.M.C.; project administration, E.-C.D., C.V. and S.M.C. All authors have read and agreed to the published version of the manuscript.

Funding: This work was supported by a grant of the Romanian Ministry of Research and Innovation, PCCDI-UEFISCDI, projects number PN-III-P1-1.2-PCCDI-2017-0833/68/2018, and PN-III-P1-1.2-PCCDI-2017-0820/67/2018 within PNCDI III.

Institutional Review Board Statement: Not applicable.

Informed Consent Statement: Not applicable.

Conflicts of Interest: The authors declare no conflict of interest.

References

1. Liu, Y.; Sheikh, M.S. Melanoma: Molecular Pathogenesis and Therapeutic Management. *Mol. Cell. Pharmacol.* **2014**, *6*, 228. [PubMed]
2. Mort, R.L.; Jackson, I.J.; Patton, E.E. The Melanocyte Lineage in Development and Disease. *Development* **2015**, *142*, 620–632. [CrossRef]
3. Ali, S.A.; Naaz, I. Current Challenges in Understanding the Story of Skin Pigmentation—Bridging the Morpho-Anatomical and Functional Aspects of Mammalian Melanocytes. In *Muscle Cell and Tissue*; Sakuma, K., Ed.; InTech: London, UK, 2015.
4. Skin Cancer Statistics. Available online: https://www.wcrf.org/dietandcancer/cancer-trends/skin-cancer-statistics (accessed on 25 April 2021).
5. Melanoma Skin Cancer Statistics. Available online: https://www.cancer.org/cancer/melanoma-skin-cancer/about/key-statistics.html (accessed on 25 April 2021).
6. Weir, H.K.; Marrett, L.D.; Cokkinides, V.; Barnholtz-Sloan, J.; Patel, P.; Tai, E.; Jemal, A.; Li, J.; Kim, J.; Ekwueme, D.U. Melanoma in Adolescents and Young Adults (Ages 15–39 Years): United States, 1999–2006. *J. Am. Acad. Dermatol.* **2011**, *65*, S38–S49. [CrossRef]
7. Olsen, C.M.; Thompson, J.F.; Pandeya, N.; Whiteman, D.C. Evaluation of Sex-Specific Incidence of Melanoma. *JAMA Dermatol.* **2020**, *156*, 553–560. [CrossRef]
8. Paulson, K.G.; Gupta, D.; Kim, T.S.; Veatch, J.R.; Byrd, D.R.; Bhatia, S.; Wojcik, K.; Chapuis, A.G.; Thompson, J.A.; Madeleine, M.M.; et al. Age-Specific Incidence of Melanoma in the United States. *JAMA Dermatol.* **2020**, *156*, 57–64. [CrossRef] [PubMed]
9. Davis, L.E.; Shalin, S.C.; Tackett, A.J. Current State of Melanoma Diagnosis and Treatment. *Cancer Biol. Ther.* **2019**, *20*, 1366–1379. [CrossRef] [PubMed]
10. Matthews, N.H.; Li, W.-Q.; Qureshi, A.A.; Weinstock, M.A.; Cho, E. Cutaneous Melanoma: Etiology and Therapy. *Codon Publ.* **2017**. [CrossRef]
11. Corona, R.; Mele, A.; Amini, M.; De Rosa, G.; Coppola, G.; Piccardi, P.; Fucci, M.; Pasquini, P.; Faraggiana, T. Interobserver Variability on the Histopathologic Diagnosis of Cutaneous Melanoma and Other Pigmented Skin Lesions. *J. Clin. Oncol.* **1996**, *14*, 1218–1223. [CrossRef]
12. Troxel, D.B. Pitfalls in the Diagnosis of Malignant Melanoma: Findings of a Risk Management Panel Study. *Am. J. Surg. Pathol.* **2003**, *27*, 1278–1283. [CrossRef]
13. Trimble, E.L. Melanomas of the Vulva and Vagina. *Oncol. Williston Park* **1996**, *10*, 1017–1023.
14. Qurrat ul Ain, Q.; Rao, B. A Rare Case Report: Malignant Vulvar Melanoma. *Indian J. Gynecol. Oncol.* **2020**, *18*. [CrossRef]
15. Boer, F.L.; Ten Eikelder, M.L.G.; Kapiteijn, E.H.; Creutzberg, C.L.; Galaal, K.; van Poelgeest, M.I.E. Vulvar Malignant Melanoma: Pathogenesis, Clinical Behaviour and Management: Review of the Literature. *Cancer Treat. Rev.* **2019**, *73*, 91–103. [CrossRef] [PubMed]
16. Ragnarsson-Olding, B.K. Primary Malignant Melanoma of the Vulva—An Aggressive Tumor for Modeling the Genesis of Non-UV Light-Associated Melanomas. *Acta Oncol.* **2004**, *43*, 421–435. [CrossRef] [PubMed]
17. Heinzelmann-Schwarz, V.A.; Nixdorf, S.; Valadan, M.; Diczbalis, M.; Olivier, J.; Otton, G.; Fedier, A.; Hacker, N.F.; Scurry, J.P. A Clinicopathological Review of 33 Patients with Vulvar Melanoma Identifies C-KIT as a Prognostic Marker. *Int. J. Mol. Med.* **2014**, *33*, 784–794. [CrossRef]
18. Wohlmuth, C.; Wohlmuth-Wieser, I. Vulvar Malignancies: An Interdisciplinary Perspective. *J. Dtsch. Dermatol. Ges.* **2019**, *17*, 1257–1276. [CrossRef] [PubMed]
19. Jamaer, E.; Liang, Z.; Stagg, B. Primary Malignant Melanoma of the Vagina. *BMJ Case Rep.* **2020**, *13*, e232200. [CrossRef]
20. Kalampokas, E.; Kalampokas, T.; Damaskos, C. Primary Vaginal Melanoma, A Rare and Aggressive Entity. A Case Report and Review of the Literature. *In Vivo* **2017**, *31*, 133–139. [CrossRef]
21. Wohlmuth, C.; Wohlmuth-Wieser, I.; May, T.; Vicus, D.; Gien, L.T.; Laframboise, S. Malignant Melanoma of the Vulva and Vagina: A US Population-Based Study of 1863 Patients. *Am. J. Clin. Dermatol.* **2020**, *217*, 285–295. [CrossRef]
22. Hu, D.-N.; Yu, G.-P.; McCormick, S.A. Population-Based Incidence of Vulvar and Vaginal Melanoma in Various Races and Ethnic Groups with Comparisons to Other Site-Specific Melanomas. *Melanoma Res.* **2010**, *20*, 153–158. [CrossRef]
23. Riker, A.I.; Zea, N.; Trinh, T. The Epidemiology, Prevention, and Detection of Melanoma. *Ochsner J.* **2010**, *10*, 56–65.
24. Scheistrøen, M.; Tropé, C.; Kaern, J.; Abeler, V.M.; Pettersen, E.O.; Kristensen, G.B. Malignant Melanoma of the Vulva FIGO Stage I: Evaluation of Prognostic Factors in 43 Patients with Emphasis on DNA Ploidy and Surgical Treatment. *Gynecol. Oncol.* **1996**, *61*, 253–258. [CrossRef] [PubMed]
25. Harting, M.S.; Kim, K.B. Biochemotherapy in Patients with Advanced Vulvovaginal Mucosal Melanoma. *Melanoma Res.* **2004**, *14*, 517–520. [CrossRef] [PubMed]
26. Baiocchi, G.; Duprat, J.P.; Neves, R.I.; Fukazawa, E.M.; Landman, G.; Guimarães, G.C.; Valadares, L.J. Vulvar Melanoma: Report on Eleven Cases and Review of the Literature. *Sao Paulo Med. J.* **2010**, *128*, 38–41. [CrossRef]
27. You, J.S.; Jones, P.A. Cancer Genetics and Epigenetics: Two Sides of the Same Coin? *Cancer Cell* **2012**, *22*, 9–20. [CrossRef]
28. Rastrelli, M.; Tropea, S.; Rossi, C.R.; Alaibac, M. Melanoma: Epidemiology, Risk Factors, Pathogenesis, Diagnosis and Classification. *In Vivo* **2014**, *28*, 1005–1011.

29. Gandini, S.; Sera, F.; Cattaruzza, M.S.; Pasquini, P.; Picconi, O.; Boyle, P.; Melchi, C.F. Meta-Analysis of Risk Factors for Cutaneous Melanoma: II. Sun Exposure. *Eur. J. Cancer* **2005**, *41*, 45–60. [CrossRef] [PubMed]
30. Bevona, C.; Goggins, W.; Quinn, T.; Fullerton, J.; Tsao, H. Cutaneous Melanomas Associated with Nevi. *Arch. Dermatol.* **2003**, *139*, 1620–1624. [CrossRef]
31. Stern, R.S.; PUVA Follow up Study. The Risk of Melanoma in Association with Long-Term Exposure to PUVA. *J. Am. Acad. Dermatol.* **2001**, *44*, 755–761. [CrossRef]
32. Mihajlovic, M.; Vlajkovic, S.; Jovanovic, P.; Stefanovic, V. Primary Mucosal Melanomas: A Comprehensive Review. *Int. J. Clin. Exp. Pathol.* **2012**, *5*, 739–753.
33. Rapi, V.; Dogan, A.; Schultheis, B.; Hartmann, F.; Rezniczek, G.A.; Tempfer, C.B. Melanoma of the Vagina: Case Report and Systematic Review of the Literature. *Anticancer Res.* **2017**, *37*, 6911–6920.
34. Stang, A.; Streller, B.; Eisinger, B.; Jöckel, K.H. Population-Based Incidence Rates of Malignant Melanoma of the Vulva in Germany. *Gynecol. Oncol.* **2005**, *96*, 216–221. [CrossRef]
35. Tasseron, E.W.; van der Esch, E.P.; Hart, A.A.; Brutel de la Rivière, G.; Aartsen, E.J. A Clinicopathological Study of 30 Melanomas of the Vulva. *Gynecol. Oncol.* **1992**, *46*, 170–175. [CrossRef]
36. Wechter, M.E.; Gruber, S.B.; Haefner, H.K.; Lowe, L.; Schwartz, J.L.; Reynolds, K.R.; Johnston, C.M.; Johnson, T.M. Vulvar Melanoma: A Report of 20 Cases and Review of the Literature. *J. Am. Acad. Dermatol.* **2004**, *50*, 554–562. [CrossRef] [PubMed]
37. Mert, I.; Semaan, A.; Winer, I.; Morris, R.T.; Ali-Fehmi, R. Vulvar/Vaginal Melanoma: An Updated Surveillance Epidemiology and End Results Database Review, Comparison with Cutaneous Melanoma and Significance of Racial Disparities. *Int. J. Gynecol. Cancer* **2013**, *23*, 1118–1126. [CrossRef] [PubMed]
38. Hassanein, A.M.; Mrstik, M.E.; Hardt, N.S.; Morgan, L.A.; Wilkinson, E.J. Malignant Melanoma Associated with Lichen Sclerosus in the Vulva of a 10-Year-Old. *Pediatr. Dermatol.* **2004**, *21*, 473–476. [CrossRef]
39. Hieta, N.; Kurki, S.; Rintala, M.; Söderlund, J.; Hietanen, S.; Orte, K. Association of Vulvar Melanoma with Lichen Sclerosus. *Acta Derm. Venereol.* **2019**, *99*, 339–340. [CrossRef]
40. Zekan, J.; Sirotkovic-Skerlev, M.; Skerlev, M. Oncogenic Aspects of HPV Infections of the Female Genital Tract. In *DNA Replication-Current Advances*; Seligmann, H., Ed.; InTech: London, UK, 2011.
41. Münger, K.; Baldwin, A.; Edwards, K.M.; Hayakawa, H.; Nguyen, C.L.; Owens, M.; Grace, M.; Huh, K. Mechanisms of Human Papillomavirus-Induced Oncogenesis. *J. Virol.* **2004**, *78*, 11451–11460. [CrossRef]
42. Crum, C.P.; McLachlin, C.M.; Tate, J.E.; Mutter, G.L. Pathobiology of Vulvar Squamous Neoplasia. *Curr. Opin. Obstet. Gynecol.* **1997**, *9*, 63–69. [CrossRef] [PubMed]
43. Swetter, S.M.; Tsao, H.; Bichakjian, C.K.; Curiel-Lewandrowski, C.; Elder, D.E.; Gershenwald, J.E.; Guild, V.; Grant-Kels, J.M.; Halpern, A.C.; Johnson, T.M.; et al. Guidelines of Care for the Management of Primary Cutaneous Melanoma. *J. Am. Acad. Dermatol.* **2019**, *80*, 208–250. [CrossRef] [PubMed]
44. Edwards, L. Pigmented Vulvar Lesions: Pigmented Vulvar Lesions. *Dermatol. Ther.* **2010**, *23*, 449–457. [CrossRef]
45. Resende, F.S.; Conforti, C.; Giuffrida, R.; de Barros, M.H.; Zalaudek, I. Raised Vulvar Lesions: Be Aware! *Dermatol. Pract. Concept.* **2018**, *8*, 158–161. [CrossRef]
46. Sand, F.L.; Thomsen, S.F. Clinician's Update on the Benign, Premalignant, and Malignant Skin Tumours of the Vulva: The Dermatologist's View. *Int. Sch. Res. Not.* **2017**, *2017*, 2414569. [CrossRef]
47. De Simone, P.; Silipo, V.; Buccini, P.; Mariani, G.; Marenda, S.; Eibenschutz, L.; Ferrari, A.; Catricalà, C. Vulvar Melanoma: A Report of 10 Cases and Review of the Literature. *Melanoma Res.* **2008**, *18*, 127–133. [CrossRef] [PubMed]
48. Genton, C.Y.; Kunz, J.; Schreiner, W.E. Primary Malignant Melanoma of the Vagina and Cervix Uteri: Report of a Case with Utrastructural Study. *Virchows Arch. A. Path. Anat. Histol.* **1981**, *393*, 245–250.
49. Hewitt, P. Sequel to a Case of Recurrent Melanosis of Both Groins and Back: The Disease Reappearing in the Brain, Heart, Pancreas, Liver and Other Organs. *Lancet* **1861**, *77*, 263.
50. Panizzon, R.G. Vulvar Melanoma. *Semin. Dermatol.* **1996**, *15*, 67–70. [CrossRef]
51. Pirlamarla, A.K.; Tang, J.; Amin, B.; Kabarriti, R. Vulvar Melanoma with Isolated Metastasis to the Extraocular Muscles: Case Report and Brief Literature Review. *Anticancer Res.* **2018**, *38*, 3763–3766. [CrossRef]
52. Campaner, A.B.; Fernandes, G.L.; de Cardoso, F.A.; Veasey, J.V. Vulvar Melanoma: Relevant Aspects in Therapeutic Management. *An. Bras. Dermatol.* **2017**, *92*, 398–400. [CrossRef]
53. Baderca, F.; Cojocaru, S.; Lazăr, E.; Lăzureanu, C.; Lighezan, R.; Alexa, A.; Raica, M.; Nicola, T. Amelanotic Vulvar Melanoma: Case Report and Review of the Literature. *Rom. J. Morphol. Embryol.* **2008**, *49*, 219–228.
54. Filippetti, R.; Pitocco, R. Amelanotic Vulvar Melanoma: A Case Report. *Am. J. Dermatopathol.* **2015**, *37*, e75–e77. [CrossRef]
55. Mukeya, G.K.; Kakoka, I.M.; Mwansa, J.C.; Kalau, W.A. Mélanome malin vulvaire: À propos d'un cas observé à l'Hôpital du Cinquantenaire de Lubumbashi. *Pan Afr. Med. J.* **2020**, *36*, 124. [CrossRef]
56. Sinasac, S.E.; Petrella, T.M.; Rouzbahman, M.; Sade, S.; Ghazarian, D.; Vicus, D. Melanoma of the Vulva and Vagina: Surgical Management and Outcomes Based on a Clinicopathologic Reviewof 68 Cases. *J. Obstet. Gynaecol. Can.* **2019**, *41*, 762–771. [CrossRef]
57. Verschraegen, C.F.; Benjapibal, M.; Supakarapongkul, W.; Levy, L.B.; Ross, M.; Atkinson, E.N.; Bodurka-Bevers, D.; Kavanagh, J.J.; Kudelka, A.P.; Legha, S.S. Vulvar Melanoma at the M. D. Anderson Cancer Center: 25 Years Later. *Int. J. Gynecol. Cancer* **2001**, *11*, 359–364. [CrossRef] [PubMed]

58. Vaccari, S.; Barisani, A.; Salvini, C.; Pirola, S.; Preti, E.P.; Pennacchioli, E.; Iacobone, A.D.; Patrizi, A.; Tosti, G. Thin Vulvar Melanoma: A Challenging Diagnosis. Dermoscopic Features of a Case Series. *Clin. Exp. Dermatol.* **2020**, *45*, 187–193. [CrossRef]
59. Pandey, G.; Dave, P.; Patel, S.; Patel, B.; Arora, R.; Parekh, C.; Begum, D. Female Genital Tract Melanoma: Analysis from a Regional Cancer Institute. *J. Turk. Soc. Obstet. Gynecol.* **2020**, *17*, 46–51. [CrossRef] [PubMed]
60. Joste, M.; Dion, L.; Brousse, S.; Nyangoh Timoh, K.; Rousseau, C.; Reilhac, T.; Laviolle, B.; Lesimple, T.; Lavoue, V.; Leveque, J. Vulvar and Vaginal Melanomas: A Retrospective Study Spanning 19 Years from a Tertiary Center. *J. Gynecol. Obstet. Hum. Reprod.* **2021**, *50*, 102091. [CrossRef] [PubMed]
61. Martin-Gorgojo, A.; Comunion-Artieda, A.; Pizarro-Redondo, A.; Bru-Gorraiz, F.-J. A Minute 'Ugly-Duckling' Pigmented Lesion on the Arm of a 60-Year-Old Caucasian Female. In *Clinical Cases in Melanoma*; Springer International Publishing: Cham, Switzerland, 2020; pp. 29–31.
62. Rogers, T.; Pulitzer, M.; Marino, M.L.; Marghoob, A.A.; Zivanovic, O.; Marchetti, M.A. Early Diagnosis of Genital Mucosal Melanoma: How Good Are Our Dermoscopic Criteria? *Dermatol. Pract. Concept.* **2016**, *6*, 43–46. [CrossRef]
63. Oguri, H.; Izumiya, C.; Maeda, N.; Fukaya, T.; Moriki, T. A Primary Amelanotic Melanoma of the Vagina, Diagnosed by Immunohistochemical Staining with HMB-45, Which Recurred as a Pigmented Melanoma. *J. Clin. Pathol.* **2004**, *57*, 986–988. [CrossRef]
64. Gautam, D.; Ahmed, M. Melanoma Detection and Classification Using SVM Based Decision Support System. In Proceedings of the 2015 Annual IEEE India Conference (INDICON), New Delhi, India, 17–20 December 2015; pp. 1–6.
65. Goldsmith, S.M.; Solomon, A.R. A Series of Melanomas Smaller than 4 Mm and Implications for the ABCDE Rule. *J. Eur. Acad. Dermatol. Venereol.* **2007**, *21*, 929–934. [CrossRef]
66. Blum, A.; Simionescu, O.; Argenziano, G.; Braun, R.; Cabo, H.; Eichhorn, A.; Kirchesch, H.; Malvehy, J.; Marghoob, A.A.; Puig, S.; et al. Dermoscopy of Pigmented Lesions of the Mucosa and the Mucocutaneous Junction: Results of a Multicenter Study by the International Dermoscopy Society (IDS): Results of a Multicenter Study by the International Dermoscopy Society (IDS). *Arch. Dermatol.* **2011**, *147*, 1181–1187. [CrossRef]
67. Lee, Y.-T. Diagnosis, Treatment and Prognosis of Early Melanoma: The Importance of Depth of Microinvasion. *Ann. Surg.* **1980**, *191*, 87–97. [CrossRef]
68. Pflugfelder, A.; Weide, B.; Eigentler, T.K.; Forschner, A.; Leiter, U.; Held, L.; Meier, F.; Garbe, C. Incisional Biopsy and Melanoma Prognosis: Facts and Controversies. *Clin. Dermatol.* **2010**, *28*, 316–318. [CrossRef] [PubMed]
69. Tadiparthi, S.; Panchani, S.; Iqbal, A. Biopsy for Malignant Melanoma—Are We Following the Guidelines? *Ann. R. Coll. Surg. Engl.* **2008**, *90*, 322–325. [CrossRef] [PubMed]
70. Dickson, P.V.; Gershenwald, J.E. Staging and Prognosis of Cutaneous Melanoma. *Surg. Oncol. Clin. N. Am.* **2011**, *20*, 1–17. [CrossRef]
71. Keung, E.Z.; Gershenwald, J.E. The Eighth Edition American Joint Committee on Cancer (AJCC) Melanoma Staging System: Implications for Melanoma Treatment and Care. *Expert Rev. Anticancer Ther.* **2018**, *18*, 775–784. [CrossRef]
72. Gershenwald, J.E.; Scolyer, R.A.; Hess, K.R.; Sondak, V.K.; Long, G.V.; Ross, M.I.; Lazar, A.J.; Faries, M.B.; Kirkwood, J.M.; McArthur, G.A.; et al. Melanoma Staging: Evidence-Based Changes in the American Joint Committee on Cancer Eighth Edition Cancer Staging Manual. *CA Cancer J. Clin.* **2017**, *67*, 472–492. [CrossRef]
73. Hou, J.Y.; Baptiste, C.; Hombalegowda, R.B.; Tergas, A.I.; Feldman, R.; Jones, N.L.; Chatterjee-Paer, S.; Bus-Kwolfski, A.; Wright, J.D.; Burke, W.M. Vulvar and Vaginal Melanoma: A Unique Subclass of Mucosal Melanoma Based on a Comprehensive Molecular Analysis of 51 Cases Compared with 2253 Cases of Nongynecologic Melanoma: Molecular Study of Vulvovaginal Melanoma. *Cancer* **2017**, *123*, 1333–1344. [CrossRef] [PubMed]
74. Coit, D.G.; Andtbacka, R.; Anker, C.J.; Bichakjian, C.K.; Carson, W.E., III; Daud, A.; DiMaio, D.; Fleming, M.D.; Guild, V.; Halpern, A.C.; et al. Melanoma, Version 2.2013: Featured Updates to the NCCN Guidelines. *J. Natl. Compr. Canc. Netw.* **2013**, *11*, 395–407. [CrossRef]
75. Smoller, B.R. Histologic Criteria for Diagnosing Primary Cutaneous Malignant Melanoma. *Mod. Pathol.* **2006**, *19*, S34–S40. [CrossRef] [PubMed]
76. Connolly, K.L.; Nehal, K.S.; Busam, K.J. Lentigo Maligna and Lentigo Maligna Melanoma: Contemporary Issues in Diagnosis and Management. *Melanoma Manag.* **2015**, *2*, 171–178. [CrossRef]
77. Saida, T.; Koga, H.; Goto, Y.; Uhara, H. Characteristic Distribution of Melanin Columns in the Cornified Layer of Acquired Acral Nevus: An Important Clue for Histopathologic Differentiation from Early Acral Melanoma. *Am. J. Dermatopathol.* **2011**, *33*, 468–473. [CrossRef] [PubMed]
78. James, W.; Elston, D.; Treat, J.; Rosenbach, M.; Micheletti, R. Melanocytic Nevi and Neoplasms. In *Andrews' Diseases of the Skin*; Elsevier: Amsterdam, The Netherlands, 2019.
79. DeMatos, P.; Tyler, D.; Seigler, H.F. Mucosal Melanoma of the Female Genitalia: A Clinicopathologic Study of Forty-Three Cases at Duke University Medical Center. *Surgery* **1998**, *124*, 38–48. [CrossRef]
80. Petković, M.; Jurakić Tončić, R. Nested Melanoma, a New Morphological Variant of Superficial Spreading Melanoma with Characteristic Dermoscopic Features. *Acta Dermatovenerol. Croat.* **2017**, *25*, 80–81.
81. Urso, C.; Rongioletti, F.; Innocenzi, D.; Batolo, D.; Chimenti, S.; Fanti, P.L.; Filotico, R.; Gianotti, R.; Lentini, M.; Tomasini, C.; et al. Histological Features Used in the Diagnosis of Melanoma Are Frequently Found in Benign Melanocytic Naevi. *J. Clin. Pathol.* **2005**, *58*, 409–412. [CrossRef]

82. Banerjee, S.S.; Harris, M. Morphological and Immunophenotypic Variations in Malignant Melanoma: Variations in Malignant Melanoma. *Histopathology* **2000**, *36*, 387–402. [CrossRef]
83. Nadji, M.; Ganjei, P.; Penneys, N.S.; Morales, A.R. Immunohistochemistry of Vulvar Neoplasms: A Brief Review. *Int. J. Gynecol. Pathol.* **1984**, *3*, 41–50. [CrossRef]
84. Xu, X.; Chu, A.Y.; Pasha, T.L.; Elder, D.E.; Zhang, P.J. Immunoprofile of MITF, Tyrosinase, Melan-A, and MAGE-1 in HMB45-Negative Melanomas. *Am. J. Surg. Pathol.* **2002**, *26*, 82–87. [CrossRef] [PubMed]
85. Cochran, A.J.; Wen, D.R. S-100 Protein as a Marker for Melanocytic and Other Tumours. *Pathology* **1985**, *17*, 340–345. [CrossRef] [PubMed]
86. Wick, M.R.; Swanson, P.E.; Rocamora, A. Recognition of Malignant Melanoma by Monoclonal Antibody HMB-45. An Immunohistochemical Study of 200 Paraffin-Embedded Cutaneous Tumors. *J. Cutan. Pathol.* **1988**, *15*, 201–207. [CrossRef]
87. Orchard, G.E. Comparison of Immunohistochemical Labelling of Melanocyte Differentiation Antibodies Melan-A, Tyrosinase and HMB 45 with NKIC3 and S100 Protein in the Evaluation of Benign Naevi and Malignant Melanoma. *Histochem. J.* **2000**, *32*, 475–481. [CrossRef]
88. Willis, B.C.; Johnson, G.; Wang, J.; Cohen, C. SOX10: A Useful Marker for Identifying Metastatic Melanoma in Sentinel Lymph Nodes. *Appl. Immunohistochem. Mol. Morphol.* **2015**, *23*, 109–112. [CrossRef]
89. D'Angelo, S.P.; Larkin, J.; Sosman, J.A.; Lebbé, C.; Brady, B.; Neyns, B.; Schmidt, H.; Hassel, J.C.; Hodi, F.S.; Lorigan, P.; et al. Efficacy and Safety of Nivolumab Alone or in Combination with Ipilimumab in Patients with Mucosal Melanoma: A Pooled Analysis. *J. Clin. Oncol.* **2017**, *35*, 226–235. [CrossRef] [PubMed]
90. Yan, J.; Wu, X.; Yu, J.; Yu, H.; Xu, T.; Brown, K.M.; Bai, X.; Dai, J.; Ma, M.; Tang, H.; et al. Analysis of NRAS Gain in 657 Patients with Melanoma and Evaluation of Its Sensitivity to a MEK Inhibitor. *Eur. J. Cancer* **2018**, *89*, 90–101. [CrossRef]
91. Hintzsche, J.D.; Gorden, N.T.; Amato, C.M.; Kim, J.; Wuensch, K.E.; Robinson, S.E.; Applegate, A.J.; Couts, K.L.; Medina, T.M.; Wells, K.R.; et al. Whole-Exome Sequencing Identifies Recurrent SF3B1 R625 Mutation and Comutation of NF1 and KIT in Mucosal Melanoma. *Melanoma Res.* **2017**, *27*, 189–199. [CrossRef]
92. Lyu, J.; Song, Z.; Chen, J.; Shepard, M.J.; Song, H.; Ren, G.; Li, Z.; Guo, W.; Zhuang, Z.; Shi, Y. Whole-Exome Sequencing of Oral Mucosal Melanoma Reveals Mutational Profile and Therapeutic Targets: WES of OMM Reveals Genomic Alterations. *J. Pathol.* **2018**, *244*, 358–366. [CrossRef] [PubMed]
93. Newell, F.; Kong, Y.; Wilmott, J.S.; Johansson, P.A.; Ferguson, P.M.; Cui, C.; Li, Z.; Kazakoff, S.H.; Burke, H.; Dodds, T.J.; et al. Whole-Genome Landscape of Mucosal Melanoma Reveals Diverse Drivers and Therapeutic Targets. *Nat. Commun.* **2019**, *10*, 3163. [CrossRef] [PubMed]
94. Rouzbahman, M.; Kamel-Reid, S.; Al Habeeb, A.; Butler, M.; Dodge, J.; Laframboise, S.; Murphy, J.; Rasty, G.; Ghazarian, D. Malignant Melanoma of Vulva and Vagina: A Histomorphological Review and Mutation Analysis—A Single-Center Study. *J. Low. Genit. Tract Dis.* **2015**, *19*, 350–353. [CrossRef]
95. Cai, Y.-J.; Ke, L.-F.; Zhang, W.-W.; Lu, J.-P.; Chen, Y.-P. Recurrent KRAS, KIT and SF3B1 Mutations in Melanoma of the Female Genital Tract. *BMC Cancer* **2021**, *21*, 677. [CrossRef]
96. Nassar, K.W.; Tan, A.C. The Mutational Landscape of Mucosal Melanoma. *Semin. Cancer Biol.* **2020**, *61*, 139–148. [CrossRef]
97. Kiuru, M.; Busam, K.J. The NF1 Gene in Tumor Syndromes and Melanoma. *Lab. Investig.* **2017**, *97*, 146–157. [CrossRef]
98. Guillot, B.; Dalac, S.; Delaunay, M.; Baccard, M.; Chevrant-Breton, J.; Dereure, O.; Machet, L.; Sassolas, B.; Zeller, J.; Bernard, P.; et al. Cutaneous Malignant Melanoma and Neurofibromatosis Type 1. *Melanoma Res.* **2004**, *14*, 159–163. [CrossRef] [PubMed]
99. Omholt, K.; Grafström, E.; Kanter-Lewensohn, L.; Hansson, J.; Ragnarsson-Olding, B.K. KIT Pathway Alterations in Mucosal Melanomas of the Vulva and Other Sites. *Clin. Cancer Res.* **2011**, *17*, 3933–3942.
100. Xiao, W.; Du, N.; Huang, T.; Guo, J.; Mo, X.; Yuan, T.; Chen, Y.; Ye, T.; Xu, C.; Wang, W.; et al. TP53 Mutation as Potential Negative Predictor for Response of Anti-CTLA-4 Therapy in Metastatic Melanoma. *EBioMedicine* **2018**, *32*, 119–124. [CrossRef]
101. Ablain, J.; Liu, S.; Moriceau, G.; Lo, R.S.; Zon, L.I. SPRED1 Deletion Confers Resistance to MAPK Inhibition in Melanoma. *J. Exp. Med.* **2021**, 218. [CrossRef]
102. Qadeer, Z.A.; Harcharik, S.; Valle-Garcia, D.; Chen, C.; Birge, M.B.; Vardabasso, C.; Duarte, L.F.; Bernstein, E. Decreased Expression of the Chromatin Remodeler ATRX Associates with Melanoma Progression. *J. Investig. Dermatol.* **2014**, *134*, 1768–1772. [CrossRef]
103. Piura, B. Management of Primary Melanoma of the Female Urogenital Tract. *Lancet Oncol.* **2008**, *9*, 973–981. [CrossRef]
104. Breslow, A. Thickness, Cross-Sectional Areas and Depth of Invasion in the Prognosis of Cutaneous Melanoma. *Ann. Surg.* **1970**, *172*, 902–908. [CrossRef]
105. Clark, W.H., Jr.; From, L.; Bernardino, E.A.; Mihm, M.C. The Histogenesis and Biologic Behavior of Primary Human Malignant Melanomas of the Skin. *Cancer Res.* **1969**, *29*, 705–727.
106. Chung, A.F.; Woodruff, J.M.; Lewis, J.L., Jr. Malignant Melanoma of the Vulva: A Report of 44 Cases. *Obstet. Gynecol.* **1975**, *45*, 638–646. [CrossRef]
107. Leitao, M.M., Jr. Management of Vulvar and Vaginal Melanomas: Current and Future Strategies. *Am. Soc. Clin. Oncol. Educ. Book* **2014**, e277–e281. [CrossRef]
108. Treatment of Vulvar Melanoma. Available online: https://www.cancer.org/cancer/vulvar-cancer/treating/vulvar-melanoma.html (accessed on 26 April 2021).
109. Gadducci, A.; Carinelli, S.; Guerrieri, M.E.; Aletti, G.D. Melanoma of the Lower Genital Tract: Prognostic Factors and Treatment Modalities. *Gynecol. Oncol.* **2018**, *150*, 180–189. [CrossRef] [PubMed]

110. Albert, A.; Lee, A.; Allbright, R.; Vijayakumar, S. Vulvar Melanoma: An Analysis of Prognostic Factors and Treatment Patterns. *J. Gynecol. Oncol.* **2020**, *31*, e66. [CrossRef]
111. Cinotti, E.; Chevallier, J.; Labeille, B.; Cambazard, F.; Thomas, L.; Balme, B.; Leccia, M.T.; D'Incan, M.; Vercherin, P.; Douchet, C.; et al. Mucosal Melanoma: Clinical, Histological and c-Kit Gene Mutational Profile of 86 French Cases. *J. Eur. Acad. Dermatol. Venereol.* **2017**, *31*, 1834–1840. [CrossRef] [PubMed]
112. Domingues, B.; Lopes, J.M.; Soares, P.; Pópulo, H. Melanoma Treatment in Review. *ImmunoTargets Ther.* **2018**, *7*, 35–49. [CrossRef]
113. Janco, J.M.; Markovic, S.N.; Weaver, A.L.; Cliby, W.A. Vulvar and Vaginal Melanoma: Case Series and Review of Current Management Options Including Neoadjuvant Chemotherapy. *Gynecol. Oncol.* **2013**, *129*, 533–537. [CrossRef]
114. Tcheung, W.J.; Selim, M.A.; Herndon, J.E., 2nd; Abernethy, A.P.; Nelson, K.C. Clinicopathologic Study of 85 Cases of Melanoma of the Female Genitalia. *J. Am. Acad. Dermatol.* **2012**, *67*, 598–605. [CrossRef] [PubMed]
115. Handolias, D.; Hamilton, A.L.; Salemi, R.; Tan, A.; Moodie, K.; Kerr, L.; Dobrovic, A.; McArthur, G.A. Clinical Responses Observed with Imatinib or Sorafenib in Melanoma Patients Expressing Mutations in KIT. *Br. J. Cancer* **2010**, *102*, 1219–1223. [CrossRef]
116. Hodi, F.S.; O'Day, S.J.; McDermott, D.F.; Weber, R.W.; Sosman, J.A.; Haanen, J.B.; Gonzalez, R.; Robert, C.; Schadendorf, D.; Hassel, J.C.; et al. Improved Survival with Ipilimumab in Patients with Metastatic Melanoma. *N. Engl. J. Med.* **2010**, *363*, 711–723. [CrossRef]
117. Cocorocchio, E.; Pala, L.; Conforti, F.; Guerini-Rocco, E.; De Pas, T.; Ferrucci, P.F. Successful Treatment with Avapritinib in Patient with Mucosal Metastatic Melanoma. *Ther. Adv. Med. Oncol.* **2020**, *12*, 1758835920946158. [CrossRef]
118. Brand, E.; Fu, Y.S.; Lagasse, L.D.; Berek, J.S. Vulvovaginal Melanoma: Report of Seven Cases and Literature Review. *Gynecol. Oncol.* **1989**, *33*, 54–60. [CrossRef]
119. Landthaler, M.; Braun-Falco, O.; Richter, K.; Baltzwr, J.; Zander, J. Maligne Melanome Der Vulva. *DMW* **1985**, *110*, 789–794. [CrossRef] [PubMed]
120. Lotem, M.; Anteby, S.; Peretz, T.; Ingber, A.; Avinoach, I.; Prus, D. Mucosal Melanoma of the Female Genital Tract Is a Multifocal Disorder. *Gynecol. Oncol.* **2003**, *88*, 45–50. [CrossRef] [PubMed]
121. Tsvetkov, C.; Gorchev, G.; Tomov, S.; Hinkova, N.; Nikolova, M.; Veselinova, T. Primary malignant melanoma of the vagina and treatment options: A case report. *Akush. Ginekol.* **2014**, *53*, 35–40.
122. Irvin, W.P., Jr.; Legallo, R.L.; Stoler, M.H.; Rice, L.W.; Taylor, P.T., Jr.; Andersen, W.A. Vulvar Melanoma: A Retrospective Analysis and Literature Review. *Gynecol. Oncol.* **2001**, *83*, 457–465. [CrossRef]
123. Schiavone, M.B.; Broach, V.; Shoushtari, A.N.; Carvajal, R.D.; Alektiar, K.; Kollmeier, M.A.; Abu-Rustum, N.R.; Leitao, M.M., Jr. Combined Immunotherapy and Radiation for Treatment of Mucosal Melanomas of the Lower Genital Tract. *Gynecol. Oncol. Rep.* **2016**, *16*, 42–46. [CrossRef] [PubMed]
124. González-Bosquet, J.; García Jiménez, A.; Gil Moreno, A.; Xercavins, J. Malignant Vulvo-Vaginal Melanoma: A Report of 7 Cases. *Eur. J. Gynaecol. Oncol.* **1997**, *18*, 63–67.

MDPI
St. Alban-Anlage 66
4052 Basel
Switzerland
Tel. +41 61 683 77 34
Fax +41 61 302 89 18
www.mdpi.com

Biomedicines Editorial Office
E-mail: biomedicines@mdpi.com
www.mdpi.com/journal/biomedicines

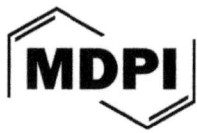

www.ingramcontent.com/pod-product-compliance
Lightning Source LLC
LaVergne TN
LVHW070450100526
838202LV00014B/1696